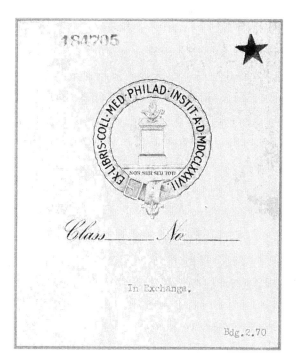

Volume 47—No. 1, January, 1954

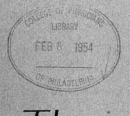

The Journal

F THE OKLAHOMA STATE MEDICAL ASSOCIATION

ANNUAL MEETING

OKLAHOMA STATE MEDICAL ASSOCIATION

MUNICIPAL AUDITORIUM OKLAHOMA CITY

MAY 10-11-12

BLISHED MONTHLY AT OKLAHOMA CITY, OKLAHOMA UNDER DIRECTION OF THE COUNCIL

ULTRASHORT-ACTING INTRAVENOUS ANESTHETIC

SURITAL sodium (thiamylal sodium, Parke-Davis) produces smooth anesthesia with rapid, quiet induction and prompt, pleasant recovery.

Detailed information on SURITAL sodium will be mailed you on request.

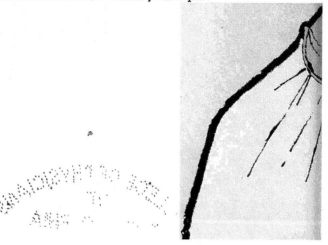

THE JOURNAL

of the

OKLAHOMA STATE MEDICAL ASSOCIATION

EDITORIALS

DEATH, THE INCOMPREHENSIBLE

On October 7th I sat at the bedside of my long time friend, Dr. Horace Reed. I observed the approaching incomprehensible separation of soul and body. In the silence of the death chamber, I suffered under the influence of more than 50 years of intimate association and the impending loss of an unbroken friendship. But to some extent, the clouds were dissipated and the light permitted to shine through when I thought what a lovable, cheerful, modest, generous, helpful, self-effacing spirit would be crossing the bar before nightfall.

In our long journey together there was never a rift. I shall miss the support of his frankness, honesty and integrity. In thought, word and deed he was devoted to the truth. In his professional life his remarkable diagnostic abilities and surgical skills were dedicated to his patients and to those members of the profession who sought his advice. All these functions he discharged without any apparent consideration of financial gain. No patient rich or poor ever left his presence without the full benefit of his knowledge as it applied to his or her individual needs. In this respect he embodied all that we treasure in the traditions of our profession.

His going leaves me in a state of wonder and uncertainty. Why can we not see beyond this narrow span and know better how to follow on? Such separations help us to realize the uncertainty of life and its immediate importance.

White I sat at Doctor Reed's bedside searching for his pulse, his faithful little terrier timidly walked to his bedside, placed her paws on my own wrist, surveyed my face with a searching eye—perhaps "all seeing" and then turned to look at her master before slipping away to her place of silent waiting.

There seemed to be a mutual comprehension of impending calamity but on my part falling short of what I would like to know about that last inescapable, incomprehensible act in the cycle of life.

THE MEDICAL SIDE OF JUVENILE DELINQUENCY

Just when the committees and councils are discussing juvenile delinquency and newspapers and magazines are dishing out large helpings for parents, school authorities and law enforcement agencies, a Metropolitan Life Insurance Company pamphlet "Understanding Your Teen Ager"[1] comes from the press. This should help all those concerned about this problem. While juvenile delinquency is a serious problem, it should not be forgotten that the teen agers who go wrong are decidedly in the minority.

Aside from hereditary influences there are many environmental factors that enter into the rising incidence of emotional instability in the adolescent as well as in the adult. The family physician, especially of the now lamented old fashioned type should have a better understanding of these varied influences than anyone else and should be able to contribute more toward their solution than anyone else with the possible of the parents. The family medical advisor employing his knowledge of emotional disorders and their causes should in an advisory capacity be of inestimable service to the parents and their children. In the changing socio-economic pattern, many people have discarded the idea of the family physician and too often try to make their own decision with reference to mental and physical health or depend upon agencies that give a relatively cold, impersonal direction too often wanting in the warmth and personal interest so necessary in the solution of such problems. All this merely for the purpose of making a plea for the old time patient-physician relationship so essential to physical and psychological stability in the family when obtainable and so helpful in the discovery of innate emotional abnormalities with measures of correction or control before serious consequences result.

REFERENCE

1. D. B. Armstrong, M.D., Metropolitan Life Insurance Co., 1 Madison Ave., New York 10, N. Y.

THE HUMAN BODY AND THE
BODY POLITIC

Apropos Virchow's cellular pathology and Russia's political philosophy it is interesting to note the following from Edward Barry's[1] *A Treatise on Consumption of the Lungs.* No doubt with political expediency in mind, the book was dedicated to his excellency John Lord Carteret Baron of Hawnes and Lord Lieutenant of Ireland.. Believing there is a lesson in this dedication for modern physicians, it is being reproduced in full:

"When persons in the highest stations, like your Lordship, are eminently distinguished for making the Good of Mankind their peculiar care, they have an undoubted right to the homage of all those who, in a more humble sphere, pursue that amiable end: While these, on the other hand, lay claim to, and think themselves in some degree entitled to their protection.

"And tho' this must often expose them to the impertinent Addresses of such who but impotently strive to promote the publick welfare; yet to one of your Lordship's candor, the sincere intention will in some measure supply the place of more successful merit, and plead an excuse for this presumption.

"The inquiries which have been made into the structure and use of the various parts of animal bodies, have been always attended with great and diffusive benefits. Several mechanic engines owe their origine to hints first taken from small machines of the same form in a human body; and some of the most curious pieces of art, and productions of nature, have been there discovered in a beautiful miniature. Sculpture, and painting, could not have arrived to such a perfection, unassisted with the previous improvements in anatomy: And the surprising contrivances that have been observed in the fabric of the ear, have not a little contributed to make music charm more powerful. The great resemblance that has always appeared between the body politic, and natural, (human body) makes the latter particularly worthy of the encouragement, and study of the greatest statesman. Thus Menenius Agrippa, by his famous Apologue deduced from the structure of the body, prevailed on the mutinous Plebeians to acquiesce in the authority of the laws. Had he been unacquainted with this sort of knowledge, the Republick, then in its infancy, might have been destroyed by civil fueds, and Rome perhaps had never been the mistress of the world. However, these advantages, my lord, tho' very considerable, are by no means equal to such as flow from a judicious exercise of the art of physic; on which often depends the safety of the best patriots, and of such who are most capable of improving all other arts, and sciences.

"Since then the due cultivation of medicine is of such use to mankind; since the most refin'd and elegant enjoyments of life grow insipid where health is wanting; since without it, we could not relish even these happy days, nor have a true flavor of the usual blessings we enjoy under your wise and auspicious administration; permit me, my lord, to lay before you, this faint essay in the Art of Healing. You make us every day more in love with life, by making us every day more happy in it, and consequently make the Art of Physic of still the greater importance.

"The universal reputation your lordship enjoys in being skill'd in every part of useful knowledge, your thorough acquaintance with the ancients, your forming your mind (where you thought the moderns imperfect) on their model, the greatest of whom made it so much their care to be versed in the Art of Physic, that it was even thought a necessary part of a polite education, make me believe I have chose the best and truest critic, as I'm sure I have the worthiest patron of the following sheets."

REFERENCE

1. A Treatise on a Consumption of the Lungs with a previous account of nutrition, and of the strure and use of the lungs. Edward Barry, M.D., London, William and John Innys at the West end of St. Paul's. 1727

VIRCHOW, COMMUNISM,
THE CELL AND THE CITIZEN

Virchow, the father of individual cellular anatomy and cellular pathology was honored by the Soviets in 1950 when their government issued a stamp bearing his likeness. But after learning more about his discovery and demonstration of the individual cell, so fundamental in medicine and so symbolic of the individual citizen in a democracy, they attempt to throw Virchow overboard.

Communists steal the science that makes atomic bombs while denying the science that suggests individual anatomy. In their philosophy, government takes the place of God, science and the free citizen.

Special Article

PRACTICAL APPLICATION OF LIVER FUNCTION TESTS IN THE MANAGEMENT OF THE JAUNDICED PATIENT

RICHARD D. HAINES, M.D.
TEMPLE, TEXAS

The jaundiced patient often presents a challenging diagnostic problem. In the analysis of a given case, it is always essential to determine two factors: (1) the extent of hepatocellular dysfunction, and (2), the degree of extra biliary tract obstruction. To assist in this analysis, a host of liver function tests have been proposed and utilized. At this time, we are not interested in the academic limitations of these tests; but, rather, to correlate the easily available tests as diagnostic aids in distinguishing cases of *medical* jaundice (patients whose tests indicate no obstruction of the extra biliary passages, but show altered liver cell function) from cases of *surgical* jaundice (patients whose tests indicate obstructed extra biliary passages and reasonably normal liver cell function). Granted, this is oversimplification of a sometimes difficult problem; yet, frequently, the primary question is: "Will this patient be benefited by surgery?"

As there is no single test to answer this question; perhaps, the problem can be solved by the judicious application and proper, at times, conservative interpretation of a group of liver function tests. As liver function tests frequently yield different results when applied to similar patient problems, their value lies in proper interpretation in the light of history and physical examination, as well as the stage and extent of the disease process. The last factor is most important in long standing extra hepatic obstruction when, as would be expected, the tests of parenchymal function are altered, depending upon the extent of associated and secondary liver cell involvement. Also, cases of non-surgical jaundice exist where liver function tests are similar to those showing extra biliary obstruction; yet, the pathological process is intra hepatic obseruction. Watson[1] has termed such cases, "cholangiolitic biliary cirrhosis." Other closely allied conditions, as xanthomatous biliary cirrhosis,

might show similar liver function patterns. Hence, before proposing the liver function tests which we employ, it is best to review the metabolic processes of hemoglobin and its breakdown products occurring normally and in the various jaundice conditions.

PHYSIOLOGY

In brief, normal hemoglobin metabolism includes the disruption of the porphyrin ring, removal of iron, and the formation of bilirubinglobin. This substance is transported via the blood to the liver where globin is separated, and bilirubin is excreted in the bile as sodium bilirubinate. Bilirubin in the colon, then, is reduced to urobilinogen. This process is illustrated in Figure 1. A portion of the urobilinogen is reabsorbed in the portal circulation; and, finally, a small amount is excreted in the urine. The normal daily range for stool urobilinogen is 40-280 mg.; while that of urine is 0-3.5 mg.[2]

The measurement of urine urobilinogen in the 2 to 4 p.m. urine, expressed in Ehrlich units (EU), is a good index of this pigment excretion. In our laboratory, the normal values for the 2 to 4 p.m. urine urobilinogen determination is less than 1 Ehrlich unit; and normal value for stool urobilinogen is 150 to 330 Ehrlich units per 100 grams of stool (Watson method).

The possibility of the existence of hemolytic jaundice is neglected too often. As it frequently enters into the diagnostic picture, it is best to consider hemolytic jaundice, first, and to obtain such laboratory data as to exclude it. Figure 2 graphically illustrates the physiological alterations prevailing. In reality, the abnormal process is *pre-hepatic. It exists as an abnormally accelerated destruction of the erythrocyte, increased hemoglobin liberation, and subsequent increase in bilirubinglobin.* (In Figure 2, this is portrayed by increase in the size of the blocks representing hemoglobin and bilirubinglobin.) In addition to the simple over-

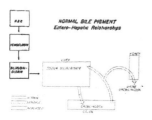

Figure 1.
Haines: LIVER FUNCTION TESTS

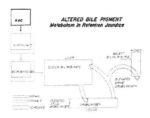

Figure 2.
Haines: LIVER FUNCTION TESTS

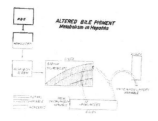

Figure 3
Haines: LIVER FUNCTION TESTS

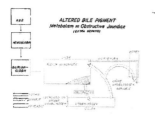

Figure 4
Haines: LIVER FUNCTION TESTS

loading of the system with surplus biliru-binglobin, there may be variable hepatic cell dysfunction since some of the cells, e v e n though intact structurally are functioning at a lower than normal rate of efficiency. No doubt, the combination of accelerated blood destruction and the temporary hepatic cell dysfunction are the factors which account for the often produced jaundice. Therefore, as would be expected, there is an increase in the delayed reacting bilirubin and a variable elevation of the stool and urine urobilinogen. Bile is not present in the urine. Fortunately, a diagnosis of hemolytic jaundice is easily established if it is seriously considered as a diagnostic possibility and pertinent evidence sought, as: splenomegaly, reticulocytosis, spherocytosis, and increased fragility of the erythrocyte to hypotonic saline solution.

There are no certain short cuts to the differentiation of hepatocellular, medical, from extra hepatic obstructive, surgical, jaundice. The importance of an accurate inquisitive history and a careful, often repeated, physical examination are of equal importance to the use of liver function tests.

The causes of hepatocellular jaundice are many; and while, occasionally, the etiology is evasive, usually, the problem is that of establishing a diagnosis of biliary cirrhosis, per sè, or that of hepatitis, either infectious or homologous serum hepatitis. In hepatitis, the primary pathology resides within the liver. The degree of cell involvement, extent of functional impairment, and amount of secondary biliary infection will determine the magnitude of bilirubinuria as well as the variations in the urine and stool urobilinogen.

In Figure 3, the altered bile pigment metabolism- is graphically depicted. In instances of severe hepatitis, the liver may be "so sick" that only small amounts of sodium bilirubinate enter the gastrointestinal tract, and the urine and stool urobilinogen excretion are within the range of value usually reserved for complete extra biliary obstruction. In these cases, the daily recording of the urine urobilinogen may gradually show an increase, and this may be the first evidence of hepatic cell function improvement.

In other instances, the disease process may be less severe. The factors determining the amount of urobilinogen excreted depend on the extent and severity of this process, as well as the functioning capacity of the liver prior to the insult, and the adequacy of therapy. (An attempt to illustrate this first factor has been made by the shaded areas in the block representing the liver.) (The variable urobilinogen excretion is illustrated by the one-sided perforated arrows.)

In extra hepatic obstructive jaundice, the site of the pathological process, as the name implies, is beyond the liver within the extra hepatic duct system. The nature of the obstruction, and in certain instances the duration of its presence, will influence the degree of the block. This will then determine the amount of recoverable stool urobilinogen. Fluctuating amounts have caused duct lithiasis to be suspected, but, also, may be evidence of duct neoplasm. Duct neoplasm, in rare instances, may disintegrate as it outgrows its blood supply, thereby, temporarily relieving the obstruction. Persistent, progressive obstruction usually indicates malignant neoplastic obstruction; however, other causes, stricture or impacted stone, must be considered. Figure 4 illustrates the altered bile pigment metabolism. Obviously, the stool and, subsequently, the urine urobilinogen will depend on the above named factors affecting the block.

LIVER FUNCTION TESTS

We have found that the consistent use of a small group of tests has yielded a high degree of diagnostic accuracy. A short statement regarding each test is of value.

Serum Bilirubin: Whether there are actually two different types of bilirubin is debatable; yet, two forms can be demonstrated, depending upon the response produced when exposed to Ehrlich's diazo reagent. The one minute form reacts promptly with the diazo reagent, and, theoretically, measures the bilirubin which has passed through the liver cells. The delayed or indirect bilirubin reacts only with the diazo reagent after the protein, with which the bilirubin is combined, is precipated by alcohol. This distinction is of value clinically in the following instances: (1). It aids in the differential diagnosis of hemolytic jaundice, as here, an elevated total bilirubin with a normal one minute bilirubin exists. (2). In some instances, it may help to differentiate hepatic from post-hepatic jaundice. Classically, one obtains an increase in the delayed reacting bilirubin in hepatitis, and an increase in the prompt reacting bilirubin in obstructive jaundice. (3). The prompt direct-reacting fraction may be elevated even when total serum bilirubin is normal, and this may be the only

PRACTICAL LABORATORY TESTS RECOMMENDED FOR DIFFERENTIAL DIAGNOSIS

Hepatocellular (Parenchymal)	Obstructive (Patency Biliary Passages)
Increased delayed reacting bilirubin	Increased prompt reacting bilirubin
Diminished cholesterol ester fraction	Bilirubinuria
Positive Hanger (Cephalin cholesterol flocculation)	Increased total blood cholesterol
Positive Maclagen (Thymol turbidity)	Increased serum alkaline phosphatase
Increased urine urobilinogen	Diminished to absent bile in duodenal contents

Table 1.
Haines: LIVER FUNCTION TESTS

INFECTIOUS (VIRAL) HEPATITIS

TESTS	7/17	7/24	7/28	12/3
van den Bergh*				
1 Minute	4.5	1.1	0.48	0.32
Total	8.8	7.8	1.8	0.78
Urine Urobilinogen				
2-4 hr. (E. Units)	0.5	5.8	14.0	
Stool Urobilinogen				
(E. Units) **	23.0		40.0	
Cholesterol *	162.0		166.0	
Ester *	58.0		87.0	
Alkaline Phosphatase				
(K. A. Units)	5.2		10.7	
Thymol Flocculation	3+		0.0	0.0
Thymol Turbidity				
(Units)	6.0		4.0	1.0
Cephalin Flocculation	2+		0.0	0.0

* mg per 100 ml.
** per 100 Gm

Table 2.
Haines: LIVER FUNCTION TESTS

HOMOLOGOUS SERUM JAUNDICE

TESTS	5/29/51	6/2/51	6/5/51
van den Bergh*			
1 Minute	2.2	0.6	0.3
Total	8.0	3.5	1.6
Alkaline Phosphatase			
(K. A. Units)	3.0		
Cholesterol	194.0		
Esters*	67.0		
Cephalin Flocculation	4+		
Thymol Flocculation	4+		
Thymol Turbidity			
(Units)	38.0	3.0	
Proteins - Total**	6.8		
Albumin	3.4		
Globulin	3.4		

* mg. per 100 ml.
** Gm. per 100 cc.

Table 3.
Haines: LIVER FUNCTION TESTS

INFECTIOUS (VIRAL) HEPATITIS

TESTS	7/15/50	7/21/50	7/24/50	2/22/51
van den Bergh*				
1 Minute	11.4	6.6	7.4	0.2
Total	25.6	14.5	12.2	0.5
Urine Urobilinogen				
2-4 hr. (E. Units)	1.20	0.5	10.1	
Cholesterol*	169.0	62.0		
Ester*	67.0	46.0		
Alkaline Phosphatase				
(K. A. Units)	4.5			
Cephalin Flocculation	3+		4+	6.0
Thymol Flocculation				4+
Thymol Turbidity				
(Units)				8.5
Proteins - Total**	6.4	5.5		
Albumin	2.6	2.5		
Globulin	4.0	2.6		
Bromsulphalein				Urine Ret.

* mg per 100 ml.
** Gm per 100 cc.

Table 4.
Haines: LIVER FUNCTION TESTS

detectable evidence of hepatic cell injury, and has been recorded in early cases of infectious hepatitis.[3]

Cholesterol and its esters: Classically, any process that tends to prompt regurgitation of bile will increase total cholesterol. As esterification of cholesteral takes place in the liver, the determination of the total cholesterol and its ester fraction may be valuable in the diagnosis of hepatic and/or post-hepatic jaundice. Severe hepatic cell dysfunction without obstruction may be associated with low values of the ester fraction with maintenance of reasonably normal total cholesterol. Among the contrainidications to biliary surgery, Snell[4] has listed a cholesterol ester fraction of less than 50 mg. per 100 ml., and a fraction below this value is certainly a poor prognostic sign.

Alkaline phosphatase: In the absence of any specific bone pathology or metabolic disease, obstruction of the hepatic bile ducts is frequently associated with marked elevation of alkaline phosphatase; and values in range of 35-45 King Armstrong units are not infrequent with complete obstruction. It is equally uncommon to find high values in diffuse parenchymal disease. In fact, in severe hepatic cell injury, such as cirrhosis with secondary post-hepatic malignant obstruction, the alkaline phosphatase may fall with a persistent high serum bilirubin.

Flocculation tests: (Cephalin-Cholesterol and Thymol Turbidity and Flocculation) Cephalin flocculation is attributed to alterations in the serum proteins. This test is usually positive in the early stages of infectious hepatitis.

Thymol flocculation is related to changes in the globulin fraction, and the turbidity has been correlated with plasma lipid levels. Thymol flocculation remains positive during the convalescent stage of infectious hepatitis, while the turbidity test may have already returned to normal. These tests also become positive in extra hepatic obstruction, but their diagnostic efficiency can be relied upon if the jaundice is of brief duration and of uncomplicated obstruction.

Urobilinogen determinations: The normal daily values for urine and stool urobilinogen have been referred to earlier. In total obstruction to the extra biliary ducts, both determinations will be exceedingly low. (Stool less than 5 mg. per 24 hours and urine less than 0.3 mg. per 24 hours.) [5,6] Increased urobilinogen excretion rates in non-jaundiced patients may be one early indication of hepatic dysfunction.

Empirically, the application of liver function tests seems ideal. Actually, this situation does not always prevail; but, from a practical, clinical standpoint, there are a number of altered functions observed frequently.

Table 1 indicates the choice of tests, and is directed toward detecting two factors mentioned in the onset: (1). degree of hepatocellular or parenchymal impairment and (2). degree of patency of extra biliary passages. One must not expect to find marked positivity of all tests in either instance; in fact, occasionally, slight positivity of one or more tests may be all that is observed. The positivity of two tests in a given case directing attention to likelihood of hepatocellular involvement and at the same time normal response of one or two tests listed under *obstructive disease* would only be of added diagnostic value. The reverse would also be true.

It might be stated in brief that the combination of weakly or strongly positive cephalin or thymol flocculation in association with depressed cholesterol esters or normal alkaline phosphatase would favor parenchymal liver disease. On the other hand, a negative cephalin and thymol flocculation combined with elevated alkaline phosphatase and increased total cholesterol would tend to indicate extra hepatic obstruction.

The last factor listed as evidence of extra biliary obstruction in Table 1 is not actually a true liver function test (determination of bile in duodenal drainage); but is a maneuver, often forgotten, but actually available to all physicians and small hospital laboratories.

When studied for evidence of infection (presence of white blood cells or bacteria) or presence of crystals, this internal secretion may lend credence to the diagnosis of a common duct stone. Likewise, when the position of the tube is checked roentgenographically, the absence of bile in the duodenal aspiration may be interpreted as strong evidence of extra biliary obstruction. Also, the presence of blood in amount greater than that expected from local trauma due to passing of the tube may be a valuable clue to the presence of a neoplasm at the ampulla of Vater. We wish to stress the value of this procedure and to suggest that it be a routine procedure in the diagnostic evaluation of any patient with marked jaundice without antecedent history of pain.

CASE REPORTS

From a practical standpoint, it is worthwhile to review a few case reports with their laboratory findings. Realizing that few cases have a "true to form" laboratory profile, it is significant to observe the usual trend of laboratory test positivity, either singularly or in combination.

Case 1. (Infectious Hepatitis) F o u r weeks prior to coming to the hospital, a 50-year-old housewife noted rather constant nausea, vomiting and moderate diarrhea. She recalled no exposure to hepatotoxic agents, but jaundice was noted 10 days prior to admission. She had lost approximately 30 pounds in weight. Physical examination revealed a chronically ill, jaundiced woman; however, no fever was noted. Her liver was not enlarged, but percussion over the right lower anterior rib cage was painful. With medical therapy (including 3,000 calorie, high protein, high carbohydrate diet; *Lipogest,* two capsules three times daily; and supplementary vitamins; plus bed rest, she improved generally, jaundice disappeared, and she gained weight.

Laboratory studies are tabulated in Table 2. It is obvious at a glance that the tests indicate only moderate hepatocellular functional derangement, evidenced by only 2 plus cephalin and thymol flocculation. There was a prompt return to normal simultaneous with the disappearance of jaundice. The original determination of the 2 to 4 p.m. urine urobilinogen was within normal limits; how-ever, this was associated with a simultaneous low stool urobilinogen (23 EU per 100 Gm. stool.) This combination of factors would indicate only small amounts of bile entering the gastrointestinal tract, presumably because of a seriously damaged liver. Later, as clinical improvements occurred, increased urine urobilinogen was detected. Apparently, this represents a case of infectious, viral hepatitis.

Case 2. (Homologous Serum Jaundice) For sudden anuria, a 72-year-old man had transurethral resection in March, 1951. During his hospitalization, one ampule of plasma was administered. (There is no information as to whether or not it was irradiated.) Following recovery from this surgical procedure, and approximately two months later, he was first seen at this institution for evaluation or rather sudden, painless jaundice of 10 days' duration. Physical examination, other than icterus, was non-contributory. There were no abdominal masses.

Laboratory studies, Table 3, indicate pure hepatocellular dysfunction. A tentative diagnosis of homologous serum jaundice was made, principally on the basis of the single feature in the case history concerning plasma administration, plus strongly positive cephalin and thymol flocculation, thymol turbidity, and normal alkaline phosphatase. With therapy, jaundice subsided promptly, and correspondence revealed that the patient was well, clinically, a month later.

Table 5.
Raines: LIVER FUNCTION TESTS

Table 6.
Raines: LIVER FUNCTION TESTS

Table 7.
Raines: LIVER FUNCTION TESTS

Case 3. (Infectious Viral Hepatitis) The patient, a 33-year-old housewife, was acutely ill when admitted. Her history was of initial nausea, vomiting, generalized myalgia, daily low grade fever, and jaundice of eight weeks' duration. Physical examination revealed fever, 100° F., pulse rate 96. Hepatomegaly was noted two fingerbreadths below the right costal margin. This region was tender to palpation.

Laboratory studies, Table 4, revealed marked jaundice and only moderately altered thymol turbidity, cephalin flocculation, and normal alkaline phosphatase in spite of low cholesterol esters and reversal of the albumin and globulin ratio. Six days later, a very marked depression of the total cholesterol and ester fraction was tabulated simultaneously with a low 2 to 4 p.m. urine urobilinogen excretion, both of which substantiates severe cellular depression. Seven months later, even though jaundice had disappeared and the patient was asymptomatic, the thymol turbidity and flocculation were abnormal. We interpreted this as severe infectious hepatitis. The future may prove the patient to have sustained liver cell injury; or, perhaps, this patient may develop cirrhosis. Unfortunately, needle biopsy was not performed.

Tables 5, 6 and 7 are typical and not intentionally chosen cases, all of surgically proved carcinoma of the head of the pancreas, in which the liver function tests show almost consistently normal parenchymal cell function. The essential historical and physical findings accompany the laboratory studies. In two instances, Tables 5 and 6, jaundice was painless. In Tables 6 and 7, the patients had easily palpable right upper quadrant tumors. In no instance was alkaline phosphatase remarkably elevated. In Tables 5 and 6, stool urobilinogen values are within the range of complete extrabiliary obstruction. Because there is little urobilinogen produced within the bowel, there is little or none in the urine even though liver cell function is probably adequate as evidenced by normal cephalin and thymol flocculation tests. All have a single common denominator—the absence of bile in the duodenal drainage. This test bears re-emphasis as a valuable diagnostic aid in the study of painlessly jaundiced individuals.

CONCLUSIONS

1. The separation of jaundiced patients into medical and surgical groups is a valid approach.

2. Laboratory studies for this differentiation are suggested, and it is emphasized that no single test accomplishes this end.

3. A combination of tests, conservatively interpreted in the light of stage and extent of disease, as well as accurate history and careful physical examination, increase ones diagnostic accuracy.

REFERENCES

1. Watson, C. J. and Hoffbauer, F. W.: The problem of prolonged hepatitis with particular reference to the cholangiolitic type and to the development of cholangiolitic cirrhosis of rivatives of hemoglobin, Blood 1:99-120, Feb. 1946.
2. Watson, C. J., Studies of urobilinogen: II Urbolinogen in the urine and feces of subjects without evidence of disease of the liver or Biliary tract, Arch. Int Med. 59; 196-205, Feb. 1937.
3. Watson, C. J.: Some newer concepts of the natural derivatives of hemoglobin, Blood 1:99-120, Feb. 1946.
4. Snell, A. M.; The management of jaundiced patients, J.A. M.A. 183:1175-1181, April 1947.
5. Watson, C. J.: Regurgitation jaundice, J.A.M.A. 114:-2427-2432, June 22, 1940.
6. Watson, C. J.: The bile pigments, New Eng. J. Med. 227:-665-672, Oct. 29, 1942.

Meet Our Contributors

Richard D. Haines, M.D., Temple, Texas, has an article in this issue of the Journal on ''Practical Application of Liver Function Tests in the Management of the Jaundiced Patient.'' Doctor Haines, who previously had an article appearing in the Journal in 1951, is with the Department of Medicine of the Scott and White Clinic.

Henry Laurens, M.D., Salina, Kans., and *Ray U. Northrip, M.D.,* Ada, are joint authors of ''The Value of Gastroscopy''. Doctor Laurens received his B.A., degree from the University of North Carolina in 1940 and received his M.D., from Tulane in 1944. From 1945-47 he served as a captain in the medical corps. His specialty is gastroenterology.

Doctor Northrip graduated from the University of Oklahoma in 1938. He practiced several years in Nigeria, Africa, and was a lieutenant commander in the Navy from 1944-46. A pathologist, he is a member of the American College of Pathologists and the Oklahoma Association of Pathologists.

Robert A. Hayne, M.D., and *Averill Stowell, M.D.,* Tulsa, and *Robert A. Martini, M.D.,* Muskogee, collaborated on the article, ''The Diagnosis and Evaluation of Treatment of the Lumbar Intervertebral Disk.'' Doctor Hayne, a neurosurgeon, is now in service. He was graduated from the State University of Iowa College of Medicine in 1940.

Doctor Stowell, also a neurosurgeon, received his A.B., from Princeton in 1934 and his M.D., from Johns Hopkins in 1938. Before coming to Tulsa, he served in the army medical corps five years and was also associated with the Cleveland Clinic, and as instructor in neurosurgery in Baltimore and New York.

Doctor Martini is a member of the Veterans Hospital staff in Muskogee. He was graduated from the University of Wisconsin in 1938 and is an orthopedist. Doctor Martini served 59 months in the medical corps in World War II, 26 of which were spent overseas.

THE VALUE OF GASTROSCOPY*

HENRY LAURENS, JR., M.D., SALINA, KANS.,
AND RAY U. NORTHRIP, M.D.,
ADA, OKLAHOMA

INTRODUCTION

Gastroscopy became an accepted method of medical practice only 10 years after its introduction into this country by Dr. Rudolph Schindler. According to Schindler the rapid development of gastroscopy in America resulted from the cooperation of roentgenologists and their appreciation of the interrelationship of gastroscopy and roetgenology.

HISTORY

The first attempts at gastroscopy were made in 1868 by Kussmaul after he watched a sword swallower. He reasoned that a tube with a lamp in it could be swallowed as easily as a sword. However, the technical problems of illumination were not solved until the early 1920's.

During the period from 1922 to 1932, Dr. Rudolf Schindler constructed a flexible gastroscope and described the endoscopic pathology of the stomach. In 1934 Doctor Schindler was invited to the University of Chicago as a visiting professor. Since then, the gastroscope has found its place in most large clinics and hospitals in America.

Since Benedict developed the operating biopsy gastroscope, the diagnosis of gastric disease is on a level equal to that of any other organ which is accessible to endoscopic examination.

INDICATIONS

The indications for gastroscopy are:
1. Some chronic ulcers.
2. Ulcer syndrome with no diagnosis.
3. To follow healing of benign ulcers.
4. Pre-operative check.
5. Differential diagnosis between gastric carcinoma and benign ulcer.
6. Differential diagnosis between chronic gastritis and gastric neurosis.
7. Gross gastric hemorrhage.

*Presented before the General Session at the Annual Meeting of the Oklahoma State Medical Association April 15, 1953.

8. Questionable narrowed antrum.
9. Post-operative stomach.
10. Atrophic gastritis.
11. Pernicious anemia.
12. Any unexplained suspected stomach disease.

Direct visualization of the gastric mucosa will sometimes reveal some form of gastritis. Some small gastric ulcers cannot be seen by the roentgenologist and are diagnosed only by gastroscopy. Gastric ulcers, in younger individuals, can often be treated medically and followed by both x-ray and gastroscopy. In addition, a biopsy of the ulcer with the operating gastroscope reveals the pathology present.

In preparing a patient for gastrectomy, it is our policy to perform a pre-operative gastroscopy. Occasionally a patient with a duodenal ulcer may have such a severe gastritis that surgery should be postponed. Also, the gastritis may be so extensive that a radical gastrectomy should be done.

The importance of pre-operative gastroscopy is illustrated by the case of a 60-year old man who had a subtotal gastrectomy for a chronic duodenal ulcer with pyloric obstruction and recent hemorrhage. A gastroscopic examination several weeks before surgery revealed only moderate hypertrophic gastritis. However, the patient refused gastroscopy the day before surgery. In the resected portion of the stomach was a shallow, acute gastric ulcer located near the edge of the line of excision. No evidence of the ulcer was found on the external surface of the stomach. If the ulcer had been diagnosed by pre-operative gastroscopy, the surgeon could have located it before determining the line of excision.

Occasionally the symptoms of a patient will cause a doctor to consider a diagnosis of psychoneurosis until a marked atrophic or hypertrophic gastritis is found by gastroscopy.

Causes of gastric hemorrhage are sometimes difficult to determine. In our series of cases (Table 4) there were two examples of gastric bleeding which were not visualized on x-ray. One was a bleeding polyp and the other an acute superficial erosion. Hypertropic gastritis may rarely produce massive hemorrhage.

The diagnosis of gastrojejunal ulcer is quite often difficult in the post-operative patient, especially in one who has not had a gastrectomy, and who presents the differential diagnosis between a recurring duodenal ulcer and a stomal ulcer. Most gastrojejunal lesions can be seen by the gastroscopist.

Atrophic gastritis and the gastric atrophy of pernicious anemia are precancerous lesions. About 10 per cent of the patients with pernicious amenia develop carcinoma. Most polyps develop in stomachs with achlorhydria and atrophic changes. Therefore, any patient who has atrophic changes in the stomach should be examined every six to 12 months.

CONTRAINDICATIONS

The contraindications for gastroscopy are absolute and relative:

1. *Absolute*
   (a) Non-cooperation of the patient.
   (b) Obstruction of esophagus or cardia.
   (c) Aneurysm of descending aorta.
   (d) Acute corrosive and acute phlegmonous gastritis.
2. *Relative*
   (a) Acute and chronic tonsillitis and pharyngitis.
   (b) Cardiac insufficiency.
   (c) Dyspnea.
   (d) Cardiospasm.
   (e) Pulsion diverticulum of esophagus.
   (f) Esophageal varices.
   (g). Kyphosis and scoliosis of thoracic spine.
   (h). Psychosis.
   (i). Hiatal hernia.

When a relative contraindication is present, careful handling of the patient will usually lead to successful gastroscopy. The flexible scope can often be passed in spite of a moderate thoracic kyphosis. If a hiatal hernia can be reduced the instrument can be passed into the stomach.

TABULATION OF EXAMINATIONS

The following tables summarize the results of gastroscopy on 171 patients at the Sugg Clinic, Ada, Oklahoma, during 1951 and 1952:

The following are case reports which reveal the importance of gastroscopy.

CASE REPORTS

(1) A 60-year-old white female entered the hospital several hours after marked hematemesis of bright red blood, soon followed by tarry stools. Past history revealed that she had had four previous similar episodes during the past 12 years, each being treated by bed rest and iron. The patient had refused surgery since no cause for the bleeding had been determined.

After admission, the RBC was 2,950,000 and Hgb. 64 per cent. All other laboratory work was normal. Free HCl following histamine was 32°. X-ray examination of the upper gastro-intestinal tract two days later revealed only a large diverticulum on the medial side of the second portion of the duodenum. Fluoroscopic examination had been difficult due to both the patient's weakened condition and the fact that she weighed 250 pounds.

Gastroscopic examination four days after x-ray revealed a large bleeding polyp on the lesser curvature of the antrum just promimal to the pylorus. Subsequent gastrotomy confirmed this, and a 1.5x1.0 cm. bleeding benign polyp was removed.

(2). A 30-year-old white female entered the hospital after the sudden onset of tarry stools and indigestion. She had been taking rather heavy doses of salicylates for rheumatism. RBC was 4,000,000 with Hgb. 80 per cent. Free HCl was 36°.

X-ray examination of the upper gastrointestinal tract was normal. Gastroscopy, however, revealed a definite small superficial hemorrhagic erosion on the lesser curvature of the antrum just proximal to the pyloric sphincter.

Following the withdrawal of salicylates the patient had no further gastro-intestinal

TABLE 1. CAUSES OF UNSUCCESSFUL EXAMINATION IN 6 CASES	
Lack of cooperation	2
Lack of cooperation and marked kyphosis	1
Lack of cooperation due to language barrier	1
Hiatal hernia	2

TABLE 2. DIAGNOSIS MADE BY GASTROSCOPY IN 171 CASES

Normal stomach	63	Superficial erosion	1
Hypertrophic gastritis	36	Prolapse of gastric mucosa	1
Atrophic gastritis	24	Pyloric obstruction	1
Superficial gastritis	4	Phytobezoar	1
Gastric atrophy associated with		Post-operative stomach	12
pernicious anemia	2	Normal gastroenterostomy	6
Tumor simulating gastritis	1	Superficial gastritis	2
Carcinoma of the stomach	11	Giant hypertrophic gastritis	1
Gastric ulcer	12	Stomal ulcer	1
		Recurrent carcinoma	1
Benign polyp	2	Gastrostomy	1

symptoms.

(3). A 47-year-old male gave a history of vague epigastric pain, indigestion, and weight loss for two years. Blood count was normal, free HCl was 68°, and the stool was negative for occult blood.

X-ray examination revealed a large ulcerated mass occupying most of the antrum, and the roentgenologist made the diagnosis of far-advanced carcinoma. The patient was therefore given a bland diet and antispasmodics. He, however, returned in nine months feeling much improved. Repeat x-ray examination revealed very little change except for more antral obstruction. Following this, gastroscopy was done and this showed very marked hypertrophic changes with large nodular, edematous folds, which no doubt represented a tumor-simulating hypertrophic gastritis. The patient continued to do well with a 10-pound weight gain in the next seven months and complete disappearance of symptoms on medical therapy.

(4). A 49-year-old white male had a gastro-jejunostomy in 1948 for a chronic duodenal ulcer with pyloric obstruction. In 1951 he had a return of ulcer symptoms with a 20-pound weight loss and occult blood in his stools.

X-ray examination revealed a chronic duodenal ulcer with some mal-function and edema of the gastro-jejunostomy. However, gastroscopy revealed a definite jejunal ulcer, and subsequent surgery confirmed this with the finding of a large chronic jejunal ulcer.

(5). A 63-year-old white male gave a history of indigestion for 10 years and of having had a perforated gastric ulcer in 1949. He was next seen in 1950, at which time x-ray revealed a duodenal ulcer. He was not seen again until February, 1953, at which time he had a marked increase in symptoms and weight loss, anemia, and occult blood in his stools. At that time, x-ray reported a large irregular filling defect in the body of the stomach, interpreted as a carcinoma. Free HCl after histamine was 75°.

Gastroscopy revealed an acute gastric ulcer on the anterior wall of the distal body and also a large brownish-black multi-lobulated lesion in the body of the stomach. A diagnosis of a bezoar was made, and after

TABLE 3. INCORRECT GASTROSCOPIC DIAGNOSES COMPARED WITH
CORRECT FINAL DIAGNOSES MADE IN 7 CASES

Incorrect Gastroscopic Diagnoses:	Correct Final Diagnoses
Infiltrating carcinoma	Retained food and secretions
Post-operative gastro-jejunitis	Recurrent scirrhous carcinoma
Recurrent carcinoma	Giant hypertrophic gastritis
Infiltrating carcinoma	Hypertrophic gastritis
Infiltrating carcinoma	Atrophic gastritis
Gastric lues	Carcinoma
Malignant ulcer	Benign ulcer

TABLE 4. INCORRECT X-RAY DIAGNOSES COMPARED WITH CORRECT
GASTROSCOPIC DIAGNOSES IN 71 CASES

Incorrect X-Ray Diagnoses:	Correct Gastroscopic Diagnoses:
Possible lesion lesser curvature	Carcinoma
Normal gastro-enterostomy	Mal-functioning stoma
Diffuse polyposis	Normal
Carcinoma of pylorus	Normal
Normal	Bleeding erosion
Carcinoma of stomach	Phytobezoar
Normal	Gastric ulcer
Carcinoma	Tumor simulating gastritis
Normal	Stomal ulcer
Normal	Bleeding polyp
Prolapsing antral polyp	Normal
Normal	Hypertrophic gastritis (36)
Normal	Atrophic gastritis (24)

a history of eating persimmons for 15 years was obtained, repeat gastroscopy was done and a definite diagnosis of a phytobezoar was made. At surgery, one large 4x5x8 cm. and two smaller 3x4 cm. bezoars were removed from the stomach, and the patient has had no further difficulty.

CONCLUSIONS

The relationship between x-ray and gastroscopic examinations is very important. Moersch and Kirkland have stated, "The close collaboration of the gastroenterologists, roentgenologist, and gastroscopist is of great importance in improving the chances of earlier diagnosis of carcinoma of the stomach."

Gastroscopy is an easy and fascinating method of examination, and with the proper preparation and psychological approach, can be done without any discomfort to the patient. Not few are those who prefer a gastroscopic examination under the proper sedation and local anesthesia to a gastric analysis.

SUMMARY

The indications and contraindications for gastroscopy are given, and the results of 171 examinations are reported.

The tables include causes of unsuccessful examinations, gastroscopic diagnosis, and a comparison of gastroscopic and x-ray diagnoses.

Five representative cases reports are presented.

REFERENCES
1. Schindler, R., Gastroscopy, The Endoscopic Study of Gastric Pathology, University of Chicago Press. Second Edition.
2. Palmer, E. D., Stomach Disease as Diagnosed by Gastroscopy, 1949. Lea and Febriger.
3. Moersch, H. J., and Kirklin, B. R., Gastroscopy and Its Relation to Roentgenology.
4. In the Diagnosis of Carcinoma of the Stomach, Gastroenterology, 7:23, 1946.

PLAN   TO   ATTEND

the

OKLAHOMA ACADEMY OF GENERAL PRACTICE

FEBRUARY 15-16 — TULSA HOTEL

TULSA, OKLAHOMA

ADMISSION SMALL CHEST FILM

L. M. PASCUCCI, M.D.

TULSA, OKLAHOMA

The decade 1930 to 1940 ushered in the era of the mass chest x-ray survey for tuberculosis. Late in the same decade the development of photoflurography made available a relatively inexpensive procedure for carrying out these mass surveys. Inasmuch as 16,000,000 or more persons are admitted to general hospitals each year[1], it was inevitable that this chest screening procedure should be considered as an addition to the routine admission blood count, urinalysis and serology. Oatway[2] conducted a hospital survey and in 1949 reported that 247 out of 4,539 hospitals already had this program in action. In New York state alone, 166 voluntary non-profit and public general hospitals had, up to 1951, incorporated the admission chest x-ray[3]. A report[4] by the Wisconsin Anti-tuberculosis Association revealed that of 110 hospitals contacted, 22 already had and 13 were planning a routine admission film. We are at the moment not aware of the number of hospitals throughout the United States employing the routine admission chest film, but it may be worthy of note that the following organizations have gone on record as endorsing the program:

The American Hospital Association

The American Medical Association,

U. S. Public Health Service,

National Tuberculosis Association,

and the

Americal Trudeau Society.

Very recently the American College of Radiology and the American College of Chest Physicians joined in support of the program.[5] In addition many state and county societies throughout the country have voiced approval and urged adoption of this program.

Our study is concerned with 3,875 out of a total of 21,703 admissions to St. John's Hospital during the period between June 1, 1951 and May 31, 1952. We are aware that this is too short a period for any worthwhile statistical analysis, but we believe that we have acquired information which will enable us to determine whether the program should be continued, and experience for making desirable modifications if continued. Obviously the value of the program hinges on its ability to demonstrate chest disease not known to the patient or doctor;

that is, its effectiveness as a screening method.

For the purpose of presentation we have selected the following categories:

1. Pulmonary and mediastinal neoplasms.
2. Inflammatory lesions.
3. Non-inflammatory lesions.
4. Miscellaneous.
5. Tuberculosis.

Only the first four classifications will be considered at this time. A subsequent report will concern itself entirely with tuberculosis.

It is quite generally recognized that the radiograph is the best method known at present for demonstrating chest tumors when there is some chance for a cure. Overholt[6] has emphasized that lung cancer can be detected when in the silent phase. Of 145 patients explored at his clinic between 1938 and 1950 for abnormalities discovered in chest surveys, 51 had lesions which proved to be neoplastic and of these, 35 were malignant. Blades[7] has stated that "successful early diagnosis of lung cancer depends almost entirely on early roentgenograms of the chest"; that asymptomatic bronchogenic carcinomata discovered on routine x-ray films of the chest are usually resectable. Boucot[8] reported an incidence of proven cancer of 0.13 per cent (24 cases) in 18,633 satisfactory photoflurograms. Many other unreported and uncounted isolated silent pulmonary growths have been discovered by extensive mass chest x-rays conducted as a community project. With extension of the program to all hospitals, coverage of the population can be broadened with undoubted resultant increase in the number of curable lung cancers detected.

Table 1 summarizes our findings in the category of pulmonary and mediastanal neoplasms. Only one half of the PFX films were checked by a routine 14x17 inch film. In 66 per cent, confirmation of the presence of a lesion was obtained; of these the lesion was unsuspected in one-half. Although only seven out of 24 were unsuspected, actually from a radiological viewpoint, we must give the procedure credit for picking up 16 out of 24 since the radiologist was not aware of the patient's symptomatology or physical findings in the known cases when he reported the small film.

The next table, Table 2 summarizes the unclassified pulmonary lesions; that is, shadows which were questionable, which could not be labeled or in which the finding of a haziness or infiltrate was reported. Of 55 such, only 21 were rechecked by large film with confirmation in 14. Of note is the fact that there were three patients with significant disease, (bronchiectasis, pulmonary metastasis and benign tumor) which were unknown to the patient or referring physician. Adding to those, the three known or suspected lesions we would then have a total of six instances of significant disease demonstrated on small films in this category.

TABLE I
NEOPLASMS

PFX Positive or Suspect—48   14x17'' Film—24
Confirmed—16   Not Confirmed—8

Known—9	Not Known—7	
Ca. of Lung	4 Hamnartoma	1 Pulmonary
Lymphoblas-	Mediastinal me-	Segment 1
toma	1 tastasis (Leio-	Inflammatory 2
Mediastinal	myosarcoma	Hilar
Path.	1 of uterus	1 Prominence 1
Malignant	Lung Metastasis	Negative Chest 4
Melanoma	(Pancreas)	1 *How Confirmed*
(Choroid)	1 Lympholastoma	1 Operation 3
Lung Metastas-	Hodgkin's	1 Bronchoscopy 2
es (Pancreas)	1 Lung Cyst	1 Known
(Prostate)	1 Substernal	1 Primary 5
		Autopsy 1
		Biopsy 3
		X-Ray 2

TABLE II
UNCLASSIFIED

PFX+ or 14x17''	Confirmation	Yes	No
Suspect—55 Film—21		14	7
Known or Suspect—3	Not Known or		
Bronchogenic cyst	Suspect		11
(operation) 1	Fibrosis &		
Pneumonia - misdiagnos-	Emphysema		4
ed ea. (Operation) 1	Atypical		
Fibrosis & Emphysema)	pneumonia)		
Substernal thyroid) 1	Bronchiectasis)		1
	(Bronchogram))		
	Benign calcific		
	tumor		1
	Tbc. inactive		2
	Metastases (Pleura		
	& parenchymal)		1
	Fibrosis		1
	Emphysema		1

The remaining categories may be considered briefly. Only seven of 25 positive or suspect inflammatory lesions were checked by large films and of these, three diagnoses of pleural effusion, and one of pneumonitis were established. However, only one pleural effusion was a surprise finding to the referring physician. Only one of 13 in the non-inflammatory category was checked by a large film probably because the diagnosis of fibrosis and emphysema did not frighten the referring physicians. The interpreta-

TABLE III
ALL CATEGORIES

		Confirmed 35	Not Confirmed 21	
		Significant Lesion		
PFX Category	14x17'' Film	Un-known	Known	
+ Neoplasms	24	16	6	9	8
O Pulmonary Lesion (Unclassified)	21	14	3	2	7
I Inflammatory Lesions	7	4	1	3	3
NI Non-inflammatory	1	0	0	0	1
M Miscellaneous	3	1	1	0	2
Total	56	35	11	14	21

tion on this 14x17 inch film was inconclusive and probably not significant. In the miscellaneous category three of six PFX films were checked and a diagnosis of silocotuberculosis was made of which the referring physician had no prior knowledge.

A summary of all categories is seen in Table 3. There is a 62 per cent confirmation by 14x17 film. Had a higher number of larger films been taken, it is very likely that the percentage of confirmations and significant pathology would be lower but still very substantial. Of significance, however, is the appreciable number of serious diseases, exclusive of tuberculosis conditions, demonstrated which were unknown to the referring physician or patient. This is a small series but Jacobson[9] with a similar program at the Los Angeles County Hospital has reported that in a hospital survey the percentage pickup of disease is 10 times as great as in the general community at large survey.

Conclusion: This preliminary report would seem to support the copious literature on the value of routine admission and hospital x-rays as a method of discovering disease not previously suspected by patient or doctor. Statistics in this small series are of no value; of more significance is the detection of four malignant and three benign lung lesions. Not detracting from the value of the method is the fact that nine additional patients with malignant lesions known or suspected by referring doctor were detected also.

REFERENCES

1. Bryant, Zella. Tuberculosis Case Findings in General Hospitals. Public Health Reports 65: 710, June 2, 1950.
2. Oatway, W. H. Jr. The Current Status of Routine X-raying in General Hospitals of the United States, Arizona Med. 6:23, 1949.
3. Siegal, W., Plunkett, R. E., and Hillehoe, H. E. Modern Hospital July, 1951.
4. Hein, John P. X-ray News-Report 24:6, November 1952.
5. Report of the Joint Committee. Diseases of the Chest 20: 709, June, 1952.
6. Overholt, Richard A. Cancer Detention in Surveys, Am. Rev. Tuberc. 62: 491-500, November, 1950.
7. Blades, Brian. Quoted in X-ray News.
8. Boucot, Katherine R. Mass Surveys on Case-Finding Techniques for Pulmonary Neoplasms. Am. Rev. Tuberc. 62: 501-511, November 1950.
9. Jacobson, G. Excerpt in X-ray News, 24:3, August, 1952.

THE DIAGNOSIS AND EVALUATION OF TREATMENT
OF THE LUMBAR INTERVERTEBRAL DISK *

Averill Stowell, M.D., Robert A.

Hayne, M.D., Tulsa, Oklahoma, Robert

A. Martini, M.D., Muskogee, Oklahoma

A great deal has been written about the diagnosis and treatment of the lumbar intervertebral disks, and this afternoon we felt that it might be interesting to discuss some of the more unusual features of this syndrome and evaluate the surgical methods of treatment. This paper will present the results of an analysis of 725 cases of suspected disk, referred to the Springer Clinic in Tulsa and to the Veterans Administration Hospital in Muskogee, Oklahoma.

You have all seen the young male who comes into the office with a complaint of severe pain in the back and one leg. Let us assume that while he was lifting a piano he noted the sudden onset of severe pain in the low back, which rapidly rediated downward into the leg. This caused him to lean over to one side when walking, and was often associated with numbness and tingling in the involved extremity. He might have had some weakness of the leg. On examination in the office you noted that the man tended to favor the painful leg in walking, that there was a marked scoliosis and reversal of the normal lumbar curve, associated with spasm of the lumbosacral musculature, that the ankle jerk was diminished or absent, and that sensory changes were found over the lateral portion of the leg and foot. If you raised his leg from the horizontal toward a 45 degree angle, you produced severe pain. You prescribed some Tolserol, bed rest on boards, and made a tentative diagnosis of protrusion or rupture of the intervertebral disk. At the end of four or five weeks, if the patient did not improve, you referred him to your orthopedist or neurosurgeon for more definite treatment.

*Presented before the Section of Neurology and Psychiatry at the Annual Meeting of the Oklahoma State Medical Association April 13, 1953.

Likewise, you have seen patients who complained of pain in both legs, associated with a relatively minor injury, and classical signs of the intervertebral disk were not present. Such patients might have pain in the inguinal region on one side, or of the great toe. They might complain of swelling of the leg or coldness of the feet. Or they might complain of numbness in the whole leg itself. The numbness occasionally is confined solely to the lateral portion of the thigh in the distribution of the lateral femoral cutaneous. Cramps on walking or on lying in bed might be the sole complaint. On examination you might note some very definite edema and cyanosis present in the lower extremity, or you might find a complete absence of evidences of sciatic nerve compression.

The x-ray findings in these cases in the first attack are usually essentially normal in regard to the intervertebral spaces, and we find no evidence of narrowing of the intervertebral space. In the more chronic disk we find evidences of localized osteoarthritis, usually involving the fourth and fifth lumbar vertebral bodies with narrowing.

Myelograms in the cases of disks are fairly reliable, although in a series of 42 consecutive cases there were 15 false-positives and three false-negatives, with a lesion found at another interspace in the false-positives or no disk found, and in the false-negatives a rupture or protrusion was found.

The next few slides will show some of the myelographic changes that are characteristic, and which may usually be called positive. Some of the more doubtful myelographic signs are also present, which may or may not indicate a protrusion of the disk.

In regard to the treatment of these cases, we feel that conservative therapy should be utilized and to the maximum degree. We feel that the most beneficial treatment in the acute disk is putting the patient to bed on boards for a period of seven days, and then having the patient in a flexion bed for a period of another seven days, perhaps utilizing leg traction during this period of time intermittently. Tolserol, Prostigmine, and other medicaments are given during this period to produce as great muscle relaxation as possible. At the end of 14 days the patient is allowed to go home with instructions to be as quiet as possible for another four weeks. At the end of this period he is re-examined and evaluated. Usually he has shown definite improvement. He is told to remain off his job for a further two-week period, and then to go back and try light work for a period of one month. If, after a three to four-month period, the patient is continuing to have pain of moderate degree, and is unable to work, we feel that surgical interference should be considered. We feel that surgery is indicated also in the acute ruptured intervertebral disk, where very positive findings, consisting of paralysis or very marked weakness, are present, and the patient has no alleviation of pain on 14 days of conservative treatment in the hospital.

In regard to the operation, we feel that a full hemi-laminectomy as advocated by W. James Gardner, is the procedure of choice. This allows a very adequate exposure, and prevents some of the complications present in other forms of disk surgery. We are able to visualize the midline disk without difficulty, as well as note a displaced disk which has moved upward from the intervertebral space or downward. Most important, we are able to spare the nerve root, and to control bleeding without damaging the nerve root. It is important to produce as little trauma to the nerve root as possible. Likewise, the more extensive operation allows a constriction of the intervertebral foramen to be visualized, and a decompression carried out if necessary. . We do not feel that the more complete operation adds to the instability of the back. The question of fusion will be discussed by Doctor Martini of the Veterans Hospital. We do not feel that routine fusion is indicated.

The causes of failure from surgery are: 1) occasionally the disk is not found or a double disk may be present. 2- a midline or bilateral disk has been noted in 6 per cent of the cases. 3) recurrence of the disk may result from insufficient curetting of the in-terspace, which is difficult in the interlaminal approach. 4) a root injury is the most usual cause of failure, while adhesions are present in approximately 25 per cent of the cases. 5) an injured facet is found in some instances.

The results in these cases are summarized. We note that there is very little difference between the results at the Springer Clinic and at the Veterans Administration Hospital. This may be due to the fact that some of the Springer Clinic group consist of compensation cases.

Our criteria, as you will note, are based on the ability of the patient to return to work, with or without pain. These. results compare very favorably with the results of other groups, and it will be noted that in approximately 80 to 95 per cent of the cases the patient is able to return to work without too much difficulty.

In this discussion of the intervertebral disk, I would like to re-emphasize certain features. First, there may be definite pain over sympathetic pathways, and it is possible in the preoperative stage to partially alleviate pain by paravertebral blocks in some cases, and in the postoperative case to often bring about a change from a poor to a fair result by paravertebral injections. Occasionally it has been necessary to do a sympathectomy when marked causalgic symptoms are present.

Likewise, in borderline cases, where a diagnosis of disk is not absolutely definite, we feel that an evaluation of the financial and physical handicaps of the patient should be one of the criteria for surgical interference. In other words, if the patient is not able to work, but has continuation of pain, we feel that surgery may well be indicated, and we are willing to accept a decrease in the percentage of cures to help these patients. In some of them no disk will be found, and they will obtain relief. In others, a small protrusion will be found, and no relief will be obtained. It is very important in these doubtful cases to evaluate both the compensation, the psychoneurotic, and the pension angles, and this is carefully done over a period of one, two, or three office visits.

We have mentioned the postoperative poor results and the causes of these. We feel that should the patient go along for a period of three to six months after operation without any definite relief with conservative treatment, and even the utilization of x-ray ther-

(Continued on Page 20)

The Problem of Nausea and Vomiting:

ITS TREATMENT WITH DRAMAMINE®

Whenever nausea, vomiting and vertigo are disturbing and complicating factors, Dramamine may be used with confidence.

Keats[1] outlines the wide list of conditions in which Dramamine (brand of dimenhydrinate) has proved valuable as follows: "It has been well established in the control of motion sickness. It has been used effectively in the prevention and treatment of seasickness, airsickness, [in the treatment of] the nausea of pregnancy, Ménière's syndrome, ... radiation sickness ... and postfenestration reactions. ... The site of action is imperfectly understood, but there is indication of an action of depressing labyrinthine function or its neural pathways, a highly selective central action, or both. Few side reactions of this drug have been noted."

The usual dose for motion sickness is 50 mg. (one tablet) taken one-half hour before departure and, if necessary, before meals for the duration of the journey. Control of nausea and vomiting of other conditions and severe motion sickness is achieved, with minimal drowsiness, by a dosage of 100 mg. every four hours.

"[Dramamine] is administered orally or rectally. ... The same doses may be administered rectally by insertion of the tablet or other suitable form. ... "[2]

Dramamine Liquid is particularly useful for children.

Dramamine is accepted by the Council on Pharmacy and Chemistry of the American Medical Association.

1. Keats, S.: Ataxic Cerebral Palsy with Akinetic Seizures: Dramatic Response to Dramamine, J. M. Soc. New Jersey 50:53 (Feb.) 1953.
2. Council on Pharmacy and Chemistry: New and Nonofficial Remedies, 1953, Philadelphia, J. B. Lippincott Company, 1953, p. 471.

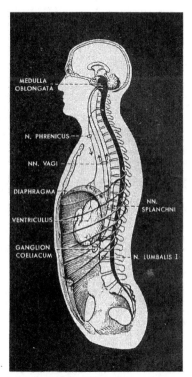

THE VOMITING REFLEX: *Vagus→ nodose ganglion→ solitary tract→ spinal cord→ cerviral, thoracic and lumbar nerves to diaphragm, cardiac sphincter, stomach, abdominal and pelvic musculature. (After Krieg, W. J. S.: Functional Neuroanatomy, ed. 2, New York, The Blakiston Company, Inc., 1953, p. 104.)*

SEARLE *Research in the Service of Medicine*

President's Page

With the beginning of this New Year the American people will be looking with interest and hope toward our national capitol.

With the convening of Congress, the Eisenhower administration will have an opportunity to prove to the country that it is an administration dedicated to the preservation of American ideals, with a sound fiscal policy and a foreign policy which will strengthen the hope of everyone for a lasting peace for the world at large.

In addition to these broad observations, American medicine will watch with interest the recommendations that will come from our newest member of the Cabinet, Mrs. Oveta Culp Hobby as Secretary of Health, Welfare and Education. In addition to Mrs. Hobby's recommendations in the field of health and welfare, close watch must also be kept on the work of the Hoover and Moulton Commissions. The Hoover Commission, which is studying the general organization and operation of the government will have as one of its prime studies the consideration of medical and health programs, including the Veterans Administration, which are now spread through 54 different agencies of government. The Moulton Commission likewise, will have an important recommendation to make to Congress as it pertains to fringe benefits in the field of medical care for the dependents of members of our military forces. This latter Commission's study and recommendations have an important bearing on the total number of physicians it will be necessary to integrate from either private practice or the interns and residents completing their postgraduate work into military service.

In addition to the action of Congress in the field of health and welfare, the medical profession should take a keen interest in bringing about the adoption of the so-called Bricker Amendment to our Constitution, which amendment would preclude international treaties to which our government subscribes, becoming the law of the land without action by Congress. It is unnecessary to point out the dangers involved in our p r e s e n t situation which the Bricker Amendment is attempting to correct. I urge that each physician who may have occasion to, contact our Senators to make his position known concerning the Bricker Amendment.

Sincerely yours,

John E McDonald M.D.

President

ACADEMY OF GENERAL PRACTICE LISTS PROGRAM TOPICS

Program has been completed for the annual meeting of the Oklahoma Academy of General Practice to be held February 15 and 16 at the Tulsa Hotel, Tulsa, Oklahoma. Speakers and titles have been announced as follows:

William F. Guerriero, M.D., clinical associate professor of obstetrics and gynecology, Southwestern Medical College of Texas at Dallas—''Carcinoma of the Cervix'' and ''Pelvic Pain.''

Horace L. Hodes, M.D., director of pediatrics, Mt. Sinai Hospital, New York—''Treatment of the Severe Forms of Poliomyelitis, and the Present Status of Measures Aimed at the Prevention of the Disease'' and ''The Antibiotic Problem and the Question of Antagonism.''

Manuel E. Lichtenstein, M.D., professor of surgery at Cook County Graduate School of Medicine, Chicago—''The Clinical Significance of the Position and Station of the Appendix'' and ''The Significance of Gall Stones to the Patient and to the Surgeon''.

Perrin H. Long, M.D., chairman of the Department of Medicine at the State University of New York, Brooklyn—''Uses and Abuses of the Antibiotics'' and ''The Etiology and Management of Longevity.''

Carlo Scuderi, M.D., associate professor of surgery at the University of Illinois, Chicago — ''Backache; From the Standpoint of a General Practioner-Diagnosis and Treatment'' and ''Treatment of Both Bone Fractures of the Leg.''

Harry Wilkins, M.D., Oklahoma City neurosurgeon—''Diagnosis of Intracranial Lesions'' and ''Emergency Treatment of Head Injuries''.

Complete program of the meeting will be mailed to O.S.M.A. members soon.

DIET MANUAL IS AVAILABLE

Of interest to physicians is the *Diet Manual* recently published by the Oklahoma Dietetic Association. Assistance in preparation of material was given by a committee of the Oklahoma State Medical Association. The *Manual* was first released at the Oklahoma State Hospital Association meeting in Tulsa in November.

The diet plans were developed primarily for the convenience of personnel in small hospitals and for clinicians who might wish to use the forms for planning and teaching dietary modifications. The manual is of loose leaf design and additional pages may be inserted. It consists of 29 pages with additional pages of tables. The terminology is simplified for the use of untrained kitchen personnel in small hospitals. A non profit project, financed by the state Dietetic Association, the price of the manual is $1.25. Individual diets in the book are available in reprint form. Among the diets included are ones for infant and pediatric care.

For the convenience of those who would like to obtain copies of the *Diet Manual*, an order blank is given below.

```
DIET MANUAL ORDER BLANK
Mail To: .........................................................
    .....................................................................
    .....................................................................
No. ordered.................................... ($1.25 each)
Check enclosed in amount of $........................
To: Oklahoma Dietetic Association
    P.O. Box 3842 N.W. Station
    Oklahoma City, Oklahoma.
```

McGREW CLINIC OPENED IN BEAVER

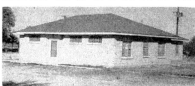

Pictured above is the new McGrew Clinic in Beaver, Oklahoma. Built by E. A. McGrew, M.D., the building consists of office space for two doctors and one dentist, and is fireproof, as dust proof as it is possible to build, and has refrigerated air conditioning. Robert M. Stover, M.D., of Miami, Okla., will be associated with Doctor McGrew when he completes his residency at the University Hospital, Oklahoma City.

Doctor McGrew's clinic has been constructed just east of the new $400,000 Beaver County Memorial Hospital, which was opened October 19. Doctor McGrew and T. D. Benjegerdes, M.D., (now of Alva) had operated the old Beaver Hospital since 1920.

COUNTY SOCIETY MEETS

Members of the Pittsburg County Medical Society met November 19 at Pete's Place in Krebs. The meeting which was well attended, had representatives from both Pittsburg and Bryan Counties.

Speakers were Representative Carl Albert who discussed problems of national legislation and O.S.M.A. President John McDonald, M.D., Tulsa, who spoke on V.A. Medical Care. Following the two speeches, there was a general discussion period. The county auxiliary Legislative Committee was represented by Mrs. E. D. Greenberger and Mrs. H. C. Wheeler.

CANCER CONGRESS

SLATED FOR BRAZIL

Physicians planning to attend the sixth International Cancer Congress in Sao Paulo, Brazil, July 23-29 are urged to make their travel arrangements immediately. Further information can be obtained from Brewster S. Miller, M.D., Director, Professional Education Section, American Cancer Society, 47 Beaver St., New York 4, N. Y.

Steamship arrangements from New York or New Orleans may be made or chartered plane via regularly scheduled airlines from Miami or New York. For those taking the chartered flight from Miami to Sao Paulo, the round trip saving will be approximately $194.00. Tentative program information can be obtained from the Executive Office or from Doctor Miller.

CLINIC OPENED IN ENID

Doctors George and Hope Ross and E. M. Robinson have opened a new clinic at 1101 East Broadway, Enid, Okla.

The one story building of steel frame and masonry construction has a unique floor plan reflecting a careful study of traffic flow. Special ''sick baby'' and ''well baby'' waiting rooms are provided.

FROM THE OKLAHOMA DIVISION AMERICAN CANCER SOCIETY

"Because it appears to be growing steadily more harassing, some remarks concerning cancer quackery are in order. They are in order, too, for the reason that from time to time the headquarters office is chided for failure to abate this or that nuisance of quackery, sometimes of local, occasionally of national concern, but always vexatious to conscientious stewards of cancer control. Cancer quackery flourishes as never before. There are fewer small-time operators than there were in grandma's time; but those in business now are in big business. Bitters, barks, and berries have given way to vaccines, scientific diets, and chemotherapy. The acetylene lights have been outmoded by high pressure direct mail advertising; the tom-tom is displaced by the press agent. The press agent is the most curious of the modern quack's gimmicks. He is not paid. He earns his living in legitimate enterprise—but usually one which involves an audience. He himself is honest, but yet not qualified to pass judgment on treatment for cancer. He is duped into playing Svengali to the quack's Trilby because he thinks he has discovered an unsung hero who has been dealt with unfairly. He defends the little fellow against the big bad wolf called organized medicine. In a word, he is a champion. He is one of the widening circle, small in number but long on decibles. In the halls of Congress, in state legisla-

tures, in newspaper columns, and on the radio, their heavy and incompetent fingers are pointed at conjured bottlenecks in science's efforts to solve this most complex of biological riddles. Their harangues have lately taken on a new, consistent, and ominous pattern: organized medicine is charged with wilfully and maliciously suppressing or ignoring evidence which promises vast benefit to cancer sufferers. If such a charge could be made out to be other than wholly irresponsible, it would follow that organized medicine is a good deal better organized than it has been in the past, when it failed to suppress insulin, sulfa drugs, penicillin, cortisone, and an impressive list of other therapeutic agents. But perhaps organized medicine is interested in hampering only the development of more effective cancer treatment; if so—it has fallen down badly in having permitted nitrogen mustard, folic acid antagonists, triethylene-phosphoramide, sex harmones, and a half-dozen radio isotopes to find a place in modern cancer therapeutics, not to mention its negligence in curbing recent surgical adcances and the development of more powerful radiations which are providing increased life and comfort to cancer victims."

From the annual report to the members by Charles S. Cameron, M D, Medical and Scientific Director, American Cancer Society.

The Diagnosis and Evaluation of Treatment of the Lumbar Intervertebral Disk

(Continued from Page 16)

apy, we should perform a re-exploration.

I would like to briefly mention the presence of fascial fat hernia, or tender nodules in the lumbar area, pressure over which will reproduce both the back and the sciatic pain. In these cases Procaine injection will often produce definite relief of the symptomatology, and we are able to remove these nodules without difficulty. It is important, however, to be sure that an intervertebral disk is not present in these cases. This is usually possible by noting no changes in the neurological examination.

Also it should be mentioned that a lumbar disk at the fourth interspace may produce only pain in the back, with very little evidence of sciatic pain and a completely negative neurological examination.

CONCLUSION

In conclusion, we feel that with a careful work-up and evaluation over 90 per cent of disk surgery can be successfully carried out and the patient returned to work.

Borderline cases should be treated surgically if his working status is not restored after six months of conservative treatment.

Fusion, as a routine measure, is not indicated in disk surgery.

A lack of typical signs and symptoms, es-

pecially sympathetic system disturbances, do not contraindicate a diagnosis of lumbar intervertebral disk.

RADIOLOGICAL SOCIETY MEETS AT LAKE MURRAY

On November 8, the 58th anniversary of the founding of x-ray by William Conrad Roentgen, M.D., the Oklahoma State Radiological Society held its fall meeting at Lake Murray Lodge near Ardmore.

Guest speaker at the meeting was Glenn Carlson, M.D., Dallas, Texas.

TULSA FORUMS POPULAR

Sponsored by the Tulsa Academy of General Practice and the Tulsa World, the public medical forums held in that city during recent months have been attracting widespread comment.

Audiences in excess of 1,000 have attended many of the forums which have been held on poliomyelitis, heart disease, and cancer. A forum on children's diseases is planned for February 16. Tulsa physicians volunteer their time to serve on the panels.

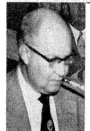

Pictured at left is Malcom Phelps, M.D., El Reno, the O.S.M.A. representative on the Oklahoma Industrial Tour. Doctor Phelps is shown reviewing his notes at a meeting of the group held in New York City.

ORAL PENICILLIN IS AT ITS BEST

 WHEN IT IS RELIABLY ABSORBED

"... the first oral preparation of penicillin which has in our experience been reliably absorbed in 100% of patients, irrespective of size and weight and using a standard dose of 300,000 units ... [it] was given irrespective of the time of meals and whether the stomach might be full or not"[1]; ... "may be given without regard to meals ..."[2,3]

2 WHEN ITS THERAPEUTIC EFFECTIVENESS IS ESTABLISHED

"The results presented indicate that the oral penicillin suspension studied by us is a satisfactory antibiotic for the treatment of some of the common infections of the respiratory tract caused by β-hemolytic streptococci" ... and uncomplicated pneumonias of childhood.[4]

Bicillin "oral suspension is palatable, was accepted without difficulty by all patients in both groups [children and adults] and was well tolerated."[2]

3 WHEN PALATABILITY ASSURES PATIENT COOPERATION

"No children of any age have been disturbed, and the palatability of the product has made its administration easy."[1]

4 WHEN STABILITY ASSURES RETENTION OF POTENCY

Bicillin is highly insoluble in water. Its aqueous suspension, ready for immediate use, is stable for 2 years at ordinary room temperature—77°F. (25°C.). Refrigeration is unnecessary.

 "The development of dibenzylethylenediamine dipenicillin is one of the important milestones in antibiotic therapy."[5]

BICILLIN ®

DIBENZYLETHYLENEDIAMINE DIPENICILLIN G

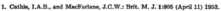

SUPPLIED: ORAL SUSPENSION BICILLIN: Bottles of 2 fl. oz.; 300,000 units per teaspoonful (5 cc.).

TABLETS BICILLIN: 200,000 units; bottles of 36.

TABLETS BICILLIN: 100,000 units; bottles of 100.

PHILADELPHIA 2, PA.

REFERENCES

1. Cathie, I.A.B., and MacFarlane, J.C.W.: Brit. M. J. 1:805 (April 11) 1953.

2. Coriell, L.L., and others: Antibiotics & Chemotherapy 3:357 (April) 1953.

3. Barach, A.L.: Geriatrics 8:423 (August) 1953

4. Finberg, L., Leventer, I., and Tramer, A.: Antibiotics & Chemotherapy 3:353 (April) 1953

5. Editorial: Antibiotics & Chemotherapy 3:347 (April) 1953.

OBITUARIES

ALLEN G. GIBBS, M.D.

1909-1953

Allen G. Gibbs, M.D., Oklahoma City, died unexpectedly November 26, 1953. He was 44.

Doctor Gibbs was President of the Oklahoma Academy of General Practice at the time of his death and had served as secretary of the organization the four previous years. He was a past vice-president of both the Oklahoma State Medical Association and the Oklahoma County Medical Society and was vice-councilor of his district. He was a member of the committee on scientific assembly of the American Academy. of General Practice.

Doctor Gibbs was born in Wilkinson county, Miss., but had lived in Oklahoma City since he was three. He graduated from Central Highschool in Oklahoma City and received both his B.S., and M.D., degrees from the University of Oklahoma. He was a member of Alpha Kappa Kappa medical fraternity. He was also a Mason and a member of the Methodist church.

During World War II, he served as a lieutenant colonel with Oklahoma's 21st evacuation hospital unit. He served three years in the South Pacific before returning to his general practice in Oklahoma City.

Besides his wife and a son 14 and daughter four of the home, 1608 Pennington Way, Oklahoma City, he is survived by his mother, four brothers and a sister.

OKLAHOMANS ATTEND COLLEGE OF SURGEONS

Oklahoma physicians registered at the American College of Surgeons annual Clinical Congress in Chicago included the following:

Floyd T. Bartheld, McAlester; Vance A. Bradford, Oklahoma City; Irwin H. Brown, Oklahoma City; A. L. Buell, Okmulgee; Lt. Ernest P. Carreau, Norman; Richard A. Clay, Oklahoma City; John Clymer, Oklahoma City; Battey C. Coker, Durant; Everette E. Cooke, Oklahoma City; D. V. Crane, Tulsa; Frank E. Darrow, Oklahoma City; H. E. Denyer, Bartlesville; Harold M. Feinberg, Muskogee; Phil Fife, Guthrie; Roy L. Fisher, Frederick; William Patton Fife, Muskogee; John Florence, Oklahoma City; Fred T. Fox, Lawton;

C. C. Fulton, Oklahoma City; Ingvald Haugen, Ada; Thornton Kell, Ardmore; Albert H. Krause, Muskogee; Ray H. Lindsay, Pauls Valley; W. Carl Lindstrom, Tulsa; F. M. Lingenfelter, Oklahoma City; Paul B. Lingenfelter, Clinton; R. E. McDowell, Tulsa; Ralph A. McGill, Tulsa; F. H. McGregor, Oklahoma City; Joseph C. Manning, Midwest City; Edward L. Moore, Tulsa;

Herman R. Moore, Norman; R. L. Murdoch, Oklahoma City; Donald Oesterreicher, Oklahoma City; Joe M. Parker, Oklahoma City; R. E. Roberts, Stillwater; J. H. Robinson, Oklahoma City; C. R. Rountree, Oklahoma City; V. M. Rutherford, Midwest City; Gregory E. Stanbro, Oklahoma City; Richard G. Stoll, Chickasha; Evans E. Talley, Enid; Edmund H. Werling, Pryor; and Harold A. White, Tulsa.

A.M.A. GROUP PLANS TRIP TO HAWAII

A party of physicians and their wives plan to take advantage of the American Medical Association's 13-day Hawaiian Holiday Tour which will follow the annual A.M.A. convention in San Francisco next June 21-25.

The party will leave San Francisco aboard Pan American Airways Strato Clippers and United Air Lines Stratocruisers at 11:45 on the night of Friday, June 25th—the closing day of the convention—and arrive in Honolulu early the next morning.

The guests will stay at the beautiful Royal Hawaiian Hotel at Waikiki Beach during their eight-day stay on the Islands.

The trip includes a motor tour of Oahu and Mount Tantalus, where the visitors will get a panoramic view of Honolulu from Pearl Harbor to Diamond Head. The doctors also plan a visit to the University of Hawaii.

The return trip, scheduled at 4 p.m., on July 3, will be made on the luxurious Matson Liner, S.S. Luline, which will dock in Los Angeles on July 8.

All of the reservations are being handled by W. M. Maloney, general agent, Room 711, 105 West Adams Street, Chicago.

Dr. George F. Lull, Chicago, secretary-general manager of the American Medical Association, said the luxurious holiday tour was arranged so that busy doctors would have an opportunity to take a brief vacation with their families after the convention business ends, and before they return to their homes. "Everything has been planned," he said, "to provide the party with a glorious vacation."

The Hawaii Medical Association will entertain the visiting physicians during their stay on the Islands.

Dr. Edwin K. Chung-Hoon, president of the Hawaii Medical Association, said in a recent letter to Dr. Lull that "a warm Hawaiian Aloha awaits every doctor and guest in the A.M.A. party." Continuing, he said:

"From the moment members of the party are greeted with fresh flower leis and Hawaiian music as they step off the plane until the Royal Hawaiian band wafts the strains of "Aloha Oe" when the S.S. Lurline leaves the dock on July 3, the visitors will be exposed to the spell of the Islands.

"In addition to beach life, sightseeing and such pastimes, doctors in the party will attend the semi-annual meeting of the Hawaii Medical Association, an organization of 518 physicians which was incorporated under the monarchy in 1856. Many doctors likely will find classmates or alumni of their medical schools, since the physicians on the Islands include graduates of all the major medical schools in the United States.

"Dr. Walter B. Quisenberry of Honolulu, general chairman of arrangements for the post-convention tour, guarantees that the scientific and social program will be different from the run-of-the mill medical convention."

Dr. Chung-Hoon added this postscript to his letter to Dr. Lull:

"Come and see for yourself. The Hawaii Medical Association anticipates extending a fond Aloha to you in person next June."

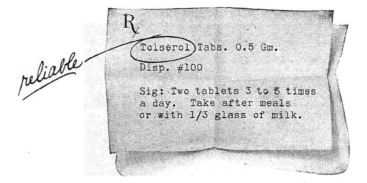
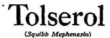

BOOK REVIEWS

MEDICAL TREATMENT OF DISEASE. Vol. VIII.

Henry A. Christian, A.M., M.D., L.L.D., Sc.D.(Hon). M.A.C.P., Hon. F.R.C.P. (Can.), D.S.M. (A.M.A.); Dale G Friend, A.B., M.S., M.D., F.A.C.P.; Maurice A. Schnitker, B.S., M.D., F.A.C.P. Co-Editors, Burgess Gordon, M.D., William J. Kerr, M.D., and Cyrus C. Sturgis, M.D., New York. Oxford University Press. 1953.

This volume in the Oxford Medicine Series represents the last contribution of the great clinician, teacher and author, Henry A. Christian, with whom Friend, Schnitker and their co-authors Gordon, Kerr and Sturgis collaborated.

In the introduction, Burgess Gordon gives the historical background of treatment showing the long continued dominance of empiricism and the appeal of fads and fancies "even in the years of our enlightenment."

He follows the pendulum into the realm of therapeutic nihilism and emerges with emphasis on the functional aspects and the more rational employment of therapeutic measures.

He states that "with the advent of the antibiotics, hormones, vaccines, and the accessory food substances, it became apparent to Dr. Henry A. Christian that treatment called for a companion book for the loose-leaf volumes and the standard textbooks of medicine. He invited Dr. Maurice A. Schnitker and Dr. Dale G. Friend to join with him in writing a book of living therapy. Dr. Christian drew from his past experience of academic and hospital practice to elucidate the value of the newer drugs and procedures. Close associations in pharmacology and clinical medicine enabled Dr. Friend to provide a happy balance of fundamental principles and practical applications in treatment. The manuscript was passed from one author to another for criticism and careful integration and was completed before Dr. Christian's untimely death."

Doctor Christian's critical and constructive guidance is obvious and his favorite dictum "that the value of treatment depends equally on the selection and termination of the regimen" is evident throughout the volume.

The simplicity implied above is best illustrated by this paragraph from the author's preface:

"This book, as the title indicates, will describe the treatment, including prophylaxis, of those diseases or diseased conditions which ordinarily fall in the province of the physician or internist. It will not consider those whose treatment usually is carried out by surgeons and specialists. Descriptions of a multiplicity of methods of treatment will be avoided. When more than one method is described, it has been done because the authors believe that not infrequently more than one method should be available to obtain best results; since individual patients often show differences in reaction to methods of treatment, sometimes one, sometimes the other proves more effective."

It is indicated that with few exceptions the methods recommended are those which the authors have employed and found useful. Apparently they have tried to choose from the new and the old those drugs and methods best suited to the disease or condition under consideration.

They have tried to employ discriminating judgment according to their experience and other available evidence.

The authors have recognized the fact that therapy today cannot become static and that they should provide for inevitable changes. The looseleaf system makes this easy and economical.

A working knowledge of diseases and diseased conditions is assumed and the space is devoted to therapy alone. Of equal importance is the assumption that a correct diagnosis will serve as the basis for treatment.

This handy, well indexed, flexible volume should be frequently fingered by the wide awake physician always in pursuit of the best for his patients.

The fact that this book devoted to treatment, shorn of all fads and fancies contains nearly 1,000 pages, shows the stupendous task confronting the physician and warrants this move toward the selective simplification of therapy.—Lewis J. Moorman, M.D.

FUNCTIONAL DISORDERS OF THE FOOT.

Frank D. Dickson, M.D., and Rex L. Diveley, M.D. J. B. Lippincott Company, 1953.

Wide neglect of feet disorders, the authors' contend, is an important justification for a book such as this. This reviewer is in hearty agreement.

The discussion of the evolution, anatomy and physiology of feet forms a sound background for the ensuing clinical descriptions. The discussion of functional disorders and their treatment is so detailed as to be prolix and repetitious.

In spite of the title, some organic diseases of the various pedal components are also discussed. Other important conditions such as gout as well as infectious and neoplasms are strangely omitted.

The authors' recommendations concerning proper footwear and the types of shoe corrections are clear and helpful as is the pictorial outline of foot exercises.—James E. Shipley, M.D.

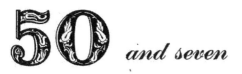 *and seven*

YEARS TREATING ALCOHOL
AND DRUG ADDICTION

In 1897 Doctor B. B. Ralph developed methods of treating alcohol and narcotic addiction that, by the standards of the time, were conspicuous for success.

Twenty-five years ago experience had bettered the methods. Today with the advantages of collateral medicine, treatment is markedly further improved.

The Ralph Sanitarium provides personalized care in a quiet, homelike atmosphere. Dietetics, hydrotherapy and massage speed physical and emotional re-education. Cooperation with referring physicians. Write or phone.

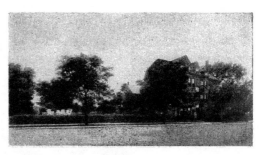

HAVE YOU HEARD?

George Kimball, M.D., Oklahoma City, attended the annual meeting of the Society of Plastic and Reconstructive Surgeons held the first week of November in Coronado, Calif.

W. W. Rucks, Sr., M.D., Oklahoma City, attended the Association of Life Insurance Medical Directors for the United States and Canada in New York.

M. H. Newman, M.D., Shattuck recently completed a course in the review of general surgery at the postgraduate medical school of New York University-Bellevue Medical Center.

H. J. Rubin, M.D., Tulsa, was recently elected to fellowship in the American Academy of Pediatrics.

Clair Liebrand, M.D., Oklahoma City, recently spent a vacation in England and the Continent.

C. J. Fishman, M.D., Oklahoma City, received the third annual B'nai B'rith Award November 15 for outstanding service in inter-faith and citizenship work.

E. C. Mohler, M.D., Ponca City, has recently been made an associate fellow in the American College of Cardiology.

J. B. Hollis, M.D., Mangum, has been named to the national committee of the American Legion on membership and post activities.

PSYCHIATRIC GROUPS MEET IN KANSAS CITY

Harold G. Sleeper, M.D., Oklahoma City, was elected councilor for Oklahoma at the annual meeting of the Mid-Continent Psychiatric Association held September 26 and 27 at the Hotel President in Kansas City, Mo.

The Mid-Continent Psychiatric Association is the official district branch society of the American Psychia-tric Association for the states of Arkansas, Kansas, Missouri and Oklahoma.

Other officers elected were: president C. J. Kurth, M.D., Wichita Kans.; vice-pres. and pres.-elect, Paul Hines, M.D., Kansas City, Mo.; secty.-treas., Frank F. Merker, M.D., Topeka, Kansas; councilor for Arkansas, Robert G. Carnahan, M.D., Little Rock; councilor for Kansas, William Rottersman, M.D., Topeka; councilor for Missouri, G. Wilse Robinson, Jr., M.D., Kansas City.

ANNOUNCEMENTS

OKLAHOMA STATE MEDICAL ASSOCIATION
May 10-11-12, 1954, Municipal Auditorium, Oklahoma City. House of Delegates, Sunday, May 9.

OKLAHOMA ACADEMY OF GENERAL PRACTICE
February 15-16, Tulsa Hotel, Tulsa, Oklahoma.

UNIVERSITY OF KANSAS SCHOOL OF MEDICINE
Postgraduate courses in surgery, January 18-21. University of Kansas School of Medicine, Kansas City 12, Kansas.

AMERICAN DAIBETES ASSOCIATION
Second postgraduate course in diabetes and basic metabolic problems. January 18, 19, 20, 1954, Mayo Clinic and Mayo Foundation, Rochester, Minnesota.

RURAL HEALTH CONFERENCE
Ninth National conference on rural health sponsored by the Council on Rural Health of the American Medical Association, March 4-6, Baker Hotel, Dallas, Texas. Pre-conference session *for doctors only* will be held Thursday morning, March 4, beginning at 10:00 a.m.

CHICAGO MEDICAL SOCIETY
Annual clinical conference, Palmer House, Chicago, Ill., March 2, 3, 4, 5, 1954.

DOCTORS IN ALCOHOLIC ANONYMOUS
Fifth annual international group, Mayflower Hotel, Akron, Ohio, May 14, 15 and 16. For information and reservation address: Doctors, Mayflower Hotel, Akron, Ohio.

1927 CLASS HAS REUNION

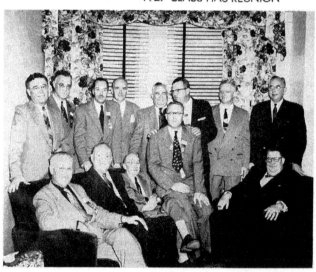

Pictured are members of the University of Oklahoma School of Medicine Class of 1827 who attended their class reunion and the Oklahoma City Clinical Society Meeting in October. Back row reading left to right: G. L. Goodman, Yukon; M. O. Hart, Tulsa; Harry Wilkins, Oklahoma City (secretary Oklahoma City Clinical Society); H. W. Harris, Oklahoma City; M. L. Saddoris, Cleveland; J. B. Miles, Anadarko; G. L. Hyroop, Oklahoma City; and W. L. Shippey, Fort Smith, Arkansas.

Front row seated left to right: N. L. Miller, Oklahoma City (president Oklahoma City Clinical Society); Coyne Campbell, Oklahoma City; J. R. Reed, Oklahoma City; C. M. Hodgson, Kingfisher; and B. D. Faris, Oklahoma City.

EDITORIALS

OLD AGE AND EMOTIONAL DISORDERS

In this issue of the *Journal* Francis J. Braceland and John Donnelly discuss "Early Detection of Emotional Disorders in Old Age."

There are many reasons why this article should have a wide reading. People who have lived long enough to have bags under their eyes have seen enough of life to warrant a variety of emotions and they are near enough to death with sufficient responsibilities to have certain misgivings, unless they are endowed with an unusual philosophy. Yet as Cicero implied, they may not be as "green as they are cabbage looking." In fact, if there is an important job to be done, it might be well to give them a booking.

Rightly and clearly the authors indicate that when confronted with problems, people over 65 react psychologically just as younger people and that they may be just as amenable to treatment. Of course, the possibility of organic changes and senility must never be forgotten. But length of years is seldom if ever the only factor.

In the light of what is said, the importance of careful analysis of each case and an earnest attempt to arrive at a proper diagnosis without too much stress upon age is obvious.

Time and sympathetic consideration in each case is of prime importance.

MEDICINE ASSAILED BY DANGEROUS TRENDS

Under present materialistic trends, it is possible that medicine may cease to be a medium of unselfish service to humanity and pass into the cold, impersonal realm of trade where financial gain becomes the governing factor?

Medicine has moved across the face of history with a simplicity of service unequalled in any other realm of human endeavor. Shall modern physicians trained and disciplined in this tradition be destroyed by the present trend toward materialistic depravity?

In the practice of medicine the road that leads to wealth is not the road to honor.

With this in mind, it is well to recount Pare's experience with one of his patients, "I did him the service of physician, surgeon, apothecary and cook. I dressed him to the end and God cured him and so I was well content with him and he with me."

To be humbly content with one's self is the physician's surest safeguard.

THE WORLD MEDICAL ASSOCIATION SPECULATIONS-ANTICIPATIONS

It may be surprising to some of our readers to know that in 1859 the Dutch Medical Association wrote to other national medical associations with the hope of gathering data and making plans for an international congress. The November issue of the *Canadian Medical Association Journal*, referring to this correspondence, quotes the following:

"In an era like ours," the letter ran, "when medical men are in such close contact with the most essential values of social life, it seems desirable that they should unite and concentrate their efforts to bring about those improvements in the organization of their profession or in its exercise, which are truly in accordance with the classical expression to their art."

Unfortunately, the plan did not materialize. Perhaps intercommunication and transportation handicaps killed the plan. If the appeal had been successful it is natural to wonder what might have happened. If the proposed international congress had convened, is it possible that a World Medical Association might have followed? Considering the above purpose, could such a world organization have averted or delayed the world confusion with which we are now confronted?

In view of the progress of the present World Medical Association, now seven years old, and its commendable purposes with reference to professional standards and worldwide human weal, it is possible that through its national constituents (national medical organizations) may become a determining factor in the sincere desire of many nations for global peace and harmony.

While it is too early to draw conclusions, the results of the 1953 World Conference on

Medical Education in London are most hopeful.

Always medicine and its ancillary agents have been able to strike across international barriers in pursuit of human welfare in both war and peace. Why should not the W.M.A. wield a potent influence? What better reason for its hearty support by all physicians and all people interested in better medicine and more peace?

SOCIAL SECURITY NOT ONLY SILLY BUT SAD

Since Bismarck first declared the policy of placing people under obligation to government, in order to get votes and to perpetuate the offices of professional politicians, civilization has been threatened by social security.

Even since F.D.R. first sent Harry Hopkins to Europe on a government mission and admonished him to look into Social Security in Germany on the theory of political expediency and through its insidious transplantation in our own government, its disturbing development and rapid growth in this country have usurped local prerogatives and states rights with disastrous effects upon personal initiative, honor and integrity. The implication that the sons of this nation's founding fathers are not capable of saving their own money and making their own way in the world amounts to a shocking insult to our worthy citizenry. It is inconceivable that the American public and the lawmakers and politicians should have so completely fallen for this annulling political philosophy.

Apparently alarmed by the implications of this octopus, President Eisenhower advocated "a pay-as-you-go-basis." Senator Taft, conscious of the inevitable and certain of ruin if the trend is not curbed and knowing that our salvation is dependent upon feeling the cost in time to correct the evil also advocated "a pay-as-you-go-system."

Though the costs are exceeding all calculations and must continue to mount, the government is considering the addition of at least another ten million to the Social Security rolls.

In many ways this socialistic trend threatens the integrity of the medical profession. What has happened in Great Britain can happen here. If complete government control should come to physicians in this country, the evil impact will be keenly felt because we have not had the same insidious indoctrination. The evil potentialities should keep us on our toes. Already our people are suffering the devastating moral and material effects we had hoped to escape.

If to date the government had spent half the sum required for social security in an educational effort to help each citizen work out his own "ham and eggs" plan and thereby retain and develop his initiative, his integrity, his skills and his self-respect, the people and the nation would be better off. Millions of outstretched hands with gimme-gimme finger movements imploring unearned security from an insecure government must be accepted as an evil omen. How much better if under a constructive educational program, the government had placed a premium upon individual frugality by making accumulated savings, within established limits, tax free to encourage individual competency and self-sufficiency.

Solomon said: "Let not thine hand be stretched out to receive and shut when thou shouldest repay."

Even under good business management, social security and old age benefits would prove fatal. Under the present confusion and uncertainty if something is not done, rapidly we may come to a catastrophic end with only "sweet Caesar's wounds" to speak for us and only our progressive incompetency under government paternalism to account for our failure. If the source of our spiritual food, the church, must be free from state control, what about the dollar, the only sourse of our physical sustenance? It says, "in God we trust," not in government control.

"MEN ARE MY TEACHERS"

If Plato could say this with such feeling, how much more surely should the physician realize that the knowledge guiding his mind and his hand in the care of the sick comes from his study of men.

Alexander Pope[1] must have had this statement from Plato in mind when he said, "the proper study of mankind is man." Pope might well have had the physician in mind when he made the above statement and prefaced it by saying, "know thyself." This should be the ambition of all good physicians.

The medical student who does not put self analysis and the study of men above material gain will fail in his service to mankind and will never fully realize the just rewards of his profession.

EDUCATION AND MEDICINE

The rapid development of medical knowledge, the marathon toward specialization and the plague of new ideologies in connection with formal premedical education have created an ever widening chasm between genuine culture and the profession of medicine. Without the humanities a full understanding of the human organism as a composite whole and the ideal patient-physician relationship is impossible. A broad general education favors satisfactory relationships from the moron to the most intellectual. After giving full credit for the gift of science it must not be forgotten that ideal medicine is largely dependent upon human relations.

In the field of medical education there is a general consciousness of deficiencies traceable to the secondary schools, the colleges and universities. The response to a questionnaire recently sent to the deans of all medical schools in Canada, the United States and the possessions reveals the almost unanimous opinion that medical students are seriously handicapped by language deficiencies. Though capped and gowned before admission to medical school, the majority are deficient in the use of the English language and therefore, in rhetorical analysis. This deficiency appears in both the spoken and written word.

The completed questionnaires indicate that medical students and physicians are becoming more and more inarticulate and less capable of satisfactory communication and with few exceptions the deficiency in part rests with the almost effortless audiovisual education.

That great advocate of better medical education, Abraham Flexner, said, "it is not so much a matter of medicine as of education." Perhaps our present fault is that too early we neglect the humanities in order to major in science. In a sense we concentrate on medicine long before we enter the medical school. This urge to get on with their special training applies to students preparing to enter other professional schools. Thus the trend is universal. The medical student feels he must make haste. The "crutch of time" is not for him; he must learn science. Unfortunately, this cutting of corners to meet the pressure of ever increasing knowledge plus the philosophy of uninhibited self expression tends to eliminate the humanities and correspondingly to lower cultural levels.

Is it not possible for the Council on Medical Education, the Association of American Medical Colleges and interested medical educators to initiate a comprehensive study of the instruction given, methods employed, and the opportunities and educational experiences of present day students anticipating the study of medicine with the hope of offering constructive recommendations.

Apropos the questionnaire sent to the deans of medical schools, a great medical editor in a recent letter said: "If more doctors could write English, medical education might be made a little smoother."

DRUG ADDICTS

Not only should physicians recognize the fact that patients under stress or from pain alone may become addicted to certain drugs, but that in the daily routine of practice, the physician himself may with less provocation, develop the habit of administering certain remedies without diagnostic and therapeutic justification. In this sense he may become a dangerous addict.

This is particularly true of the past few decades because of fabulous new drugs. There is no way to estimate the volume of unnecessary vitamins channeled through the innocent oesophagus or the hypodermic needle, violating the sacred functions of conservative organs. The sulfa drugs suffered a similar vogue paralleling the swift run of cold vaccines. Now comes the breathtaking therapeutic marathon of antibiotics. What can we do to make this remarkable run relatively safe and sane.

These few examples familiar to all practicing physicians, should at least sound a warning against over-enthusiasm with reference to certain drugs and unstudied and unscientific administration. Indications and contra-indications should be carefully considered and rigidly observed. even after allowing for all limitations in knowledge and physical facilities from the remote country community up to the fully equipped medical center, there is room for improvement. In the light of their respective knowledge and opportunities, all physicians must account for their sins. Both those of ommission and commission.

THE HIGHWAY TOLL AND
THE MEDICAL PROFESSION

Of the making of cars there is no end and of the craze for speed there is no cure. As a result our nation moves on merciless wheels with a casualty list that is appalling. The mounting death toll is inevitable, unless improved safety measures can be devised.

Since physicians must bind up the highway wounds and sign the death certificates, as in other disabling and life taking conditions they should consider all possible preventive measures and advise accordingly.

All patients of undetermined susceptibility, receiving narcotics and antihistaminics should be advised not to drive a car. All patients given to psychological blackouts from any cause should be admonished not to take the wheel. This group includes the epileptics, those in whom fainting spells are easily provoked and possibly diabetics subject to insulin shock. All nervous patients, obviously lacking coordination under the pressure of responsibility, all alcoholics and grave cardiac cases including those known to have had coronary attacks, should be urged not to drive.

These precautions added to the present accepted safety measures should materially reduce the highway hazards. This is only one of medicine's many obligations to society.

BOOK REVIEW

RUDOLPH VIRCHOW, Doctor, Statesman, Anthropologist. Erwin H. Ackerknecht. University of Wisconsin Press, Madison. 1953. Price $5.00.

The author of this story has rendered a great service by depicting the personality and recounting the varied interests and accomplishments of this exceptional man.

After a brief but interesting account of Virchow's life and family background he gives detailed accounts of his achievements as physician, statesman and anthropologist.

Most physicians know that "one hundred years ago a thirty-year-old pathology professor in the small Bavarian University of Wuerzburg ventured for the first time the idea that the basic units of life are the self-reproducing cells of living bodies and that pathology has to study primarily cell changes. This idea, named later "cellular pathology," has dominated biology and pathology up to this very day; and when the creator of cellular pathology died fifty years ago, the whole medical world bowed at his grave.''

But not many know that in addition to being the father of cellular pathology, Virchow worked incessantly for general medical advancement, political and socioeconomic reforms. He sought to identify medicine with virtually all human interests and to show that it is a significant factor in the advancement of civilization. He was not drawn into politics by personal ambitions but by convictions which made his battles for reforms in government seem obligatory.

For physicians who have not had time to follow medical history this book will appear as a revelation. Reading it is much like digging for facts in the ruts of Troy, Babylon or Baalbeck.

Even though Virchow died more than a hundred years ago, he cut out a pattern that present day physicians might follow with profit. He was an indefatigable worker, a profound scholar, an exacting scientist, a genuine individualist, a great democrat, devoted to freedom of thought and action. He championed the interests of the poor and oppressed and did all he could to advance public health in all its phases. Not only was he interested in politics but he held political appointments and took an active part in political reforms. He was a bitter antagonist of Bismarck. It is good to note that his influence and activities so harrassed this hard man of "blood and iron" that he sought to rid himself of the "little professor" by challenging him to a duel. Fortunately, the scientist had sufficient sense and dignity to decline. The author indicates that the tremendous public ovations to Virchow were directed as much at the opposition leader (Bismarck) as at the scientist.

This story of Virchow's life should help to awaken the medical profession of today and alert its members to the fact that humanitarian philosophies, political reforms and medical safeguards now so badly needed cannot be realized without militant champions from their ranks.

By way of emphasis I quote from the preface of *Cellular Pathology*: "I insist on my rights, and therefore I respect the rights of others. This is my standpoint in life, in politics, in science. We owe it to ourselves to defend our rights, because this is only guarantee of our individual development and of our influence on the community."

Space will not permit the enumeration of his many scientific discoveries, his public health and political achievements and his contributions in the field of anthropology. All of these call for a careful reading.

—Lewis J. Moorman, M.D.

Scientific Articles

PROSTATIC SURGERY

D. W. BRANHAM, M.D.

M. E. JACOBSON, M.D.

OKLAHOMA CITY, OKLA.

The surgical treatment for prostatism is becoming less hazardous. Twenty years ago a mortality rate of approximately 10 per cent was found in a study of 220 patients treated by the various types of prostatic surgery at the University of Oklahoma Hospitals. Complications were frequent and convalescence was prolonged. The use of antibiotics, blood transfusions, and Foley catheters among other medical and surgical advances has markedly decreased mortality and morbidity following prostatic surgery. Comparisons of old studies with current results are encouraging not only as a guide for advice to patients whom we are seeing this year, but also as a hope for future improvements.

The present study is an analysis of 384 recent cases of prostatic obstruction treated in Oklahoma City. Nearly all of these cases were admitted to the hospitals in 1951. One-third were charity patients treated at the University of Oklahoma Hospitals; the remaining two-thirds were consecutive private patients treated in two private hospitals in Oklahoma City. The entire group was operated by the same group of urologists using the standard transurethral, suprapubic or retropubic procedures. The perineal approach is rarely used in this vicinity for radical removal of the prostate in cases of early carcinoma. Thirty-six per cent of the patients were submitted to transurethral surgery and the remainder, 237 patients, 64 per cent, were operated by open methods. Of

*Presented before the Oklahoma Urological Association, February 28, 1952, Oklahoma City, Okla.

the latter, 140 were operated by suprapubic route and 97 were removed retropubically. The majority of patients were operated without preliminary bladder drainage. In only four patients were cystostomies performed. The so-called two stage operative procedure for the removal of the hyperplastic prostate has become almost obsolete.

AGE: There were only six patients in the series who were under the age of 50. Most of the patients ranged from 78 to 80 years of age; two were over 90 years of age. It is of interest to note that the latter two individuals had a rather uneventful recovery from their surgery. There seemed to be little relation between the age of patients and the operative hazards so far as mortality was concerned. In the study of the records of those patients who died, fatal cases were from 60 to 85 years of age.

CARCINOMA: Carcinoma of the prostate in this series, averaged approximately 10 per cent which is below the accepted figure for such pathology in other studies. In most instances the diagnosis of carcinoma of the prostate is made by clinical examination prior to hospitalization. In many patients who were found to have been so diagnosed, considerable improvement in bladder function was noted after a short interval of catheter drainage, administration of estrogens or the performance of orchiectomy obviating the necessity of surgery.

MORTALITY: There were seven postoperative deaths, a mortality rate of 1.8 per cent. There was a slight increase in incidence of deaths in the University Hospital as compared to those noted in private institutions. Undoubtedly the higher death rate observed in charity patients was due to the more advanced degenerative pathology in patients common to such institutions. The relation of operative procedure to the cause of death was not significant. Four patients died who were operated by open methods of surgery and three succumbed following transurethral resection. Some form of vascular accident was the predominant cause of death in most instances. One patient died from coronary occlusion, another from a cerebrovascular accident, a third from pulmonary embolism and a fourth from mesenteric thrombosis. There was only one instance of fatal pyelonephritis that followed suprapubic removal of the gland and in two patients massive pneumonia developed postoperatively following transurethral resection. Severe infection was the chief cause of death following prostatic surgery before the era of antibotics. Today both local and systemic infections which previously complicated operative procedures have become a rarity because of the general use of antibiotics.

HEMORRHAGE: This is still the most troublesome complication in prostatic surgery, despite the various methods advanced to control bleeding. It occurred in 35 cases, nine plus per cent, and in 11 patients was of sufficient magnitude at the time of surgery to necessitate packing the prostatic fossa. There were no deaths directly due to hemorrhage.

POST-OPERATIVE HOSPITALIZATION: The average number of days required for all patients to be discharged from the hospital was 15 plus days. Charity patients stayed in the hospital slightly longer than private patients, 16 days as compared to 13 days in private institutions. The private patients who were submitted to transurethral surgery left the hospital in the shortest period of time, nine plus days. Many of these patients probably could have been dismissed from the hospital sooner but for the fact that their home was some distance from the city and would be without adequate medical care in event of late complications.

SAUPRAPUBIC URINARY DRAINAGE: In 22 patients, five per cent, this annoying complication occurred. In most instances of prolonged bladder fistulas the drainage ceased spontaneously within two or three weeks following surgery. In eight instances transurethral resection of remnants or tabs of prostatic tissue left in the bladder neck were necessary to induce closure of the draining sinus. It appears from the records that patients who had retropubic operative procedures seem to have had more trouble from prolonged urinary drainage than those convalescing from the suprapubic method. In this locality most of the surgeons perform complete bladder closure with urethral catheter drainage. When suprapubic drainage was used and the suprapubic catheter was removed within a few days following surgery, the sinus closed rapidly and did not seem to be a factor in the prolongation of convalescence.

EPIDIDYMITIS: Twelve patients, three per cent, developed epididymitis while in the hospital following removal of the gland. In three of these patients epididymitis occurred despite bilateral vas ligation that had been performed before surgery. Epididymitis was not a serious factor in convalesence in any instance. Undoubtedly epididymitis may be eliminated to some degree if vas ligation is performed routinely, preferably before surgery.

INCONTINENCE OF URINE: This is a post-operative complication difficult to evaluate statistically from study of hospital records. Many patients who had such surgery suffered from some degree of incontinence for a variable length of time; sometimes for a few days but not infrequently for a protracted time. The majority of patients who had incontinence ultimately regained control as the healing process in the vesical neck progressed. Permanent incontinence seems to be a rarity. From a study of the records incontinence of urination seems to be severe enough to merit notation and in two it appeared to be of sufficient magnitude to be described as severe.

SUMMARY: It is evident from the review of these records that great progress has been made in the surgical treatment of vesical nesk obstruction due to hyperplasia of the prostrate. This may be based on several factors; better selection of operative procedures, improved surgical techniques, antibiotic therapy and better utilization of newer systemic supportive measures in the form of blood and fluid balance. These and other refinements in surgical management have contributed to a lower mortality, a lessened hospital stay and fewer complications compared to past years.

EARLY DETECTION OF
EMOTIONAL DISORDERS OF OLD AGE

FRANCIS J. BRACELAND, M.D. SC.D.

JOHN DONNELLY, M.D., D.P.M.

HARTFORD, CONNECTICUT

"Intelligence and reflection and
judgment reside in old men and,
if there had been none of them,
no states could exist at all."

Cicero (*De Senectute* XIX)

The cogency of Cicero's words is brought home to us when we note the ages of the men who were called upon to make the vital decisions in the recent war and of some of those who still guide the ship of state in the nations of the free world. Premiers, monarchs, presidential advisors, and emissaries, they are for the most part prodigious workers, alert, keen, intelligent and of good judgment, and they point up the paradoxical situation which obtains in the present day when men are forced to retire from industry and business at 65, while they are sought for positions in government and the judiciary, some of them to enter the most productive period of their lives. This latter fact would seem to call for a re-examination of present-day attitudes toward the older age groups.

The vicissitudes of, and the attitudes toward, the aging and aged are of great interest to the physician, especially to the general practitioner, for it is to him that the senescent and their families will turn for advice, not only because they know him best but also because they trust him most. Apparently his interest will have to grow apace for, if present-day census figures are to be believed and the present population course continues, by 1980 nearly 50 per cent of all the people in the United States will be 55 years and over.[1] It follows, then, that the practice of medicine as we proceed

*Presented before the Section on Neurology and Psychiatry at the Annual Meeting of the Oklahoma State Medical Association April 13, 1953.

through the century will require a knowledge of gerontology. There are signs of it already, especially in psychiatry, for the incidence of major psychiatric illness in this age group is even now taxing to the utmost the available treatment sources and demonstrating the urgent need for new approaches to early diagnosis and appropriate therapy.

The urgency of the situation becomes even more obvious when it is noted that the conventional attitude taken by physicians to the mental symptoms of the older age group has been altogether too lugubrious.[2] Historically, these disorders have been regarded uncritically as all being manifestations of organic change and, therefore, irreversible and beyond treatment. In the light of present-day knowledge, this medical and psychotherapeutic nihilism[3] is hardly justifiable.

It has been customary to classify the psychiatric syndromes of later life from several different viewpoints; as neuroses or psychoses depending upon the type and severity of the clinical picture; as organic or functional depending upon the presumed cerebral pathology; or as involutional or senile depending upon the occurrence of onset before or after the 65th year. Isolating those cases where evidence of definite neurological pathology, such as arteriosclerosis, tumors, atrophy, etc., is demonstrable, the age of 65 has been the magic number chosen by custom; below this, diseases are usually regarded as involutional and beyond this age they are thought of as senile. Clearly, such a criterion has little value scientifically and is the relic of a rule adapted in the past for socio-economic[4] reasons.

Reference to any standard textbook of psychiatry reveals that there is usually a division of the so-called senile conditions into two main groups: (a) simple deterioration, defined as an accentuation of normal aging; and, (b) functional syndromes, the neuroses and the psychoses. The descriptions of these latter disorders commonly state that each differs little clinically from the corresponding conditions of earlier age groups. It is our belief and experience that a great number of these reactions in the elderly respond as readily to therapy as do the conditions in the younger persons. For example, because the circumstances of age are especially likely to promote insecurity, anxiety and agitation are prominent in the depressive reactions of older people and, clinically, it is difficult, if not impossible, to differentiate such states occurring in the late involutional period from those of the older age groups. The only reliable criterion is the presence of definite intellectual deficit in the latter, for both groups respond to the same treatment.

A careful examination of the literature reveals unanimity in the conclusion that the cerebral pathology revealed by autopsy cannot be directly correlated quantitatively or qualitatively with the type of psychiatric clinical picture or with the degree of severity of the individual syndromes.[5,6,7] There is no one-to-one ratio between symptomatology and extent of cerebral lesions. Correlation of the clinical aspects and of postmortem findings leads to the conclusion that patients hitherto classified together as senile may be divided into three main groups: (1) Those in whom the disturbances are essentially of psychogenic origin, though minimal degenerative processes may be present. (2) Those suffering from emotional disturbances, not actually an integral part of the organic changes but which are psychological reactions to the results of such changes. (3) Those in whom the cerebral degenerative pathology is of such magnitude that the neurologic basis on which the personality structure has been organized is gravely disrupted, thus predicating little hope of improvement. There are gradations between the groups and it is obvious that patients in the first two groups may progress to the third.

Of late there has been an increasing tendency to diagnose psychosis with arteriosclerosis when a functional picture concides with the presence of alterations in the retinal or peripheral vessels; yet, retinal arteriosclerosis may be correlated with cerebral vascular pathology in only about 30 to 40 per cent of individuals.[8,9] Simon et al,[10] studied the lipoprotein level in groups of patients diagnosed as psychoses with cerebral arteriosclerosis and in normals of the senile age group and found little significant difference. The conclusion was drawn at autopsy that cerebral atherosclerosis played only an insignificant role in the production of the psychotic picture.

The question will arise, then, as to what accounts for the mental picture. Rothschild, among others, has stressed the decisive influence of psychological, extra-cerebral, somatic and environmental factors in the production of these disorders.[11,12,13,14] He has also emphasized the importance, as an etiological factor, of the vulnerability of the pre-morbid personality. Early recognition of the psychodynamic elements and application of effective measures to correct them would yield results perhaps as extensive and as gratifying as those achieved from the corresponding approaches to the psychiatric ills of young people. It cannot be too strongly stressed that elderly people react to the difficulties which they encounter just as do persons at other ages and that they too can be helped to resolve their problems.

DEFENSES AND SYMPTOMS

It is known that among the early signs of senescence are lapses of memory. Not only may there be failure of recall of recent events, new acquaintances, etc., but sometimes the initial symptom recognized by the patient is the inability to recall the name of someone with whom he is relatively familiar. Great care must be taken, however, to differentiate pathological memory loss from the lapses of memory which are due to attention defects and which are the lot of most of us at various times.

Mistakes in judgment and a certain carelessness in detail are common in early senescence and there may be less acute appreciation of the problem or the topics under discussion. The individual may be aware of an increasing tendency for the direction of conversation to wander with a trend toward circumlocution. It is said that, as we get older, our bodies get shorter and our anecdotes get longer. Whether or not the individual is aware of these feelings may have some effect on his status; they are certainly noticed by others whose reaction in turn may lead him to responses of a defensive nature. The threat to his security or his self-esteem may be met by either a conservative or an aggressive reaction, that is, withdrawal from all situations likely to make his difficulties obvious, or seeking for occasions to prove to himself or to others that he is as capable as ever.

Some of the manifestations of the effort to maintain the status quo may be a constriction of interests, a staunch adherence to methods and patterns long familiar, a rigidity of outlook and suspiciousness of change. There is, consequently, an over-evaluation of the past and an increasing depreciation of the present. Daily activities become more and more restricted and more routine. With this there may be accentuation of the characteristic modes of reaction, so that any threat to the life system will produce a response greater than that merited by the stimulus: irritability, hasty judgments, the tendency to blame others, the false interpretation of events, exaggeration of minor offenses, all of these increase and provoke still greater insecurity, so that more overt anxiety may be engendered.

The basis of the aggressive type of defense is essentially a denial of loss. With consciousness of the decline in one or more spheres of power, whether in competition with younger rivals at work, in the sexual field, or in any area where gratification is needed, opportunities are sought to demonstrate his continued vigour. Tasks requiring physical strength, endurance, or superior performance may be undertaken by the individual so that excessive demands are self imposed. The hostility may show itself divertly in attitudes toward members of the family or colleagues at work. Even if this aggressiveness does not achieve conscious and overt expression, however, it may result in anxiety manifested in somatic or mental symptoms. Likewise, the sexual drives, giving rise to fantasies, conflicts, and unacceptable sexual activity, may produce guilt and anxiety, all the more so because the culture in which we live tends to deprecate even normal sexual activity in elderly persons.

Somatization of anxiety may occur in any of the physiological systems with complaints of palpitation, breathlessness, tremors of the head and extremities, loss of appetite, indigestion, diarrhea, headaches, frequency of micturition, and insomnia, etc. The mental symptoms may include such complaints as loss of power of concentration, feelings of tension and nervousness, or feelings of impending danger. Not only may there be lack of desire to leave the home or to undertake normal activities, but there may also be actual fears of going into open streets, of crowds, of subways, etc. These phobias represent the inadequate resolution of conflicts in which sexual or aggressive drives are unsatisfactorily repressed and the object or situation feared symbolizes the occasions in which there may be temptation to gratify these drives.

In the conditions mentioned so far, the individual is still relating himself to the environment but, if there is loss of opportunity for gratification, there are feelings of aimlessness and lack of purpose with complaints of general fatigue representing loss of adequate motivation and of interest in external objects. Or he may completely withdraw and focus attention on himself, thus engendering hypochondriacal symptoms. Whereas in anxiety states there are somatic accompaniments of anxiety, in hypochondriasis no evidence, upon medical examination, can be found to justify the intense preoccupation with bodily function. It has been stated that the most common focus is on the gastrointestinal tract with emphasis on eating, digestion, and bowel function, and it has been suggested that the factors responsible for this include not only the impairment of the physiological functions involved but also a regressive psychological defense by which gratification is sought on an infantile level.[15] However, any system may be the center of hypochondriacal symptoms and the medical practitioner may be called upon to deal with complaints of disorders of the excretory, cardiovascular, respiratory, or musculo-skeletal systems. Characteristic are the self-concern, the egocentric preoccupation and, with due allowance for the age of the patient, the absence of sufficient evidence of physical disease to account for the symptoms.

Hypochondriasis in pure form without evidence of marked alteration in mood is frequently encountered but simple neurotic depression and severe psychotic melancholia also occur just as frequently and the differentiation can be extremely difficult. Therefore, when the opinion has been reached that the origin of the physical complaints is essentially psychogenic, special attention must be directed to detecting the presence of depression. Dissatisfied with the life they envisage before them, deprived of their self-esteem, and consciously or unconsciously holding themselves responsible for their failure, aging persons are liable to develop conditions in which self-destructive tendencies are prominent.

For example, a serious illness or the death of the marital partner may produce disruption in the established patterns of the individual, threatening the very foundations on which adjustment has hitherto been built. Loss of gradification of dependency needs and even loss of motivation for life itself may result but, above all, if there has been ambivalence towards the partner, strong guilt feelings may be aroused with consequent melancholia of psychotic proportions. In the initial stages, the presenting symptoms may be apathy, loss of interest and of initiative, retardation, or confusion; there may be either hypochondriasis or agitation, with preoccupation with the question of whether the individual had been, by commission or omission, a contributing factor to the suffering or demise of the deceased. Within a very short time this preoccupation may be replaced by self-recrimination, usually accompanied by marked depressive feelings. At the root of this concern, of course, lies repressed hostility which is unconsciously deemed to have caused the illness or death of the partner and which leads to the development of feelings of guilt.

In general, patients are aware of being depressed but, nevertheless, one must be alert for those occasions when no complaints of depression are made and when careful inquiries are necessary to elicit its presence. Such conditions, if allowed to progress, may develop all the signs of psychotic depression with hypochondriacal delusions, marked anxiety and agitation, delusions of degradation in the spheres of health, wealth, and worth, and intense feelings of guilt as a result of which self-destruction becomes a sacrificial expiation.

A special clinical picture during later life that appears to occur in individuals in the higher executive class is the development of depressive reactions in those who, judged by the normal worldly standards, have recently attained success such as promotion in their occupations and in whom one would expect to find contentment and satisfaction. The

psychodynamics of these depressions include such factors as increased responsibility with heightened fears of inadequacy, feelings of being alone with no one to depend upon, and consequent mixed feelings about the position achieved. Such personalities have long been driven to seek the success which symbolizes for them the final resolution of insecurity, only to find the search has been in vain. This presents an area for research in the field of industrial psychiatry in terms of recognition of the types of personality which are best suited for the very highest level of executive direction and of those who perform most efficiently in less exalted positions.

The considerable variation in the relative incidence of arteriosclerotic and senile conditions, as revealed by the figures from different hospitals, illustrates the difficulty of present-day classifications. As an etiological factor, it is probable that arteriosclerosis has been too greatly emphasized. Classically, these illnesses present a fairly well-defined clinical picture commencing as early as the fifth decade. There is a history of headaches, tetany, dizziness, paresthesia, or other somatic symptoms accompanied by the general feeling of ill health. There are few essentially psychiatric symptoms, however, until a major episode ensues with a convulsion or with evidence of focal cerebral damage.

Subsequently, there occurs some restoration of function but more episodes follow, after each of which the level of improvement attained is less than that existing prior to the episode. Dating from the initial attack, there may appear any of the functional features indicated earlier; anxiety states, hypochondriasis, depressive reactions, confused episodes, paranoid outbursts, lability of effect, all may be seen. Physicians are quite familiar with the irritability, anxiety, or depression experienced by hitherto very active individuals when, following illness or operation involving parts of the body other than the head, they become dependent on others for all their needs. Functional symptoms in such patients arise as the reactions to the impairment of function, to the threat to life, and to the fears of dependency which physical illness entails.

Although the incidence of delirious conditions is relatively higher in patients in whom the presence of definite arteriosclerosis is clear and, although toxic factors may produce similar pictures in others, Cameron[16] has demonstrated the operation of psychodynamic elements in the production of such states, pointing out that delirium occurs especially on retiring at night and remits in the morning. He was able to provoke similar disturbances by placing patients in darkened rooms. He demonstrated that impairment of the ability of such patients to orient themselves without frequent visual aid aroused insecurity and produced an elevation of the blood pressure with the onset of the delirious state. The possibility of the development of these episodes should be borne in mind when older patients show a restlessness at night, perhaps with a proclivity to wandering out of doors after dark. There is a marked impairment of memory, and a tendency to disorientation, manifested in disordered time sense, in the inability to identify those with whom they have recently become acquainted, and in the tendency to become anxious in unfamiliar surroundings. Many of these patients are able to adjust satisfactorily when managed in the home but are unable to do so when circumstances have necessitated change of residence. Thus, when it has been deemed neither practical nor advisable for the elderly person to live alone, transfer to the home of the children or to the hospital may, in fact, provoke an acute delirium.

In conclusion, the evaluation of the incipient signs of psychopathological processes in later life is rendered difficult because of the intimate relationship of organic and psychogenic symptoms. Clear-cut affective conditions, depression, anxiety, elation, apathy, when they constitute the central complaint, present no abstruse problem in diagnosis; but somatic symptoms, which bulk so largely, require that the physician be constantly vigilant. Axiomatic as it is that the aging body is more liable to pathological change, it is very important to remember that the normal changes of senescence, physical, social and cultural, are particularly conducive to emotional stress which may manifest itself in exactly the same symptomatology; it is important because such conditions are amenable to psychiatric therapy.

REFERENCES

1. Rusk, H A., Geriatrics: 6, 3, 1951
2. Roth, M and Morrisey, J D, J. Ment. Sci : 98. 410. 1952
3 Cameron, N, Neuroses of later Maturity, Mental Disorders of Later Life. Ed. O. J. Kaplan. Stanford University Press, 1945.
4. Lawton, G., Problems of Aging: Ed. E V. Cowdry, Baltimore; Williams and Wilkins Co., 1942.
5. Rothschild, D and Sharp, M L, Dis. Nerv. Syst.: 2. 49, 1941
6. Robinson, G. W., Jr., J AMA 116, 2139. 1941
7. Wexburg, L. E., Mental Health in Later Maturity. U. S Publ. Health Repts. Suppl. 168. 1942
8. Wagener, H. P., Med. Clin. of N. A.: 7, 1923
9. Alper, B. J. Arch. Neur. Psychiat.: 60, 1948.
10. Simon A. et al., Am J. Psychiat.: 108, 9, 1952.
11. Rothschild, D, Dis. Nerv. Syst.: 8, 1947.
12. Rothschild, D., Geriatrics: 2, 1947
13. Rothschild, D., Am. J. Psychiat.: 100, 1947.
14. Boyd, D A., Jr., and Braceland, F. J, Med. Clin. of N.A.: 34, 1950.
15. Hamilton, G., Problems of Aging: Ed E. V. Cowdry. 2nd Ed. Williams and Wilkins Co., 1942.
16. Cameron, D E., Psychiat Quart.; 15 1941.

THE CLOSED METHOD OF LAUGE-HANSEN FOR TREATMENT OF FRACTURES OF THE ANKLE*

DAVID C. RAMSAY, M.D.

ADA, OKLAHOMA

Neils Lauge-Hansen of Randers, Denmark, recently has presented a very complete contribution on fractures of the ankle.[1, 3] He gives much historical background, experimental-surgical studies, and analysis of a large number of x-rays of ankle injuries. This study of 228 cases forms the basis for a new clinical approach to the problem of fractures of the ankle which he terms "Genetic Reduction", the subject of this paper.

The terminology used in the original writings of Lauge-Hansen is slightly different than that used in most English literature on the subject. The current English terminology is applied rather loosely and I have decided to retain the original as given by Lauge-Hansen to facilitate reference to his work and avoid an illusion of originality for this interpretation. Lauge-Hansen's terminology with commonly used English equivalents is given in Figure I.

The mechanism of production of ankle fractures has been demonstrated very clearly by Lauge-Hansen's carefully worked out experimental-surgical investigation. He has found that the type of injury depends on two basic factors. The first is the position of the foot at the moment of injury which is nec-

*Presented at the General Session of the Annual Meeting of the Oklahoma State Medical Association April 14, 1953, at Tulsa, Oklahoma.

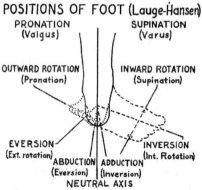

POSITIONS OF FOOT (Lauge-Hansen)

PRONATION (Valgus)   SUPINATION (Varus)

OUTWARD ROTATION (Pronation)   INWARD ROTATION (Supination)

EVERSION (Ext. rotation)   INVERSION (Int. Rotation)

ABDUCTION (Eversion)   ADDUCTION (Inversion)

NEUTRAL AXIS

GENETIC DIAGNOSIS BY STAGES				
Type of Fracture	Supination—		Pronation—	
	Adduction	Eversion	Abduction	Eversion
Stage 1	*Lateral malleolus (or lateral ligaments)	Tibio-fibular diastasis	Medial malleolus (or deltoid ligament)	Same as Pron.-Abd. type (R.-same)
Stage 2	Medial malleolus (high-oblique) (2 stages only)	*Lateral malleolus (long, spiral-oblique)	Tibio-fibular diastasis and dorsal lip (sm. fragment)	Tibio-fibular diastasis
Stage 3	Note: * denotes character-istic fibu-	Dorsal lip of tibia (Variable size)	*Lateral malleolus (short, straight, oblique, at joint)	*Fibular fracture (short, spiral, oblique, 6-9 cm. prox.)
Stage 4	lar fracture for each type	Medial malleolus (or deltoid ligament)	(3 stages only)	Dorsal lip of tibia (Variable size)

Figure I
TERMINOLOGY OF FOOT POSITION
(after Lauge-Hansen)

Note: Parenthetical equivalent term used in
English Literature.
Pronation is ''valgus' as applied to clubfoot
Outward rotation is the ''pronation'' of flat-
foot
Eversion is usually termed ''external rota-
tion''
Abduction (hindfoot) is ''everted or valgus
heel''
Supination is ''varus'' as applied to clubfoot
Inward rotation is ''forefoot supination''
Inversion is usually termed ''internal rota-
tion''
Adduction (hindfoot) is ''inverted or varus
heel''

Figure II
*THE GENETIC DIAGNOSIS
OF ANKLE FRACTURES*

Note: The characteristic x-ray feature of each
type is the fibular fracture indicated by*. First
stage of Supination fractures and first two
stages of Pronation fractures *may* be present

with only ligament injury, therefore negative
x-rays will result.

Conversely malleolar fractures usually mean
major ligamentous damage as well. Ligament
status should be determined to complete diagnosis
so that proper genetic reduction may be selected.

A. Low fracture lateral malleolus or lateral
ligament rupture, plus or minus oblique
fracture base of medial is *Supination-adduction type.*
B. Tibio-fibular diastasis plus or minus spiral
oblique fractures of fibula at and just
above joint line is *Supination-eversion type*
(40-70%)
C. Low fracture medial malleolus or deltoid
ligament rupture plus or minus tibio fibular diastasis and small fracture fragment
on dorsal lip (may be *only* x-ray finding),
finally straight, oblique fibular fracture at
joint is *Pronation-adduction type.*
D. Low fracture of medial malleolus or deltoid
ligament rupture plus or minus tibio-fibular
diastasis and high (6-9 cm.), short, spiral,
oblique fibular fracture (may be only x-ray
finding) is *Pronation-eversion type.*

essary to take up the slack in all of the ligaments of the foot joints. This converts the
foot into a rigid lever arm by which extreme
force can be applied to the bones forming
the ankle mortise or to the ligaments responsible for the integrity of the joint. The second factor is the direction in which abnormal, forced movement is applied to the foot
to produce the injury. Combinations of these
two basic factors determine the basic type,
and to these qualitative factors is added a
quantitative one, namely, the amount of force
applied. This latter factor determines the
various stages of the basic types of injury
which occur in definite order, characteristic
of the basic type.

The four basic fracture types of Lauge-
Hansen are:

1. Supination-adduction fracture.
This injury occurs when a foot in
maximal supination is subjected to abnormal, forced adduction. It occurs in
two stages.

2. Supination-eversion fracture.
This injury is produced when a foot
in maximal supination is subjected to
forced eversion. It occurs in four
stages.

3. Pronation-abduction fracture.
This injury is produced when a foot:

in maximal pronation is subjected to forced abduction. It occurs in three stages.

4. Pronation-eversion fracture.

This injury occurs when a foot in maximal pronation is subjected to forced eversion. It occurs in four stages.

In the course of his experimental-surgical studies, Lauge-Hansen demonstrated that when a maximally supinated foot is subjected to inversion force, the lesion produced is confined to the lateral ligaments in varying degrees. Pronation-inversion injuries were found to result in supramalleolar fractures of the tibia and fibula. The inversion mechanism of injury is therefore excluded from a discussion of fractures of the ankle joint proper.

The genetic diagnosis of ankle injuries by stages according to Lauge-Hansen is presented in tabular form in Figure II.

Genetic reductions should be done under adequate spinal or general anesthesia as successful reduction depends on complete re-laxation. For all type fractures the thigh is held vertically with the patella facing straight up so that a constant position of the leg will be a point of reference during the reduction maneuvers. A snug plaster boot is applied with the reduced position carefully guarded during application. Bony union is usually complete in eight to ten weeks. The after care for all fracture types is the same except where it must be individualized for a particular case. Genetic reduction should be performed as soon as possible following the injury, as marked swelling prevents adequate manipulation. Certain compound fractures do not lend themselves to this method because of the swelling which is to be expected and the opportunity for internal fixation which is present.

Supination-Adduction Fracture (Figure III)

A maximally supinated foot subjected to forcible adduction sustains injury due to stress directed in a medial and superior direction. Stage one is produced by avulsion of the distal fibula, producing a transverse fracture of the lateral malleolus below the joint line or rupture of the lateral ligaments. Stage two results from shearing force exerted by the medial portion of the talus against the medial malleolus which is fractured

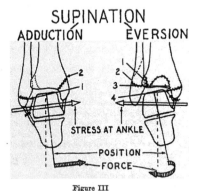

SUPINATION
ADDUCTION   EVERSION

STRESS AT ANKLE

POSITION

FORCE

Figure III

SUPINATION FRACTURES OF ANKLE

Left—Supination-adduction type
  Position *of* foot—Supination
  Force *to* foot—Adduction
  Stress *at* ankle—Medial, slightly superior
Right—Supination-eversion type
  Position *of* foot—Supination
  Force *to* foot—Eversion (External rotation)
  Stress *at* ankle—Rotatory, lateral and transverse.

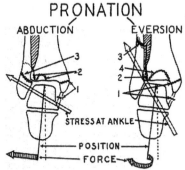

PRONATION
ABDUCTION   EVERSION

STRESS AT ANKLE

POSITION

FORCE

Figure IV

PRONATION FRACTURES OF ANKLE

Left—Pronation-adduction type
  Position *of* foot—Pronation
  Force *to* foot—Abduction
  Stress *at* ankle—Lateral and superior
Right—Pronation-eversion type
  Position *of* foot—Pronation
  Force *to* foot—Eversion (External rotation)
  Stress *at* ankle—Rotatory, lateral and almost vertical.

through its base and obliquely upward· allowing medial subluxation of the ankle joint.

Genetic reduction is performed by grasping the heel from its plantar aspect with the right hand in a right ankle injury while the left hand holds the midfoot. The foot is moved in an anterior and lateral direction, the hindfoot abducted, and the whole foot dorsiflexed into the final position of slight eversion, which is the normal position of the pronated foot in dorsiflexion.

Supination-Eversion Fracture (Figure III)

A maximally supinated foot subjected to forcible eversion (external rotation in the axis of the leg) is injured by a rotation stress directed laterally. Stage one is a diastasis of the distal tibio-fibular joint by wedging of the talus against the lateral malleolus. Stage two is a long, curved, oblique fracture of the fibula in the frontal plane beginning just above the joint anteriorly and extending proximally and medially for three to five centimeters. This lesion is produced by torsion of the fibula. Stage three is a fracture of the dorsal lip of the tibia of variable size produced by shearing force of the now unimpeded talus against the posterior margin of the tibia. Stage four is a fracture of the medial malleolus or a rupture of the deltoid ligament by avulsion.

Genetic reduction of the supination-eversion fracture is performed by grasping the right midfoot with the right hand. The left hand holds the heel on its posterior aspect. For stage one or other undisplaced fractures of this type, the foot is simply pronated, inverted, and dorsiflexed. If reduction is necessary to restore anatomical relations, the foot is supinated, everted, and plantarflexed to clear soft tissue from the fractured surfaces. Reduction is accomplished by moving the hindfoot in an anterior direction, inverting (internally rotating) the forefoot and finally pronating and dorsiflexing the whole foot. The hindfoot is molded into adduction as the plaster sets.

Pronation - Abduction Fracture (Figure IV)

A maximally pronated foot subjected to forcible abduction is injured by lateral and superior stress. Stage one consists of a fracture of the medial malleolus or rupture of the deltoid ligament by avulsion force. Stage two consists of tibio-fibular diastasis and fracture of a small fragment of the dorsal lip of the tibia by the wedging action of the talus. Stage three is a short, straight· oblique fracture of the fibula in an essentially transverse plane. It occurs just above the joint and may be comminuted.

Genetic reduction of the pronation-abduction fracture is performed by grasping the foot as in the supination-eversion fracture. For undisplaced fractures, the foot is simply adducted at the hindfoot, inverted (internally rotated) slightly, and dorsiflexed. When reduction is required, soft tissue is disengaged by slightly exaggerating the deformity in pronation, eversion (external rotation), and plantar flexion. The foot is then moved in an anterior direction, inverted internally rotated slightly, and dorsiflexed. The hindfoot is adducted and the forefoot is pronated while the cast is applied.

Pronation-Eversion Fracture (Figure IV)

When a maximally pronated foot is subjected to eversion or external rotation forces, a lateral and almost vertical stress is produced. Stage one consists of a fracture of the media malleolus or rupture of the deltoid ligament by avulsion identical with stage one of the pronation-abduction fracture. Stage two is a tibio-fibular diastasis extending high into the interosseus membrane, produced by wedging of the talus against the distal fibula. Stage three consists of a short, curved, oblique fracture of the fibula six to nine centimeters proximal to the malleolus by torsion from rotation of the talus in an unstable mortise. Stage four consists of a dorsal lip fracture of the tibia of variable size by shearing action of the freely movable talus. The foot is subluxated posterolaterally.

Genetic reduction of a pronation-eversion fracture is performed by grasping the foot as in the supination-eversion and pronation-abduction types. Stage one and other undisplaced fractures are treated as their counter-parts in the pronation-abduction types. When reduction is necessary the fracture is opened to clear soft tissue by slight pronation· eversion and plantar flexion. The foot is then moved in an anterior direction, inverted (internally rotated), the hindfoot is adducted and the whole foot dorsiflexed. The forefoot is slightly pronated as the cast is applied.

In a series of 27 consecutive cases treated personally the differences in the percentage incidence as compared with Lauge-Hansen's series of 228 were noted as in Table I.

TABLE I

Types	Lauge-Hansen 228 cases	Author 27 cases
Pronation-abduction	5%	22%
Pronation-Eversion	7%	15%
Supination-Adduction	16%	26%
Supination-Eversion	70%	37%

No explanation for the difference and the much more even distribution between the types in the personal series was discovered but it probably reflects the statistical difference in the size of the two series.

In the personal series, 21 cases were undisplaced and uncomplicated and presented no difficulties whatsoever in therapy. Six cases, however, were displaced sufficiently that they probably would have been subjected to open reduction and internal fixation prior to the adoption of the closed method of Lauge-Hansen. All of these fractures healed in virtually anatomical position in eight to ten weeks, and the patients were able to walk in the original walking boot in one to two weeks. Although it is too early to judge final results with the oldest case being less than two years after injury and the most recent four months, so far all have good motion and stable ankle mortises. There were two unsuccessful cases, each of which illustrates a valuable point. A 38 year old cowboy with a pronation-eversion fracture in the fourth stage was seen early in the series and refused to have adequate anesthesia. The reduction was attempted under local infiltration of the fracture hematoma, and it was thought that the reduction was successful. The displacement recurred, however, and he was finally treated, after much discussion, by open reduction and internal fixation of the medial malleolus three days after injury. The second case was that of a 74 year old woman who was seen with a severely comminuted fracture into the joint. The injury was misdiagnosed by x-ray as an explosion type fracture. At open operation a supination-adduction type fracture was found. This fracture probably could have been treated successfully by genetic reduction if the diagnosis had been correct. The preliminary study of these cases indicates that the results equal those of open operations. Surgery is avoided and the patients are ambulated earlier. Mobilization following removal of the cast appears to be easier than following open operation.

SUMMARY

1. Lauge-Hansen's interpretation of fractures involving the ankle joint provides diagnosis according to the mechanism of injury and classification according to genetic diagnosis determines the appropriate genetic reduction.

2. Adequate x-ray and clinical examination results in accurate genetic diagnosis of the great majority of ankle fractures due to indirect violence. Ankle injuries due to direct violence are uncommon.

3. Proper positioning according to the principles of genetic reduction results in excellent stability allowing painless, early ambulation. Heretofore, weight bearing occasionally caused pain and/or loss of position even in originally undisplaced ankle fractures treated by less stable methods.

4. Genetic reduction, a closed method performed without instruments under adequate anesthesia, results in anatomical reposition which is stable in a snug walking boot applied immediately post-reduction and worn eight to ten weeks. A preliminary study of 27 personal cases revealed that 25 have excellent early anatomical and functional results. Failure of the method is noted immediately and open operation can then be performed. In the unsuccessful cases in the personal series, one was failure of adequate reduction and retention due to inadequate anesthesia and the other was opened electively when misdiagnosed as an explosion type fracture.

5. Genetic reduction, in my experience, has reduced very drastically the indications for open reduction. I now reserve the open method for those cases in which the genetic reduction fails, severely compounded fractures, and severely comminuted explosion type fractures for which the method is not recommended by Lauge-Hansen himself. It is my hope that interest may be aroused in this approach to the treatment of fractures of the ankle.

REFERENCES

1. Lauge-Hansen, N.: Fractures of the ankle: Analytic historic survey as basis of new experimental roentgenologic and clinical investigations, Arch. Surg. 56:259 (March) 1948

2. Lauge-Hansen, N.: Fractures of the ankle: Combined experimental-surgical and experimental-roentgenologic investigations, ibid. 60:957 (May) 1950

3. Lauge-Hansen, N : Fractures of the ankle: Clinical use of genetic roentgen diagnosis and genetic reduction, ibid. 64:488 (April) 1952

President's Page

Recently, President Eisenhower and his Secretary of H.E.W., Mrs. Oveta Culp Hobby, gave the American people, the medical profession, the hospitals, and the insurance companies, as well as non-profit pre-health plans, a bird's eye view of their program for the subsidizing of certain health care programs.

President Eisenhower's health message to Congress dealt in generalities and it was assumed that Mrs. Hobby at her subsequent meeting with leaders in the health and insurance fields would be more specific but to date there has been no outline given of the legislation to be introduced into Congress. Mrs. Hobby and her advisors, when quizzed by representatives of the medical profession and others on the points of whether or not her legislation would follow the Wolverton Bill of the last Congress, declined to either affirm or deny.

Subsequent to the meeting with Mrs. Hobby, the Board of Directors of the American Medical Association issued a very cautious statement concerning their attitude to the proposals, which, I believe, was prudent on their part. Until such time as the legislation proposal to accomplish the contemplated ends can be carefully reviewed, American medicine should refrain from taking a definite stand.

This suggested cautiousness should in no way be accepted as tacit approval as it is difficult to envisage a government program that can achieve better success in any field than private endeavor except in military and civilian defense. Likewise, we must again remember that the Supreme Court has already laid down the dictum that whatever the government subsidizes, it can control.

The Republican party program in this session of Congress in all fields of governmental endeavor will be watched with great interest and will have tremendous bearing upon the coming Congressional and Senatorial elections. Medicine must not hide its head in the sand as to health legislation.

Sincerely yours,

John E. McDonald, M.D.

President

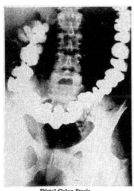

Distal Colon Stasis

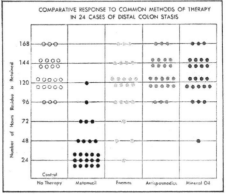

COMPARATIVE RESPONSE TO COMMON METHODS OF THERAPY IN 24 CASES OF DISTAL COLON STASIS

Management of
Distal Colon Stasis with Metamucil®

The "irritable colon" resulting in distal colon stasis is a hard-to-manage by-product of many abdominal or stress conditions.

Roentgen evaluation of the commonly used methods to combat colonic stasis has shown the value of Metamucil because of its lack of irritation and its high degree of effectiveness[*] in this most prevalent type of stasis.

Metamucil is the highly refined mucilloid of Plantago ovata (50%), a seed of the psyllium group, combined with dextrose (50%) as a dispersing agent. It produces smooth fecal bulk necessary to incite the normal peristaltic reflexes, without causing irritation, straining, impaction or interference with the digestion or absorption of vitamins.

The average adult dose is one teaspoonful of Metamucil powder in a glass of cool water, milk or juice, followed by an additional glass of fluid if indicated. This amount of fluid is essential for the production of "smoothage."

It is supplied in containers of 4, 8 and 16 ounces. Metamucil is accepted by the Council on Pharmacy and Chemistry of the American Medical Association.

SEARLE *Research in the Service of Medicine*

*Barowsky, H.: A Roentgenographic Evaluation of the Common Measures Employed in the Treatment of Colonic Stasis. Rev. Gastroenterol. *19*:154 (Feb.) 1952.

OKLAHOMA ACADEMY OF GENERAL PRACTICE WILL HOLD
SIXTH ANNUAL MEETING IN TULSA FEBRUARY 15-16

Complete program has been announced for the annual meeting of the Oklahoma Academy of General Practice which will be held in Tulsa February 15 and 16 at the Tulsa Hotel.

Physicians throughout the state are invited to attend the program which will include papers by six top flight guest speakers.

Another feature of the program will be a symposium at 1:45 the first day, Monday, February 15, on ''Emergencies in Every Day Practice,'' with all guest speakers participating.

An outstanding program has been planned for the dinner Monday night, February 15, at which time E. T. Cook, M.D., Anadarko, will be inaugurated at 1954 President of the organization.

An innovation at the annual meetings of the Academy is the breakfast held the second morning of the meeting, at which time approximately 50 prizes are awarded to those in attendance. The annual meeting for election of officers and other Academy business will be held immediately following the breakfast.

Roundtable luncheons will be held each day.

Twenty-seven commercial exhibitors have contracted for space at the meeting.

A luncheon and style show and other entertainment is planned for the ladies attending the meeting.

Complete scientific program is as follows:

MONDAY, FEBRUARY 15, 1954

8:00 a.m. to 9:00 a.m.
Registration
9:00 a.m. to 9:30 a.m.
William F. Guerriero, M.D.
''Carcinoma of the Cervix''
9:30 a.m. to 10:00 a.m.
Harry Wilkins, M.D.
''Diagnosis of Intracranial Lesions''
10:00 a.m. to 10:30 a.m.
Visit Your Exhibitors
10:30 a.m. to 11:00 a.m.
Manuel E. Lichtenstein, M.D.
''The Clinical Significance of the Position and Station of the Appendix''
11:00 a.m. to 11:15 a.m.
Visit Your Exhibitors
11:15 a.m. to 11:45 a.m.
Horace L. Hodes, M.D.
''Treatment of the Severe Forms of Poliomyelitis and the Present Status of Measures Aimed at the Prevention of the Disease''

11:45 a.m. to 12:00 noon
Visit Your Exhibitors

12:00 noon to 1:30 p.m.
Roundtable Luncheon

1:30 p.m. to 1:45 p.m.
Visit Your Exhibitors

1:45 p.m. to 3:45 p.m.
Symposium—''Emergencies in Every Day Practice'' Guest speakers participating

3:45 p.m. to 4:00 p.m.
Visit Your Exhibitors

4:00 p.m. to 4:30 p.m.
Perrin H. Long, M.D.
''Uses and Abuses of the Antibiotics''

6:30 p.m.
Dinner

TUESDAY, FEBRUARY 16, 1954

7:30 a.m. to 8:30 a.m.
Breakfast
8:30 a.m. to 9:30 a.m.
Annual Business Meeting
9:30 a.m. to 10:00 a.m.
Visit Your Exhibitors
10:00 a.m. to 10:30 a.m.
Carlo Scuderi, M.D.
''Backache: From the Standpoint of a General Practitioner—Diagnosis and Treatment''
10:30 a.m. to 11:00 a.m.
Visit Your Exhibitors
11:00 a.m. to 11:30 a.m.
William F. Guerriero, M.D.
''Pelvic Pain''
11:30 a.m. to 12:00 noon
Visit Your Exhibitors
12:00 noon to 1:30 p.m.
Roundtable Luncheon

1:30 p.m. to 1:45 p.m.
Visit Your Exhibitors
1:45 p.m. to 2:15 p.m.
Manuel E. Lichtenstein, M.D.
''The Significance of Gall Stones to the Patient and to the Surgeon''
2:15 p.m. to 2:30 p.m.
Visit Your Exhibitors
2:30 p.m. to 3:00 p.m.
Horace L. Hodes, M.D.
''The Antibiotic Problem and the Question of Antagonism''
3:00 p.m. to 3:30 p.m.
Carlo Scuderi, M.D.
''Treatment of Both Bone Fractures of the Leg''
3:30 p.m. to 4:00 p.m.
Perrin H. Long, M.D.
''The Etiology and Management of Longevity''

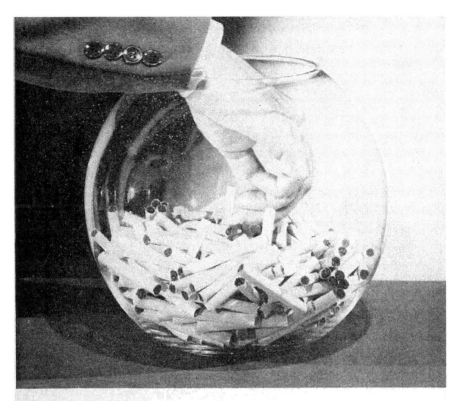

Which filter-tip cigarette is the most effective?

IN continuing and repeated impartial scientific tests, smoke from the new KENT consistently proves to have much less nicotine and tar than smoke from any other filter cigarette—old or new.

The reason is KENT's exclusive Micronite Filter.

This new filter is made of a filtering material so efficient it has been used to purify the air in atomic energy plants of microscopic impurities.

Adapted for use as a cigarette filter, it removes nicotine and tar particles as small as 2/10 of a micron.

And yet KENT's Micronite Filter, which removes a greater percentage of nicotine and tar than any other filter cigarette, lets through the full flavor of KENT's fine tobaccos.

Because so much evidence indicates KENT is the most effective filter-tip cigarette, shouldn't it be the choice of those who want the minimum of nicotine and tar in their cigarette smoke?

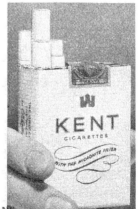

Kent with the exclusive Micronite Filter

"KENT" AND "MICRONITE" ARE REGISTERED TRADEMARKS OF P. LORILLARD COMPANY

ALL STATE PHYSICIANS MAY ATTEND CONFERENCES

Four practitioners' conferences remain to be held during the present school year at the University of Oklahoma School of Medicine through the Postgraduate Instruction Program made available to the physicians of Oklahoma by the Office of Postgraduate Instruction at the School.

All physicians in the state are invited to attend the conferences which are held at the auditorium at the School of Medicine at 7:30 p.m. Notices are mailed to physicians the first of each month. Any physician not receiving notices of the conferences is asked to contact the Office of Postgaduate Instruction at the School.

Aim of the conference is to present up-to-date postgraduate seminars on timely topics in medicine. From time to time, clinical teaching material available in the University Hospitals or the Research Foundation Hospital is presented to stress important medical points.

Remaining schedule of conferences is as follows:

February 18—Gall Bladder Disease

March 18—Atopic Dermatitis

April 15—Poliomyelitis

May 20—Diagnosis and Treatment of Congestive Failure.

INDUSTRIAL HEALTH TO BE CONFERENCE TOPIC

Health problems of the worker and his family will be discussed at the 14th annual Congress on Industrial Health, to be held February 23-25 at the Brown Hotel, Louisville, under the sponsorhip of the American Medical Association's Council on Industrial Health.

The role of industry in the maintenance of the health of the nation will be the subject of the opening general session on Wednesday morning, February 24. The keynote will be that industry and medicine are partners, it was announced by Dr. Carl M. Peterson, Chicago, secretary of the council.

In the afternoon, a clinic on health programs for executives will be presented. The value of screening examinations also will be discussed.

The President's award to the physician making the outstanding contribution to employment welfare of the handicapped in 1953 will be presented at a dinner which will be co-sponsored by the Jefferson County Medical Society.

On Thursday morning, February 25, the problems of a small plant operator will be considered. The National Safety Council's small business and associations committee will assist. This will be followed by a presentation of how a plant can prepare for emergencies.

The Louisville Chapter of the American Red Cross will participate in the program.

In the afternoon, a joint session with the A.M.A.'s Council on National Emergency Medical Service will discuss community preparations to meet a disaster. A report will present the working of such a plan in Vicksburg, Miss. The program will cover atomic bombing and bacterial, chemical and psychological warfare.

A preliminary conference with chairmen of state medical committees on industrial health will be held on Tuesday, February 23. One of the subjects will cover what American medicine should strive for in its relations with labor and management. Group conferences on subjects related to industrial health also will be held.

In the evening, a dinner will be given in honor of two retiring members of the Council on Industrial

Health, Dr. Anthony J. Lanza, New York, chairman, and Dr. Clarence D. Selby, Detroit.

MEDICAL SOCIETIES AROUND THE STATE

Newspapers' reports received by *Journal* press time indicate that several county medical societies have elected 1954 officers at recent meetings. Counties not listed below are urged to send reports of their meetings and new officers to the Executive Office for publication in a later edition of the *Journal*. Readers are reminded that because of publication deadlines, information in this issue includes only that received before January 1.

KIOWA-WASHITA

J. B. Tolbert, M.D., Mountain View, is the 1954 President of the Kiowa-Washita Society. He was elected at a meeting held in Cordell and the following additional officers were also named: Aubrey Stowers, M.D., Sentinel, Vice-President; and Wilson Mahone, M.D., Hobart, Secretary-Treasurer. Program at the meeting was presented by John Miller, assistant vice-president of the trust department of the First National Bank and Trust Company of Oklahoma City.

OKLAHOMA

Installed recently as President of the Oklahoma County Medical Society was Henry G. Bennett, Jr., M.D., Oklahoma City, son of the late President of Oklahoma A. and M. College. Other new officers are: Donald W. Branham, M.D., President-Elect; Bert E. Mulvey, M.D., Vice-President; and Elmer Ridgeway, Jr., M.D., Secretary-Treasurer, all of Oklahoma City.

CLEVELAND-McCLAIN

George A. Wiley, M.D., Norman, has been elected President of the Cleveland-McClain County Medical Society, Curtis Berry, M.D., was named Vice-President and a Secretary and Treasurer will be elected later.

PAYNE-PAWNEE

Newly elected officers of the Payne-Pawnee County Medical Society are: Harold R. Sanders, M.D., Stillwater, President; E. O. Martin, M.D., Vice-President; and Clifford W. Moore, M.D., Stillwater, Secretary-Treasurer.

JACKSON

E. A. Abernathy, M.D., Altus, is the new President of the Jackson County Medical Society. W. E. Mabry, M.D., Altus, was re-elected Secretary.

COMANCHE-COTTON

W. F. Lewis, M.D., Lawton, was elected President of the Comanche-Cotton Society. Other new officers include Charles Graybill, M.D., Vice-President; and G. G. Downing, M.D., Lawton, Secretary-Treasurer.

FROM THE OKLAHOMA DIVISION, AMERICAN CANCER SOCIETY . . .

IMPROVEMENTS IN THE LAST TEN YEARS

The following table, based on Metropolitan Life Insurance Company data, vividly shows the decline in cancer death rates among white women during the period from 1940-42 to 1950-52. It demonstrates that in the last 10 years, 10,000 additional women are being saved yearly as a result of improved methods of detection and treatment and a better educational program.

Age Group	Percentage of Decline
25-34	17.9
35-44	22.6
45-54	11.3
55-64	15.5
65-74	9.4

The over-all decline in women from the ages of one to 74 is 12.6 per cent.

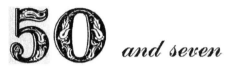
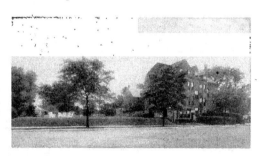

HAVE YOU HEARD?

Ira Pollock, M.D., Oklahoma City, recently was accepted as a member of the American Board of Surgery.

Melvin Hicks, M.D., formerly director of the Hughes County health department, has accepted a residency in Akron, Ohio.

Evelyn Rude, M.D., Enid, has recently completed a residency in Brooklyn. Before taking a residency, she spent two years in Saudi-Arabia where she was employed as physician by the Arabian-American Oil Company.

Sam A. McKeel, M.D., was recently presented with a plaque by the Ada Lions Club which read "Presented by Ada Lions Club to Dr. Sam A. McKeel, beloved member, in appreciation of a life which builds up and dignifies Lionism."

Charles E. Baker, M.D., University of Oklahoma graduate, has opened his office in Granite.

Violet Sturgeon, M.D., Hennessey, has been elected to the board of trustees of Oklahoma Baptist University. Doctor Sturgeon is the first woman to be named to the board of trustees of O.B.U.

Earl Lusk, M.D., Tulsa, has been elected president-elect of the Tulsa Academy of General Practice. 1954 President is L. A. Munding, M.D.; Vice-President, Lowell. Stokes, M.D.; and Marshall O. Hart, M.D., was re-elected secretary-treasurer.

APPLICATIONS URGED

FOR SCIENTIFIC EXHIBITS

Applications for Scientific Exhibits for the Annual Meeting to be held in Oklahoma City May 10, 11, and 12, should be submitted to the Executive Office before March 1, 1954.

Complete information and application forms have been sent to those who had scientific exhibits at the last meeting which featured such exhibits, to secretaries of county medical societies, the Medical School, the larger hospitals and research groups. However, requests for applications are welcomed by the Scientific Exhibits Committee from any physician who contemplates the preparation of a scientific exhibit.

The entire scientific program will be held in the Zebra Room of the Municipal Auditorium, Oklahoma City. Space for scientific exhibits will be located between two sections of the commercial exhibits but will be separate from the commercial exhibits. Space assignments will be made on the basis of the applications received and each applicant will be advised promptly of the action of the committee in regard to his application.

For further information, application forms and regulations, write: Scientific Exhibits Committee, Oklahoma State Medical Association, 1227 Classen Drive, Oklahoma City, Oklahoma.

ATTEND

Oklahoma Academy of

General Practice

Tulsa Hotel—Tulsa, Okla.

February 15-16

OBITUARIES

CHARLES O. LIVELY, M.D.

1869-1953

Charles O. Lively, M.D., pioneer Oklahoma physician, died November 24, 1953, in a Pawnee hospital.

Doctor Lively was born March 8, 1869, in Kentucky. He attended Louisville University and practiced medicine for more than 50 years coming to Durant in 1898. He practiced in Bryan county until 1924 when he came to Ralston where he practiced until about 15 years ago when he was injured in an automobile accident. He had been bedfast much of the time since.

He is survived by his widow of the home and a half-brother who lives in Kentucky.

MEDICAL EDUCATION PROBLEMS

TO BE TOPIC OF CONFERENCE

Postgraduate medical education needs, and how these best can be met by medical schools, will be considered at the 50th annual Congress on Medical Education and Licensure in the Palmer House, February 7-9.

The meeting will be sponsored by the American Medical Association's Council on Medical Education and Hospitals, with the cooperation of the Federation of State Medical Advisory Boards of the United States and the Advisory Board for Medical Specialties.

Three panel discussions will be built around a preliminary report of a survey on postgraduate medical education undertaken by the Council on Medical Education and Hospitals. These panels will consider the objectives of such education, how to achieve these objectives and the needs of such programs — faculty, facilities and finance.

"The survey has brought out the views of doctors on their postgraduate education needs," said Dr. Edward L. Turner, Chicago, secretary of the council. "It will be the aim to combine these with the opinions of medical school facilities so as to provide a comprehensive and correlated program."

Dr. Edward J. McCormick, Toledo, president of the American Medical Association, who will be one of the principal speakers, will stress the importance in undergraduate medical education of instruction in fundamental professional ethics, public relations and medical practice.

TULSA HOST TO PUBLIC

HEALTH CONFERENCE

The thirteenth annual meeting of the Oklahoma Public Health Association was held at the Mayo Hotel, Tulsa, December 3, 4, 5, 1953. Program chairman was Kirk T. Mosely, M.D.

Program topics included "Health Facilities and Program in Oklahoma and How We Can Utilize Them," "Joint Sessions with the Oklahoma Advisory Health Council," "Rural School Health," and sections for physicians, nurses, sanitarians, health educators, veterinarians, clerks and others interested in any phase of health as it relates to the individual or to the community.

RURAL HEALTH TOPIC
OF NATIONAL CONFERENCE

The roles of community planning, cooperative efforts, nutrition and insurance in the maintenance of healthful conditions in agricultural areas will be discussed at the ninth annual National Conference on Rural Health in Dallas, Tex., March 4-6.

The conference, sponsored by the American Medical Association's Council on Rural Health, will be held in the Baker Hotel. It will be participated in by physicians and by farm, community and education groups, including agricultural extension workers, from all parts of the country.

Dr. Edward J. McCormick, Toledo, O., president of the American Medical Association, will be the speaker at the closing session. Also participating in that program will be Dr. Joseph I. Greenwell, New Haven, Ky., who at the Clinical Session of the A.M.A. in St. Louis last December was named as the "General Practitioner of the Year."

Dr. Carll S. Mundy, Toledo, acting chairman of the Council on Rural Health, speaking at the opening session, will sound the conference keynote—"Let's Put More 'U' in CommUNITY."

There will be panels on community programs, nutrition and health insurance. Presentations will be made by Mrs. Charlotte R. Bensen, Raleigh, N. C., health education consultant of the Medical Society of North Carolina; Dr. John B. Youmans, Nashville, dean of the Vanderbilt University School of Medicine and member of the A.M.A. Council on Foods and Nutrition, and Lambert Schultz, Chattanooga, staff executive of the group department, Provident Life and Accident Company. J. P. Schmidt, Columbus, O., professor of rural sociology at the University of Ohio, will be the discussion leader for all three panels, each of which will have three other participants.

State committees on rural health will hold a pre-conference meeting with the A.M.A. Council on Rural Health on Thursday morning, March 4. The topics will include prepaid insurance and the physician's responsibility to his community.

A.M.A. PUBLICIZES
OKLAHOMA FILM

"School Health in Action"—a sound and color film produced for the Oklahoma State Department of Health with the cooperation of the Oklahoma State Medical Association, was recently publicised in an A.M.A. Secretary's Letter and in the American Medical Association News Notes.

The film explains how a typical town in Oklahoma recognized its school health problems, and, through community effort, launched a plan to solve them. Service charge for the film ordered through the A.M.A.'s Committee on Medical Motion Pictures is $2.00.

Announcements

OKLAHOMA ACADEMY OF GENERAL PRACTICE. February 15-16, Tulsa Hotel, Tulsa, Oklahoma.

OKLAHOMA STATE MEDICAL ASSOCIATION. May 10-11-12, Oklahoma City, Municipal Auditorium.

MEDICAL AND SURGICAL POSTGRADUATE CONFERENCE. Scott and White Clinic, Temple, Texas, March 1, 2, 3, 1954. Registration forms are available from the office of the Assistant Dean, University of Texas Postgraduate School of Medicine, The Temple Division, Temple, Texas.

X-RAY ANATOMY. Course will be opened February 16 for 10 weekly sessions at the University of Oklahoma School of Medicine. This course will be conducted by Dr. Ernest Lachman, Professor and Chairman of the Department of Anatomy, Consultant Professor of Radiology at the University of Oklahoma School of Medicine. This course will consist of a systematic review of the field of x-ray anatomy, laying the foundation for an understanding of the appearance of the normal on film and screen.

TUMOR CONFERENCE. Third annual conference at Midwestern University, Wichita Falls, Texas, March 31, 1954 sponsored by the Wichita County Medical Society Clinic, Texas State Department of Health and the American Cancer Society.

INTERNATIONAL ACADEMY OF PROCTOLOGY. April 8, 9, 10, 11, 1954. Palmer House, Chicago, Sixth Annual Convention. Programs are available upon request to the Executive Office of the International Academy of Proctology, 43-55 Kissena Blvd., Flushing, New York.

RECENT ADVANCES IN CARDIOLOGY. Baylor University College of Medicine and the University of Texas Postgraduate School of Medicine announce a course on recent advances and current problems in cardiology February 15-19 in Houston. Visiting lecturers will include Robert H. Bayley, M.D., Professor of Medicine, University of Oklahoma.

SIXTH ANNUAL NEUROPSYCHIATRIC MEETING. Veterans Administration Hospital, North Little Rock, Arkansas February 25 and 26, 1954. No registration charge. Further information may be obtained by writing to Dr. Ewin S. Chappell, Director, Professional Education, Veterans Administration Hospital, North Little Rock, Arkansas.

A.M.A. CLINICAL MEETING
HOUSE OF DELEGATES ROUNDUP

The House of Delegates of the American Medical Association, meeting at the Jefferson Hotel in St. Louis during the Seventh Annual Clinical Session took important policy actions on social security, voluntary health insurance, medical ethics and unethical practices, medical education, hospital accreditation, military affairs and a wide variety of subjects affecting both physicians and the public. James Stevenson, M.D., O.S.M.A. Delegate from Tulsa, served on the reference committee on industrial health.

Highlights of the opening House session on Tuesday was the announcement that Dr. Joseph I. Greenwell of New Haven, Kentucky, had been selected by a special committee of the A.M.A. Board of Trustees as the 1953 "General-Practitioner of the Year."

The Tuesday program also included addresses by Dr. James R. Reuling of Bayside, New York, Speaker of the House of Delegates, and Dr. Chester Keefer of Boston, Special Assistant to Mrs. Oveta Culp Hobby, United States Secretary of Health, Education and Welfare. Annual reports were presented by Dr. George F. Lull, Secretary and General Manager of the A.M.A.; Dr. Dwight H. Murray of Napa, Calif., Chairman of the Board of Trustees, and by the standing and special committees of the House of Delegates.

Approving a recommendation by its Reference Committee on Legislation and Public Relations, the House passed a resolution reaffirming its opposition to the compulsory coverage of physicians under the Old Age and Survivors Insurance provisions of the Social Security act and advocating passage of the Jenkins-Keogh bills now pending in Congress. These bills were described as providing for "the development of a voluntary pension program which is equitable, free from compulsion, and satisfies the retirement needs of physicians."

The same committee report urged continued action to obtain passage of the Bricker Amendment (S. J. Res. 1) and approved the principles of legislation which would reduce or remove the limitation on the deduction of medical and dental expenses for income tax purposes. It also opposed any further extension of the "Doctor Draft" Law beyond the present expiration date of June 30, 1955.

The House acted to accelerate the development of voluntary health insurance by passing a resolution requesting the Council on Medical Service to proceed immediately with a special study of the problems of catastrophic coverage and coverage for retired persons. The Council was asked to present its findings and recommendations to the House not later than the 1954 Clinical Meeting. The resolution pointed out:

"There are two large groups of citizens for whom improved coverage could be offered under present prepaid medical care plans, namely: (a) those individuals who suffer catastrophic or long-continued and highly expensive illness and whose financial resources are not adequate to meet the cost thereof and (b) those citizens who have retired and are living on small incomes and who are not eligible under presently existing public or private plans."

Another resolution on voluntary health insurance, adjudged to be emergency business by the Reference Committee on Insurance and Medical Service and then passed by the House, stated that "the American Medical Association condemns all insurance contracts which classify any medical service as a hospital service." The

REGISTERED AT MEETING

According to the Daily Bulletin of the A.M.A. Clinical Session in St. Louis, the following Oklahomans were among those registered:

George S. Bozalis, M.D., Oklahoma City
John F. Burton, M.D., Oklahoma City
Beverly C. Chatham, M.D., Chickasha
William H. Cook, M.D., Chickasha
Charles D. Cunningham, M.D., Ardmore
John A. Cunningham, M.D., Oklahoma City
Robert Kendall Endres, M.D., Alva
C. J. Fishman, M.D., Oklahoma City
Marion K. Ledbetter, M.D., Tulsa
E. O. Martin, M.D., Cushing
John McDonald, M.D., Tulsa
Howard B. Shorbe, M.D., Oklahoma City
Winfred A. Showman, M.D., Tulsa
James Stevenson, M.D., Tulsa

O.S.M.A. REPRESENTED
AT PR CONFERENCE

Attending the sixth annual A.M.A. public relations conference preceding the clinical session in December was Executive Secretary, Dick Graham.

Topics discussed were. Facing Up to PR Facts, Making a PR Program Work, What Motivates the Public's Feelings Toward Medicine, Seling Our Economic System: How Others Do It, Mending Our PR Fences and What's in Store in '54.

resolution reaffirmed previous actions of the House defining pathology, radiology, anesthesiology and physiatry as medical services.

To clarify misunderstandings among physicians regarding the rules and regulations of the Joint Commission on Accreditation of Hospitals, especially as they concern the role of the Department of General Practice in a hospital, the House adopted the folowing resolution:

"That this House of Delegates of the American Medical Association request the Joint Commission on Accreditation of Hospitals to publish an article, or series of articles, in the Journal of the American Medical Association and other official publications circulating among the medical and hospital professions, to acquaint the medical-hospital profession with the regulations, bylaws and their interpretations, and

"That the Commission clarify the methods by which an aggrieved hospital or its staff may appeal a decision with which they are not in agreement."

In the field of medical education the House was "pleased to note" that a fourth grant of $500,000 had been made by the American Medical Association to the American Medical Education for financial aid to the nation's medical schools, and that the number of contributors now is more than double the total in 1952.

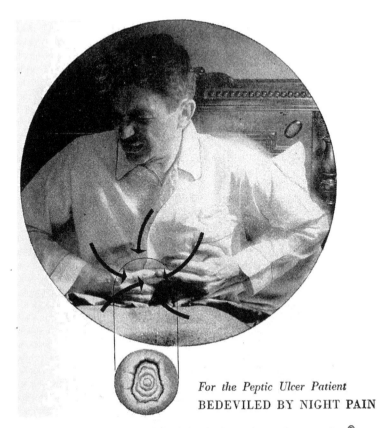

For the Peptic Ulcer Patient
BEDEVILED BY NIGHT PAIN

A M P H O J E L®

ALUMINUM HYDROXIDE GEL

AMPHOJEL helps patients sleep by neutralizing acid promptly . . .
promoting pain relief through the night. A double dose at bedtime
will effectively control "night pain" in most patients.

AMPHOJEL is a double gel—one *reactive*, for immediate buffering of
gastric acid; the other, *demulcent*, for prolonged coating of the
gastric mucosa—protection for the granulation tissue in the ulcer crater.

Available: Suspension: Bottles of 12 fl. oz.

Tablets: Boxes of 30 (5 gr.), bottles of 100
            Boxes of 60 (10 gr.)

Wyeth
®
Philadelphia 2, Pa.

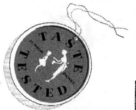
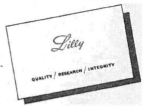

Editorials

The A. D. A. Forecast

The American Diabetes Association publishes the *A.D.A. Forecast* which is a magazine for patients and it might be said for physicians who undertake the management of this condition.

Before insulin the forecast was difficult and usually dark. Now it is relatively good especially if the patient can be given an intelligent grasp of the disease and all its implications. The forecast for the individual patient depends largely upon his power to grasp the full significance of his condition and the great importance of his full cooperation with the attending physician. A notice of the publication appears on another page in this issue of the *Journal*.

A few years ago the editorial columns of the *Journal* carried a notice of this publication and recommended that it should be brought to the attention of all practicing physicians and placed in the hands of all literate diabetics.

"What Luck?"

Though this might well be the physician's abiding question with reference to his daily work, it really is the angler's greeting. Fortunate is the doctor who has heard it echoing across the water and has learned its meaning while otherwise oblivious to the world's demands.

Spring is here. Reverie overrides the New Year resolutions. I am dreaming. Far from the world's fish markets comes the sweet smell of a freshly lined creel. I catch the glint of a speckled trout or the iridescent gleam of a rainbow through the moist greenery in the creel. I see ". . . a few shining pebbles from the bed of the brook, a few ferns from the cool green woods and a few wild flowers from places that you remember." I hear the song of the mountain steam as it laves my limbs and sends my blood aloft. I feel the thrill of the rod as it yields to the strike, responds to the run, levels with the leap and holds its spring until the battle is won.

The spell of the primitive is upon me. I'm headed for far-away silent places where sun and stars above limitless horizons hold whispering converse over the incomparable gifts of nature. I see sweet smelling wooded slopes, aspen clad morains and musical streams tumbling down to the mountain meadows for a peaceful pause in placid pools where fanning fins are never still. Once one has packed into high mountain fastnesses, the call of spring is irresistible.

Physicians long in the harness, primed by preaching, disciplined by duty, cursed by custom, and held by habit need a vacation. If you are made of ordinary human stuff and the call comes you will listen. Perhaps you will go. The Great Fisherman would approve. Izaak Walton would agree. Henry Van Dyke would acquiesce and Grover Cleveland would vote aye.

The road is open. If you can find a place where no plane has crashed, where no cars have collided and no dudes have resided, you are lucky.

Get out your rod and your red bandanna, and fling your troubles upon the wind and let time fly. Simon Peter said, "I go a-fishing: and they said we also will go with thee."

Who is a Medical Technologist

The importance of this question to all practicing physicians is emphasized by the following definition:

"A medical technologist is one who, by education and training, is capable of performing, under the supervision of a pathologist or other qualified physician, the various chemical, microscopic, bacteriologic and other laboratory procedures used in the diagnosis, study and treatment of disease."

These functions formerly belonging to physicians alone are now performed by the members of a relatively new profession. Medical technologists organized as the American Society of Medical Technologists registered by the Board of Registry of Medical Technologists of the American Society of Clinical Pathologists. The profession is ancillary to the medical profession and while it has made important diagnostic services more readily available, increasing the physicians competency and conserving his time, it has in no way lessened his responsibility to the patient. Though the technologist carries out the techniques and performs all the tests, the attending physician is responsible to the last detail for every procedure. His protection is dependent upon the qualifications and certified competency of the technologists. Thus it is imperative that all physicians keep these facts in mind. The Hippocratic Oath and the modern Code of Medical Ethics makes this incumbent.

If this is true of all physicians who directly or indirectly make use of the services of medical technologists, how much more important that physicians, medical clinics, clinical laboratories and hospitals employing medical technologists determine the qualifications of all laboratory technicians. Only those who have fully met the high standards of the Board of Registry under the auspices of the American Society of Clinical Pathologists should be considered fully competent. These only are graduates of schools approved by the Council on Medical Education and Hospitals under the American Medical Association. Though "The Registry of Clinical Laboratory Technicians" was discussed in the *Journal of the American Medical Association* March 30, 1940[1], it seems wise to call the situation to the attention of our readers. The proper designation is Medical Technologists (M.T.-A.S.C.P.), the latter indicating registration under the authority of the American Society of Clinical Pathologists.

This Issue of The Journal

For years with cautious conservatism your

1. J.A.M.A. Vol. 114, No. 13, page 1296 (March 30) 1940.

Editorial Board with the help of Miss Mary Lou Crahan, Editorial Assistant, and the cooperation of the Executive Office, has tried to improve the appearance, readibility and usefulness of the *Journal*.

Certain changes having become necessary, the Board in cooperation with representatives of The Transcript Company, Norman, our new publishers, decided to employ 10 point type throughout, and to alter departmental headings conforming to modern trends in good journalism.

Perhaps of greater importance are the plans for more careful preparation of manuscripts, more meticulous editing with accuracy, clarity and brevity ever in mind. The Board bespeaks your criticism and cooperation.

Important Lecture:

From the University of Edinburgh to the University of Oklahoma

On March 22 at four o'clock in the afternoon Dr. Douglas Guthrie of Edinburgh will lecture on the history of the microscope in medicine. His title, "The Pursuit of the Infinitely Small."

In his splendid text on the history of medicine, Doctor Guthrie quotes Mr. Churchill as having said, "The longer you can look back, the further you can look forward." This being the case we should attend this lecture and look back. In so doing we may better understand how the infinitely small may help to explain the appallingly large.

All physicians are invited. The main auditorium in the Medical School Building.

Europe Grand Tour

The California Medical Association announces its first annual Grand Medical Tour of Europe which is open to physicians in all states. The tour, which will be held April 5 to May 5, will include France, England, Italy, Holland, Belgium, Germany and Switzerland. Further information may be obtained from John Hunton, Executive Secretary, California Medical Association, 450 Sutter, San Francisco 8; Calif.

Scientific Articles

Treatment of
DISSEMINATED COCCIDIODOMYCOSIS
with Stilbamidine (Case History)

M. C. GEPHARDT, M. D. and T. J. HANLON, M. D., Muskogee

Previous methods of treatment for systemic infections with coccidioides immitis have been unsatisfactory. The reports on the usefulness of stilbamidine in the treatment of sytemic blastomycosis suggested trial in a case of coccidiodomycosis.[1, 2] Personal communications from Clarence L. Robbins, M. D., of Tucson, Arizona, and John H. Seabury, M. D. of New Orleans, Louisiana, furnished the details for the administration of stilbamidine. The drug was made available through the courtesy of R. C. Pogge, M. D. of Cincinnati, Ohio.

Case Report

A 33-year-old white oil field hand and farmer (L.E.D.) first developed persistent fever from his disease in November, 1950. This was while employed in oil field work near Bakersfield, California. His grandmother died of the disease in 1946 after a short illness. His diagnosis was established in February, 1951, with cervical lymph node biopsy material. The patient was told the diagnosis and was given a poor prognosis. Supportive therapy was started.

He was first seen by one of the authors in June, 1951. By this time there was progressive weight loss. Also, small skin nodules with chronic drainage had developed. These occurred on the right hand, leg, and foot, both cervical areas, and on the left hip. Weakness and fatigability were bothersome. There had been a right eye injury unrelated to the fungus disease.

On this examination the blood pressure was 98/72 with a normal temperature, pulse,

THE AUTHORS

Maurice C. Gephardt M. D. and Thomas Joseph Hanlon, M. D. of Muskogee are joint authors of "Treatment of Disseminated Coccidioidomycosis with Stilbamidine". Doctor Gephardt was graduated from the University of Oklahoma and practiced in Illinois before coming to Oklahoma. Doctor Hanlon is on the staff of the Veterans Administration Hospital in Muskogee.

and respiration. He was a thin, chronically ill appearing white male. Skin lesions were present on tip of nose, right cheek, right shoulder, right hand, and left buttocks. They were violacious in color, crusted, slightly indurated, and non-tender. Two soft masses, 2 cms. in diameter, were present in the scalp. One was just anterior to the vertex and one in the occipital region. They seemed to involve the external table of the calvarium. There was an open wound in the left cervical region at the site of a previous biopsy. In the middle of this wound there was a lymph node about 1 cm. in diameter.

Scrapings from the nose lesion and sputum examination on wet smear showed bodies resembling Coccidioides immitis. Culture of sputum was negative. Gastric washings showed many spherules on wet smear resembling the fungus. Complement fixation tests by the Army Medical Center, Department of Bacteriology, were negative to histoplasma antigens, but positive to Coccidioides antigen to a dilution of 1:1280. Collodion agglutination test for histoplasma antibodies was negative. Pathological examination of the lymph node showed the fungus. (Figure 1)

Roentgen films showed enlarged paratracheal and hilar lymph nodes with an appearance of diffuse fibrosis and infiltration of the lung. Heart shadow was normal. The skull showed multiple, irregular areas of bone destruction with a moth-eaten appearance in the frontal, parietal, and occipital regions. (Figures 2 and 3). Similar areas of bone changes were found in the shaft of the left tibia and fibula and in the right tibia. (Figure 4). These were interpreted as being due to a fungus infection.

After two days in the hospital he returned to his home physician. About two months later a drainage appeared near the top of his head. In July, 1952 he returned because of a throbbing right frontal headache that had been present for one week. No motor incoordination or sensory changes had been noted. There had been anorexia with 10 pounds weight loss in the week before this admission.

Physical examination this time showed a weight of 130 pounds, temperature 99.4° F., pulse 80, and blood pressure 110/70. He appeared chronically ill but was alert, orientated, and cooperative. There was the draining lesion on the vertex of the skull with a serous discharge. The soft nodule in the occipital region was still there. The nose and neck lesions were healed. Cervical, axillary,

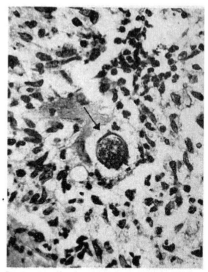

Fig. 1. Magnification 1500X. Section of lymph node obtained June, 1951, showing cell of coccidodes immitis.

epitrochlear, and inguinal lymph nodes were small, shotty, discrete, and non-tender. No localizing neurologic findings were found. Other findings, including no papilledema,

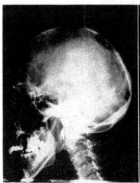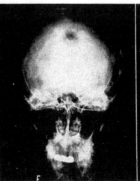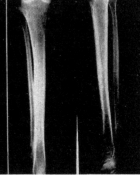

Fig. 2 Left alteral view of the skull shows areas of bone destruction in the posterior, frontal, and parietal regions. Margins of lesions are of "punched out" character with no evidence of bone reaction. June, 1951.

Fig. 3. A PA view of the skull shows areas of bone destruction in the posterior, frontal, and parietal regions to the left of the sagittal suture. Margins of lesions are of "punched out" character with no evidence of bone reaction. June, 1951.

Fig. 4. Multiple small cystic lesions are shown involving the left tibial and fibular cortices. The upper lesion of the tibia in profile on the lateral view demonstrates short margins. The lesion of the lower fibula expands the cortex and is surrounded by a small zone of a reactive bone. Again there is no periosteal reaction.

were unchanged from the previous evaluation.

Urinalysis was normal. Hemogram showed RBC 4.90, hemoglobin 14.5 grams, hematocrit· 48, sedimentation rate of 23 mm/hr (Wintrobe), and WBC of 5,000. Spinal puncture showed a pressure of 14.0 cm. of water. The fluid was cloudy with WBC 1250/cmm (polymorphonuclears 16 per cent and lymphocytes 84 per cent) ; globulin markedly increased; total protein 182 mgm per cent; normal serology and collodial gold; and no growth of fungi on culture. Sputum was negative on wet smear and culture for fungi. Skin test with cocciodin, 1/100 dilution was negative. Roentgenograms at this time · showed no significant change from those the year before except some increase in digital impressions of the skull films suggesting increased intracranial pressure.

Shortly after admission the patient developed persistent nausea and vomiting. A Miller-Abbott tube was passed to administer the desired nutrients and drugs. In a three day period, the nausea and vomiting disappeared. After this the patient's appetite and general condition gradually improved. He was kept on aureomycin hydrochloride for nearly two months until he experienced G.I. distress. The spinal fluid test before discharge showed a WBC of 380/cmm. (polymorphonuclears 56 per cent and lymphocytes 44 per cent), sugar of 25 mgm per cent, marked increase in globulin and total protein of 201 mg per cent. He was discharged September 12, 1952 until stilbamidine could be obtained.

On November 18, 1952, the patient was recalled to the hospital for stilbamidine treatment. Since the previous discharge he had had no new symptoms. He had gained weight to 141½ pounds. The temperature, pulse, and respiration were normal. Blood pressure was 100/70. The lesion on the vertex of the skull was not draining; the depression was still there. Other findings were unchanged from time of previous hospitalization. Urinalysis, Kahn, hemoglobin, hematocrit, and WBC were normal. Sedimentation rate of 25 mm/hr was obtained. Blood chemistries were: NPN 34, serum calcium 9.7, serum phosphorus 3.2, alkaline phosphatase 1.2 units, and total protein 6.6 per

cent. Spinal fluid results were: WBC 400 (12 per cent polymorphonuclears-, 64 per cent lymphocytes, and unidentified cells 24 per cent; total protein 657 mg per cent, collodial gold 5544444444; and Kolmer negative. Bone lesions in the skull, tibia and fibula were unchanged since July 10, 1952. Arms, shoulders, and hands showed no bony abnormalities of significance. Chest film showed progressive clearing of the bilateral miliary lymphadenopathy. All x-ray findings were interpreted as compatible with diagnosis of coccidioidomycosis.

Treatment

To minimize the reported toxic neuropathy due to stilbamidine great care in its preparation and administration were observed.[3,4,5,6] The stilbamidine vial and an intravenous fluid bottle were wrapped in aluminum foil before making the solutions. After dissolving the stilbamidine, the desired amount was diluted in the 200 cc. of physiologic saline in the parenteral fluid bottle. This solution was given intravenously by slow drip in a darkened room. The dosage schedule was 50 mg. the *first* day, 100 mg. the *third* day, 150 mg. the *fifth* day, and on *alternate days* thereafter until 12 *full* doses were given. Total amount of stilbamidine given was 1950 mgm. (1.95 grams) over a 27 day period.

The spinal fluid at time of discharge this time showed WBC 650/cmm. (Lymphocytes 73 per cent, polymorphonuclears 12 per cent, and unidentified cells, 13 per cent) and total protein 680 mg per cent. X-ray films of bones showed no change during the course of treatment. No evidence of sensory changes over trigeminal distribution were apparent.

Return visits on February 4, 1953 and July 10, 1953 interrupted his farming. All sinus tracts had remained healed with residual scarring. Numbness of the lips, bridge of the nose, and malar prominences developed after the February visit. This subsided slowly and by September 10, 1953 there was only slight hypesthesia of the upper lip. The skin lesion between the base of the thumb and index finger of the right hand was still present. No other skin lesions were identified. Believing that this might be a focus of fungi that were not accessible to drug therapy, this was excised.

Microscopic Examination: "The epidermis exhibits a marked hyperkeratosis. Within the dermis there is an active granulomatous inflammatory reaction chacterized by the proliferation of numerous mononuclear inflammatory cells including epitheloid type cells. There are also multinucleated giant cells, many of which are characteristic Langhan's type. Within an occasional one of these giant cells there is a spherule characterisitc of coccidioides immitis."

Spinal puncture nine months after the showed a normal pressure, WBC of 100 lymphocytes, total protein 780 mgm per cent, a marked increase in globulin, collodial gold of 5555555430, and negative serology. Sedimentation rate was 40 mm/hr.

Summary

A case of disseminated coccidioidomycosis which has been under medical observation since November, 1950, is reported. Treatment during that time was supportive until July, 1952, when two months of aureomycin
hydrochloride was given. This was done in a desperate attempt to avert a chronic meningitis due to the fungus. There was clinical improvement but no objective changes. A course of stilbamidine (1.95 grams in 27 days) was given with appropriate precautions approximately two years from the onset of the illness. There is improvement in the spinal fluid WBC but still evidence of persistence of the meningeal invasion 12 months from time of stilbamidine treatment. Further treatment with this drug is indicated and planned.

REFERENCES

1. Schoenbach, E. B., Miller, J. M., Ginsberg, M., and Long, P.: Systemic Blastomycosis Treated with Stilbamidine, J.A.M.A. 146:1317, 1951.

2. Schoenbach, E. B.: The use of Aromatic Diamidines for the Treatment of Systemic Fungal Disease, transactions of the New York Academy of Sciences 14:272, 1952.

3. Sen Gupta, P. C.: Cerebral Lesions in Dogs Following Injections of 4-4'-diamidinostilbene, Transcactions Royal Society of Tropical Medicine and Hygiene, 40:508, 1947.

4. Henry, A. J.: The Instability of Stilbamidine, British Journal of Pharmacology 3:163, 1948.

5. Schoenbach, E. B. and Grenspan, E. M.: The Pharmacology, Mode of Action and Therapeutic Potentialities of Stilbamidine, Pentamidine, Propamidine, and other Aromatic Diamidines. A Review, Medicine 27:345, 1948.

6. Satl, M. H.: Post-Stilbamidine Neuropathy with Reference to the Retention of the Drug in the Body, Annals of Tropical Medicine, 43:4, 1949.

REPORT FROM AMERICAN CANCER SOCIETY

Since the close of World War II, the American Cancer Society has been the pioneer and pace maker in cancer research support in the U. S. In 1946 when the Society made its first large appropriation of $2,500,000 for research, other agencies — both governmental and voluntary — were spending only an additional $500,000. This and ensuing research allocations by the Society stimulated expansion of cancer research support by other agencies, until today the other agencies spend over twice as much annually for cancer research as the Society, even though the Society's allocation has increased every year.

Money for cancer research grants has been allocated, out of contributions obtained during the annual Cancer Crusade of the Society, as follows:

1945	979,047.42
1946	2,503,934.50
1947	2,996,714.44
1948	3,297,973.03
1949	3,471,424.15
1950	3,474,069.23
1951	3,746,591.91
1952	4,109,546.00
1953	4,950,000.00
Total	$29,529,300.68

ANEURYSM of the MITRAL VALVE

SAM N. MUSALLAM, M. D. and MARSH McCALL, M. D.

Even though aneurysms of the valves of the heart have been recognized for a long time, being noted with the first description of malignant endocarditis, they remain rare anatomical findings.

In a review of the literature we have been able to find only three cases of aneurysm[1,2,3] of the mitral valve reported during the last quarter of a century and none in the American literature.

Ogle[4] in 1858 reported a case of aneurysm of the mitral valve and declared that he had observed all together 10 instances of cases of true and false aneurysm of the various valves of the heart which he could find in the "Transactions of the Pathological Society of London."

Osler[5], in his textbook (1908), discussed aneurysms in detail and expressed that in the case of mycotic aneurysm emboli in all probability pass to the vasa vasora and cause weakening of the wall. The intima splits and in this way a small aneurysm is formed. Any artery may be affected. About aneurysm of the valves, he stated that weakness of the tissue of the valve results from erosion, from mycotic ulceration or from softening of an atheromatous focus; that involvement of mitral segment is not so common as the aortic and the anterior valve more frequently than the posterior.

Aschoff[6], in discussing aneurysm of the valves, differentiated between thromboendocarditis simplex and thromboendocarditis septica (ulcerosa). He remarked that while thromboendocarditis simplex usually runs a superficial course, there are cases in thromboendocarditis ulcerosa where the whole valve tissue is destroyed through the effect of micro-organisms. The ulcers in the latter are bigger and more irregular in contrast to changes occurring with thromboendocarditis simplex. By contact extension the muscular walls are affected. The chordae tendineae may be destroyed. Occasionally a whole valve may be separated from the papillary muscle. Thinning of the valvular tissue due to ulceration with thrombi on top causes

THE AUTHORS

Sam N. Musallman, M.D. has recently moved to Oklahoma City from New York City. He was born in Lebanon and received his M.D. from the American University of Beirut. He practiced in Haifa, Palestine before coming to the United States. Marsh McCall, M.D., co-author of "Aneurysm of the Mitral Valve," is attending physician and chief of the adult cardiac clinic of the Beekman-Downtown Hospital, New York City.

protrusion of the valves. The mitral valves protrude mostly towards the auricles and the aortic valves towards the ventricles. These various aneurysms might finally perforate and result in acute insufficiency.

Thus it seems easy to understand why an aneurysm of a heart valve develops if one discovers any of the above mentioned causes and considers the dynamics of the heart in the development of such an aneurysm. But in our case no such cause could be detected. The questionable etiology, the rarity of this pathological problem and the size of the aneurysm, make our case worthy of being reported.

We have collected seven mitral aneurysms described in the literature since 1871, [1,2,3,7,8,9,10] and compared them with our patient. The data are shown in Table I.

Report of Case

I.L.W #55998, a 49-year-old Chinese female, born in the United States, was admitted July 21, 1951 to Beekman-Downtown Hospital at 11:30 P.M. because of unconsciouness of four hours duration. The husband stated that she had had "heart disease" since childhood. Edema of the legs was noted six months prior to admission and one or two injections of a mercurial diuretic had been administered weekly. She had no history of rheumatic fever, luetic infection or diphtheria. Family and personal history were otherwise irrelevant.

Physical examination revealed a poorly developed and undernourished Chinese fe-

TABLE 1: Summary of data of seven cases of mitral aneurysm from the literature as compared with data from our case.

AUTHOR	SEX	AGE	RHEUMATIC HISTORY	CARDIAC ENLARGE.	RHYTHM	MURMURS	ACUTE OR MAL. ENDO-CARDITIS	VEGETATIONS	ANEURYSM Size	ANEURYSM Location	ANEURYSM Perforation
Simon 1871	M	16	—	+	RSR	—	+	Mitral Valve	Pea	Aortic Cusp (Ant. Val.)	+
Bouilly 1872	M	58	.....	.....	RSR	Systolic Apical	.....	.....	Hazel Nut	Right (Ant.)	+
Lepine 1873	M	46	?	+	RSR	Systolic Apical	+	Mitral Valve	5-6 M.M.+	Ant. Cusp & Aortic Valve	+
Peyrot 1874	M	20	——	—	RSR	Systolic	+	...	Big Pea	Free Edge ?Mitral	+
Whimster 1928	F	15	+	+	RSR	Systolic Apical Sys. & Pre. Sys. Aortic	+	Aortic & Mitral Valves	¼"	Aortic Cusp (Ant.)	+
Pichon & Bidou 1932	F	20	.....	?	RSR	Diastolic Apical Double Aortic	+	Aortic & Mitral Valves	Filbert	Large Leaflet (Ant.)	+
Soulie & Porge 1937	M	37	+	+	Sinus Tachy.	Double Aortic Diastolic Sternal Edge	+	Aortic & Mitral Val. Muriform	Large Marble	Large Leaflet (Ant.)	+
McCall & Musallam 1953	F	49	.....	+-+	Auric. Fib.	Double Apical	——	.....	Walnut	Left Cusp (Post)	+

male in deep coma with Grade III cyanosis. Temperature 96° F (rectal); pulse 46 per minute, irregular. Skin was cold and moist. Both pupils were contracted and equal. The neck was soft with no adenopathy. Chest was emaciated and narrowed; lungs revealed moist rales. Heart was enlarged to right and left of sternum; sounds were of poor quality; rhythm was totally irregular with apex rate about 80 per minute. Diastolic and systolic murmurs were heard over the apex. Blood pressure was unobtainable. Abdomen was soft, liver and spleen were not palpable. There was Grade II edema of both a r m s and legs. An electrocardiogram taken on admission (Fig. 1) revealed r i g h t axis deviation, vertical electrical position of heart with extreme clockwise rotation, atrial fibrillation and multifocal ventricular extrasystoles. Unfortunately, the patient expired a short while after admission. Thus further studies, chest x-ray and stethographic tracings could not be done. Autopsy was performed 10 hours after death.

Autopsy Findings (Gross protocol)

Body of a poorly developed, undernourished Chinese woman, 49-year-old; height 5'4"; weight 90-95 lbs. Pupils were round and dilated equally. No evidence of external injury or violence. No adenopathy. Brownish discoloration on both lower extremities.

Abdomen: No free fluid. No pathology

in G.I. tract, gallbladder and ducts, liver and spleen.

Thorax: 300 cc of clear fluid in the right chest; no adhesions. There was a thrombosis in branch of the right pulmonary artery with collapse of the right middle lobe. Other parts of the lungs were fully crepitant.

Heart: the apex was at the sixth intercostal space in the anterior axillary line. There was a generalized enlargement of all chambers, mainly the auricles. When the left auricle was cut open to expose the mitral ring, a soft smooth aneurysmal dilatation of the left mitral leaflet, the size of a walnut, was readily seen filling the mitral ring (Fig. 2). The convex surface of this mass faced the auricular cavity; its concave surface, which can easily hold a walnut, faced the ventricular cavity. Chordae tendineae were attached to the edge of this dilated valve. When inspected from the ventricular cavity it resembled a "parachute". No thrombus or blood was found in it. The surfaces were smooth and there was a small rent 6 to 7 mm. at the apex of this dilated valve flap. The edges of this rent were ragged. It seemed to be a point of rupture that occurred antemortem. There were no vegetations or evidence of scarring macroscopically. The mitral ring was normal, so was the other mitral leaflet. The aortic

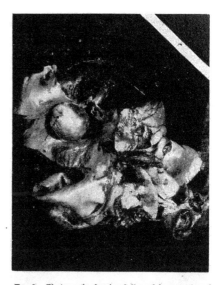

FIG. 2: Photograph showing left auricle opened and partly excised to expose the aneurysm, which is seen bulging into the auricular cavity and practically filling the mitral ring. Left ventricle is cut open. Note thick wall and enormous enlargement of left auricle. Arrow points to perforation at apex of aneurysm.

ring, valve cusps and aorta seemed normal. There were no vegetations, ulcerations or atheromatous changes anywhere. The coronaries were wide and patent.

Nothing grossly abnormal was found in the liver, spleen, pancreas and suprarenals. There were no infarcts. The kidneys revealed multiple small cysts, but capsules stripped easily. No infarcts were seen grossly.

Uterus: Was infantile and ovaries atrophied.

Head: Was restricted.

Microscopic
(Description by Dr. Gregory Brown)

Left Mitral Leaflet: Section shows a complete "parachute" (aneurysm of leaflet). The point of rupture shows the ragged and frayed edges of the cusp as in a mechanical tear. The essential changes in the whole flap are those of thickening and fibrosis. The leaflet consisted of a plain hyalinized fibrous tissue without calcium. Cellularity beyond scattered fibrocytes is poor. This vas-

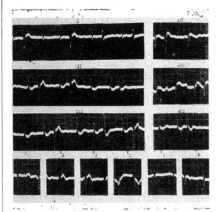

FIG. 1: Twelve lead electrocardiogram showing right axis deviation, vertical electrical position of the heart with extreme clockwise rotation, atrial fibrillation and multifocal ventricular extrasystoles.

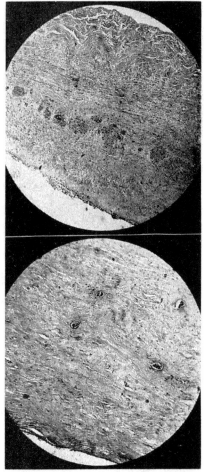

FIG. 3: Microphotograph of a section through left mitral leaflet (aneurysm). Plain hyalinized fibrous tissue accounts for thickening. The "vascular residua" of healing, i. e., vessels of capillary caliber are seen to advantage.

FIG. 4: Microphotograph of a section through the right mitral leaflet which shows the same thickening by hyalinized connective tissue. The small, thick walled arterioles of musculo-elastic type probably represent stigmata of R.F. (?), i.e., signs of healed rheumatic disease.

cularity is quite marked at the base. Here the vessels are of course larger and uniformly show fibrotic thickening which in-

volves all layers. Myocardium fanwise from the ring is likewise insidiously streaked with fibrous tissue, i.e. a healed lesion. Even further out small serving vessels in the myocardium are thickened and often show peri-adventitial fibrotic changes (Fig. 3).

Right Mitral Leaflet: Changes strikingly similar to the left leaflet are found in this section. The same thickening and hyalinized connective tissue was found. There is a random scattering in the leaflet of small thick walled arterioles of the musculo-elastic type. Here too, at the base, arteries of larger type show the distortion, adventitial and peri-adventitial scarring (Fig. 4).

Papillary Muscle: Section of a stout, squat and thickened papillary muscle to which the mitral leaflet was attached shows the same vascular changes as described above. Medium sized and smaller vessels show the same eccentric intimal fibrotic thickening and the same peri-adventitial hyalinized fibrous tissue. There were no typical Aschoff's bodies and none show the Aschoff's cells of the earlier lesions. All are residua of former acute changes.

Left Auricle: Section of the left auricle shows similar changes restricted to the vascular fields.

Branch of Pulmonary Artery: Section shows the thrombus described in the gross. It is practically a ball plug and leaves little of the lumen patent. It has firm anchorage to the wall and is now being invaded by a trajectory of small capillaries and accompanying fibroblasts. Parenchyma generally shows the effects of long standing stasis in the lesser circuit (Pulmonary) i.e. thickening, beading of alveolar walls and heart failure cells in the sacs.

Discussion

We have presented a case of aneurysm of the left mitral leaflet. As compared with seven cases collected from the literature our case seems to differ from the others in the following points:

1. Our aneurysm seems to be the largest yet described.

2. All other cases except that of Bouilly (1872) reported aneurysm secondary to acute or malignant endocarditis. There was

no evidence of such endocarditis in this patient.

3. All previous cases except that of Peyrot, who did not mention which valve was affected, were on the right (anterior or aortic) cusp. Ours was on the left.

4. All other reported aneurysms were strictly affecting a part of the valve, Peyrot's, for example, the free edge. Our case may well be described as aneurysmal valve rather than aneurysm of the valve, as the whole valve was dilated to form the aneurysm.

5. Our aneurysm was the size of a walnut bulging into the mitral ring, causing full stenotic effect in life with its auscultatory signs and electrocardiographic changes. The signs of mitral insufficiency can be explained partly by the fact that the mitral leaflets could not close properly due to the aneurysm and partly by the rupture of the latter at its apex.

6. We have failed to demonstrate any evidence of malignant endocarditis, ulcerations or atheromatous plaques in any part of the heart to act as a cause of the aneurysm.

Summary

A patient with aneurysm of the mitral valve has been presented. The etiology could be congenital weakness of the valve, possibly due to congenital endocarditis which is known to occur[11]. An endocarditis in infancy or early childhood, or an old arrested rheumatic fever could not be definitely excluded.

REFERENCES

1. Whimster, W. S.: A case of aneurysm of the mitral cusp. Lancet, 2:653 (September 29, 1928).
2. Pichon, E. and Bidou, S.: Anevrysme cardio-cardiaque sur la grande mitrale. Archives des maladies du coeur, des vaisseaux et du sang, 25:296 (May 1932).
3. Soulie, P and Porge, J.: Anevrysme de la valvule mitrale au cours d'une endocardite maligne. Archives des maladies du coeur, des vaisseaux et du sang, 30:491 (July 1937).
4. Ogle, J. W.: True and false aneurysmal pouching of the cardiac valves. Trans. of the Path. Society of London IX, PP 117, 123 (February 1858).
5. Osler, W.: Modern Medicine, Vol. IV (1908).
6. Aschoff, L.: Pathologische Anatomie, Vol. II, PP 26-29 (1923).
7. Simon, T.: Ein fall von aneurysma der mitral klappe. Berlin, Klin. Woschenschr. 37 (1871).
8. Bouilly, M.: Anevrysme de la valvule Mitrale; Souffle d'insuffisance. Bulletin de la Societe anatomiquo de Paris, 47:287 (1872).
9. Lepine, R.: Endocardite ulcereuse; anevrysmes valvulaires; Atherome aortique: Bulletin de la Societe anatomique de Paris; 43:411 (1873).
10. Peyrot, M.: Endocardite aigue; Anevrysme de la valvule mitrale Bulletin de la Societe anatomique de Paris, 49:260 (1874).
11. White, P. D.: Heart Disease, 4th Ed: 325 (1951).

ADMITTING PATIENTS TO CEREBRAL PALSY INSTITUTE

Physicians desiring to admit patients to the Cerebral Palsy Institute at Norman are reminded that an appointment must be made for the child at the diagnostic clinic monthly at Crippled Children's Hospital, Oklahoma City. Appointments may be made by writing the Oklahoma Commission for Crippled Children, 402 Baptist Bldg., Oklahoma City. Letters should give the child's name and age, parents' name and address, and state whether or not the child has ever been a patient at Crippled Children's Hospital or ever been seen in a clinic there or throughout the state sponsored by the Crippled Children's Commission. If so, the type clinic it was, and the identification number given the child at that time should be included in the letter. Following examination at Crippled Children's Hospital, the recommendation is made to the Crippled Children's Commission.

The following training facilities are available at the Cerebral Palsy Institute:

(1) Physical Therapy — training of large muscle groups of the body, usually associated with ambulation training.

(2) Occupational Therapy — training of the smaller muscle groups of the body, usually associated with the upper extremities-self help activities such as feeding, dressing, etc.

(3) Speech Therapy — training to initiate speech where there is none, improve enuciation, pronunciation, etc.

(4) Academic Schooling — for the benefit of those children who have been in school in the home community and in the case of those who have not had the advantage of school, evaluation of the children for possible school work.

Clinical Pathologic Conference

HOWARD C. HOPPS, M. D. and STEARLEY P. HARRISON, M. D.

DOCTOR HOPPS: Dr. Harrison will discuss the clinical aspects of our case this afternoon. The factual data presented to him is identical to that which has been provided to each of you in mimeographed form and no pertinent clinical information, available from the patient's chart, has been withheld. The case does pose an unusually difficult diagnostic problem ‑with many complexities. Our first problem is to unravel these as best we can from the clinical standpoint, then to review the autopsy findings and see to what extent we can make a clinical pathologic correlation.

Protocol

Patient: 52 year white male.

Chief Complaints: 1) Pain in RUQ of abdomen

2) Nausea

3) Cough

Present Illness: The patient was first seen in University Hospitals in the OPD some 10 months before admission. At this time he stated that he had not been well for nine years having had moderate shortness of breath and easy fatigability. For the past two or three years there had been definite exertional dyspnea together with slight orthopnea and pedal edema occurring in late afternoon. During these two years he also had intermittent "pain and soreness" in the right upper abdominal quadrant. This dull pain occurred one to three times daily and was not associated with meals or exercise. He denied food intolerances. His bowel habits were regular. He had noticed bright red blood in his stools for several years—this he attributed to "piles". During the past two years he had lost 30 pounds in weight. At the time of this first OPD visit his blood pressure was

Presented by the Departments of Pathology and Medicine, The University of Oklahoma School of Medicine.

recorded as 133/88. There were a few medium moist rales scattered over both lung fields. The heart was normal to percussion and auscultation. The liver extended six fingerbreadths below the costal margin in the right midclavicular line; it was moderately tender. At that time urinalysis revealed 2+ glycosuria. He was given an appointment to return in one week for further studies. However, he did not return until nine months later (one month before admission). At his second OPD visit he gave a history essentially similar to that recorded previously. During the intervening nine months all of his symptoms had gradually increased. He had become even weaker and had lost more weight (exact amount not known). He had begun to notice a fullness in the RUQ of the abdomen. Physical examination at that time showed that the lung fields were clear to percussion and auscultation. His liver had further enlarged and extended to the umbilicus in the midline. There was 1+ pitting edema of the feet and ankles. The urine contained a trace of glucose. A chest x-ray at this time was reported: "Heart is of normal size, shape and position. Costophrenic angles are free. An area of fibrosis involves the upper half of the right lung field. Remaining lung fields are clear. X-ray findings would suggest a minimal tuberculosis, activity questionable. Sputum studies are indicated and another film in one month." He was scheduled for several laboratory studies, but again failed to keep his appointments.

One month later he returned to the emergency room in extremis. He was unable to give a history, but his wife stated that 10 days previously the pain in the RUQ had rather suddenly become much worse. He was much more dyspneic and within a day or two began to have a persistent cough productive of small amounts of sputum (character not known). He also had been

64

nauseated frequently and had vomited several times during the last two or three days. He had eaten nothing for the past week. The day before admission he had become irrational.

Past History: He had drunk whiskey rather heavily during the depression but not in recent years.

Family History: No history of diabetes, tuberculosis or other hereditary or familial diseases.

Physical Examination: T. 102.4° (R), P. 130, R. 40, BP 60/?. The patient was well developed, rather poorly nourished and very acutely ill. The skin was cold and clammy. Lips and nail beds appeared dusky. There were a few spider hemangiomata scattered over the chest and shoulders. He responded to vigorous stimuli but talked irrationally. There was a pronounced increase in the anterior-posterior diameter of the chest. Respiratory excursions were unequal with very little expansion of the right side. There was dullness to percussion over the entire right posterior lung field (most marked in basilar regions) with associated marked increase in tactile fremitus. Numerous fine and medium moist rales were heard over the entire right chest and there were occasional rhonchi. The percussion note of left chest was normal, and there were a few scattered, basilar, fine, moist rales here. The trachea was in the midline. Heart sounds were distant and largely obscured by loud respiratory sounds. The heart was of normal size to percussion. The abdomen was scaphoid. There was marked guarding by the patient, thus hampering examination. In the epigastrium and RUQ there was tenderness to deep pressure and questionable rebound tenderness. An ill defined epigastric mass was palpable and this was felt to be continuous with liver margin which extended just below the level of the umbilicus in the right midclavicular line. Rectal examination was negative. A cursory neurological survey was reported as within normal limits.

Laboratory Data: Urine examination for glucose and acetone bodies was negative. The hematrocrit was 41 per cent. Hb. was 12 gm. per cent with 4.3 m. RBC's/cu.mm. Leukocytes numbered 10,750/cu.mm. with 89 per cent neutrophils (40 per cent stab

forms), 10 per cent lymphocytes and 1 per cent monocytes. The sedimentation rate was 48.5 mm. in one hour. NPN was 158 mg. per cent. A fasting blood sugar was 317 mg. per cent. Serum amylase was 39 mg. per cent. The CO_2 combining power was 31.36 vol. per cent. A blood Mazzini done at the first OPD visit was negative. An electrocardiogram disclosed auricular fibrillation with a rapid ventricular rate (135 per min.) There was "no definite evidence of myocardial infarction."

Clinical Courses: The patient was given nasal oxygen, demerol and penicillin (100,-000 u.q.4 h.). During the first 12 hours he received 1500 cc. plasma and 500 cc. whole blood, together with 2000 cc. of other parenteral fluids. However, his blood pressure never rose over 74/52 and gradually he became more cyanotic. Gastric suction was started with an initial recovery of 1500 cc. of thick green fluid. The patient went into coma. Thirty units of regular insulin I.V. failed to affect any change. He was then given 0.6 mg. and 0.4 mg. of digitoxin I.V. six hours apart. Despite all efforts his course was rapidly downhill and he died 20 hours after admission.

Clinical Diagnosis

DOCTOR HARRISON: As is so often the case the first lesson to be learned here concerns the importance of a good history in evaluating a difficult diagnostic problem such as this one. Many times it's the little details which are crucial not a simple statement such as, bowel habits were regular with the exception of one or two or three occasional appearances of red blood in the stool. In this case questioning was dropped at this point — that was just the place where it should have started.

This patient, first seen at the age of 52, presented himself with some very commonplace and apparently inconsequential symptoms. The most important thing is the fact that the patient dated his symptoms back nine or 10 years — to the age of about 41 years. At that time something caused him to be more easily fatigable and short of breath. Those, as I say, are commonplace symptoms, but they do suggest a few possibilities, e.g. early cirrhosis, early heart disease, some chronic fibrosing pulmonary disorder, or perhaps severe anemia. Then we jump seven or eight years to the next significant statement, that for the past two or three years there had been exertional dyspnea with orthopnea and pedal edema. At this time he would be 49 or 50 years of age. Especially the orthopnea turns our attention again to some cardiac disorder. The intermittent pain and soreness two or three times a day in the RUQ of the abdomen, not related to anything in particular, would also fit into the pattern of congestive heart failure. Many times patients with congestive failure will have tenderness in the RUQ, and sometimes they describe this as pain. This complaint could also fit with cirrhosis. We find that the bowel habits were regular, but that the patient had had some red blood in the stools, assumed to be from hemorrhoids. Since hemorrhoidal bleeding may be a manifestation of increased portal pressure, this brings up the question of cirrhosis again. We must presume the statement of regular bowel habits to exclude diarrhea, tenesmus, the presence of pus or mucus or any other significant change which might reflect an intestinal lesion accounting for this bleeding. At least tentatively we'll have to accept hemorrhoids as the most likely source of blood in the stool.

At this point we note a statement that there had been a 30 pound weight loss in two years; this we certainly must bear in mind. It is stated that the liver was tender and enlarged, the margin extending six fingers below the right costal margin. That this hepatic enlargement might be from congestive failure is not a reasonable supposition when we consider that the patient had a normal blood pressure and that the heart was normal to physical examination. At about this point in the patient's course first mention is made of glycosuria—2+ sugar in a single urine specimen. Presumably further studies were planned to continue the investigation, but the patient did not keep his appointment and was not seen again for nine months. His weight loss had continued and he had begun to be aware of his enlarged liver from a feeling of fullness and discomfort in his RUQ. He did have one plus edema of his feet and ankles. Again a urine specimen contained a trace of glucose.

Physical examination of his chest was negative and the heart shadow was normal on x-ray. There was an area of fibrosis found in the right upper lung field, suggestive of tuberculosis. Appropriate follow-up studies were recommended but again the patient failed to keep his appointment and again we are left up in the air. It was one month later that he was admitted to the hospital in extremis. Ten days before this admission there occurred a rather sudden increase in the abdominal pain, and I'm inclined to believe that this was severe pain. Then he became dyspneic, and within a day or two began to have a persistent cough, (That's the first mention we have of that) and some nausea with vomiting. For the two or three days immediately before he was admitted he hadn't eaten anything. He became irrational, semi-comatose, and was brought to the hospital. This brings to mind again diabetes, and I should have mentioned before, in regard to the positive urine sugar tests, that diabetes can produce an enlarged liver and can, of course, cause weight loss. Uncontrolled diabetes can give a very disturbed general metabolic picture. There is a great deal to be desired in the history that is not here if we are to consider diabetes as playing a major role in this man's disease. At the time of last admission rectal temperature was 102.4°, pulse 130, presumably regular, respiration 40, and BP 60/?. The skin was cold and clammy and there was some cyanosis. A few scattered spider hemangiomata were described which were not mentioned before. Respiratory excursions were unequal, with very little expansion on the right side. There was dullness to percussion, most marked in the basilar regions and marked increase in tactile fremitus. Rales were present in both lungs, more noticeable in the right. We know that this dullness to percussion is not from pleural effusion since we have increased tactile fremitus and we assume that these findings indicate pneumonia. The heart was normal in size to percussion. An electrocardiogram revealed auricular fibrillation at a rate so rapid that it might not have been easy to detect by physical examination. I don't think that this is of major consequence, but rather a reflex disturbance, — not arising from primary heart disease.

Back to the physical examination, it's often a problem to learn much from palpating the abdomen of a comatose or semi-comatose individual. There was marked guarding and a questionable mass in the epigastrium, assumed to be part of the liver, or at least continuous with the markedly enlarged liver.

Turning to the laboratory data it's rather surprising that, after the illness which has been described to us, the patient has a 4.3 million red count, a hematocrit of 41 per cent, and 12 gm. per cent Hb. Although his white count was but questionably elevated he had an increased percentage of neutrophils, 40 per cent of which were stabs. Certainly this shift in white count is additional evidence of an active pyogenic process, to go along with fever and findings of pneumonia. The NPN was 158 mg. per cent. We have had no previous report of proteinuria casts, etc. — nothing to suggest previous kidney disease, but here now is evidence of uremia in this man who has been in a state of profound shock for from seven to 10 days. Urinalysis did not reveal sugar or acetone. Serum amylase was 39 mg. per cent which is quite low, a value that we might expect to see in late pancreatitis where extensive pancreatic destruction had occurred. Additional evidence of pancreatic insufficiency is found in the several instances of glycosuria which would indicate some degree of diabetes for nearly a year. During his last admission the patient's blood sugar was 317 mg. per cent. During this short, terminal hospitalization efforts were made to effect some change in the very low blood pressure. Transfusions with whole blood and plasma, together with other fluids, 4,000 cc's in approximately 12 hours, failed to have much effect. Neither did insulin intravenously nor digitoxin.

To summarize the pertinent findings in this individual, we have evidence of some liver disturbance without jaundice at any time, without ascites, and without much indigestion. We have evidence of pancreatic insufficiency — we have evidence of pulmonary disease, both chronic (by x-ray) and acute (terminal). We have at least terminal renal insufficiency without sufficient information to be sure that this was not an exacerbation of some chronic disease.

However, I believe that his terminal shock state can explain the elevated NPN. We have very suggestive evidence that some acute abdominal process provoked the terminal events, an acute abdominal crisis such as may occur in pancreatitis. As a matter of fact, this terminal picture includes all of the essential features for a diagnosis of pancreatitis. We might assume here that the patient's recurrent pain was from the pancreas, although admittedly somewhat atypical in character. With a very large liver, persistently enlarged from the vary earliest observation of the case, one would be justified in giving consideration to a primary neoplasm of the liver, but as we have remarked, there was no ascites — not even at the time of death. He had no findings which would be strong evidence of portal hypertension and he certainly had plenty of time to develop such changes. At no time is mention made of the spleen in this case, so we can infer that at least marked splenomegaly was not a feature. His blood picture, particularly his lack of anemia, seems to me additional evidence against neoplastic disease of the liver. If we assume that the patient had tuberculosis of the lung, which I'm inclined to do, we must consider the possibility of a large tuberculous process involving the liver. This is rare and I don't believe that this was the cause of hepatic enlargement.

Can we relate these findings to a single major disease? This is what I shall try to do. For my first choice I'm going to consider pulmonary tuberculosis with secondary amyloidosis involving principally the liver, infiltrating and enlarging it to produce so-called lardaceous liver, with involvement also of the pancreas and probably the spleen and kidneys. I believe that an acute intraabdominal crisis, similar to acute pancreatitis, with peritonitis and ileus was the terminal event and was the cause of shock. Finally, of course, terminal pneumonia complicated the picture.

Clinical Discussion

QUESTION: Could one consider hemochromatosis without bronzed pigmentation of the skin, and if so, would this fit the picture?

DOCTOR HARRISON: I think this is worth considering. It would certainly help to explain this atypical diabetes, and would go along with the other findings too.

QUESTION: Could the terminal abdominal episode be secondary to thrombosis of portal vein?

DOCTOR HARRISON: I doubt it. Our history is not entirely adequate but I'm inclined to think that the abdominal episode happened very quickly, too precipitously to be explained by vascular occlusion. Also, he lived for 10 days after this episode during which time we would have expected somewhat different signs and symptoms to have developed.

Pathologic Findings

DOCTOR HOPPS: Doctor Harrison has done a very skillful job in resolving this problem. He has concluded that the patient had some condition which lasted for a long time and which involved the pancreas to produce considerable pancreatic deficiency and which involved also the liver. He mentions both amyloidosis and hemochromatosis as possibilities. This man had hemochromatosis, which had produced cirrhosis of the liver and had also lead to much damage of the pancreas. This latter was reflected in a rather characteristic type of diabetes — a form notoriously difficult to control. The question was raised about bronzing of the skin. In most of the textbooks the situation is wrongly stated. The inference is given that bronze diabetes is a synonym for hemochromatosis. If one evaluates the cases of hemochromatosis that have been described in the literature to find which of these patients had clinical diabetes and which of them also had recognizable bronzing of the skin, one finds that this particular combination of signs and symptoms occurs in considerably less than half of patients with hemochromatosis. So "bronzed diabetes", representing a patient with a complexion like an Indian and outspoken diabetes, is found in the minority of those with hemochromatosis.

At the time of autopsy we could see no evidence of bronzed discoloration of the skin. When the abdominal cavity was opened the liver was found to extend 12 cm. below the costal margin in the right mid-clavicular line. There was no excess of fluid in the abdominal cavity and no evidence of peritonitis or other inflamatory process. The pleural cavity contained some fibrous adhesions in the left apex that could well have been the result of old tuberculosis. There was no evidence of active tuberculosis. The right pleural cavity was completely obliterated by easily separable fibrinous adhesions. This right lung did not collapse at all. It weighed 1960 gm. and was very dense. It presented the typical picture of red to gray hepatization and there was an area of beginning suppuration. Cultures made from this obvious lobar pneumonia revealed *Klebsiella pneumoniae* (Friedlander's bacillus). That's a very serious condition, as you know. It carries a high mortality rate, a very high mortality — especially if it isn't recognized and treated. Friedlander's lobar pneumonia, with suppuration, can easily account for abdominal manifestations. As in this case, intestinal obstruction often is a medical problem, in terms of being a reflex paralytic ileus. You might think that this lobar pneumonia was a rather peculiar complication, but it is not; it fits in with the diagnosis of hemochromatosis. Hemochromatosis, as you know is an inborn error of iron metabolism in which an iron-containing pigment, predominantly hemosiderin, piles up in great amounts not only in reticuloendothelial cells, but in epithelial cells too, especially the parenchymal cells of the liver and pancreas, setting up a low grade chronic inflammatory reaction which characteristically leads to a peculiar pigmentary cirrhosis and atrophy with interstitial fibrosis of the pancreas. It affects the reticuloendothelial system and the function of many other organs too. It certainly causes decreased resistance to infectious disease and persons with hemochromatosis frequently succumb to some infectious disease that is a little out of the ordinary — infections that are often produced by organisms which are not highly pathogenic for normal persons. The spleen was enlarged to 450 gm., which is not quite large enough to lead to ready palpation. The liver weighed 2640 gm., which is nearly twice normal. There was an increased resistance to sectioning and both capsular and cut surfaces gave a pebble-grained appearance which grossly indicated uni-lobular cirrhosis. The kidneys were considerably enlarged, weighing 300 and 270 gm. respectively, and there was marked parenchymatous degeneration. I agree with Doctor Harrison that the azotemia was probably pre-renal and related to hypotension. These were the main findings except for the heart. The heart weighed 400 gm., representing slight hypertrophy. There were rather marked changes here in terms of parenchymatous degeneration, i.e. degenerative changes of muscle fibers. Fat stains of the cardiac muscle revealed a very marked degree of fatty change within the individual muscle fibers. These changes would explain the terminal myocardial failure and hypotension, on a toxic basis and would also explain auricular fibrillation.

Our final pathologic diagnosis was:

Hemochromatosis with marked involvement of liver, producing cirrhosis, and pancreas, producing diabetes mellitus

Lobar pneumonia, right (*K. penumoniae*) with early abscess formation and with fibrinous pleuritis and pericarditis

Septic splenitis, acute

Parenchymatous degeneration of kidneys, marked

Fatty change of myocardium, marked.

On TV Programs

Faculty members of the University of Oklahoma School of Medicine have been participating in a series of TV programs on two Oklahoma City television stations.

Presented by the Oklahoma Medical Research Foundation, one series of programs is televised on WKY-TV at 2:30 p.m. Sunday.

A series of programs on Family and Child Health is televised on KWTV from 11:45 to 12:00 noon on Wednesdays.

Elected To Fraternity

The following faculty members and students at the University of Oklahoma School of Medicine have been elected to membership of the Alpha chapter of Alpha Omega Alpha, honorary medical fraternity:

Loyal Lee Conrad, M. D., Assistant Professor of Research Medicine; Onis G. Hazel, M. D., Clinical Professor of Dermatology and Syphilology; William G. Rogers, M. D., clinical Professor of Gynecology; Harry Wilkins, M. D., Professor of Surgery; and Robert N. Barnes, Shelby D. Barnes, William Hathaway, John W. Johnson Jr., and William Tex Stone, all senior medical students.

Have You Heard?

NEW OFFICERS of the Oklahoma Academy of General Practice elected at the annual meeting in February are: President-elect, Earl Lusk, M. D., Tulsa; Vice-President, Roy Anderson, M. D., Cordell; Secretary-Treasurer, Elmer Ridgeway, Jr., M. D., Oklahoma City (re-elected); Director, Mark Holcomb, M. D., Enid; Delegate to the American Academy of General Practice, Malcom Phelps, M. D., El Reno (re-elected); and Alternate, E. A. McGrew, M. D., Beaver. E. T. Cook, M. D., Anadarko, is serving as President.

J. E. BROOKSHIRE, M. D., Tulsa, was recently pictured on the cover of Akdar Shrine News as a Shriner of more than 50 years. He is believed to have been active in the Shrine longer than any member in Akdar.

LEROY LONG, M. D., Oklahoma City, has endowed an annual award for the freshman medical student with the highest rating in anatomy. The student will receive the latest edition of Callander's "Surgical Anatomy".

WARREN B. POOLE, M. D., has recently moved from Oklahoma City to Lubbock, Texas. His address is 3020 34th St., Lubbock.

Association. Activities

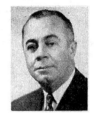

PRESIDENT'S LETTER

The 83rd Congress is now in session. It becomes the duty of the American doctor to again acquaint himself with bills introduced concerning the health and welfare of the people of this nation.

The President-Elect, Doctor Walter B. Martin, a member of the Board of Trustees of the American Medical Association, was called upon to make a statement for American medicine to the Committee on Interstate and Foreign Commerce of the House of Representatives. Doctor Martin made a very complete statement covering the efforts of medicine to furnish better and more complete medical care of the sick. He pointed out the progress of our educational facilities and the aid of organized medicine to research. This support has produced the best health care in the world. This statement will appear in the *Journal of the American Medical Association* in the very near future. I recommend that everyone read it carefully, because of the vast amount of factual material that is so vital to our understanding of the subject. It will help us to give intelligent answers to the inquiring public.

In spite of the organized and widespread efforts of the profession, there appears to be need for improvement. The man in the street is still clamoring for what is apparently something not available to him at this time. This demand is evidenced by the new bills that have been introduced. There are requests for more complete coverage by health insurance companies and more federal aid to the needy—for increasing the Social Security benefits, even to include the physician—assistance is asked for dependents of military personnel, to rehabilitate the handicapped, to increase veterans care, and to further aid families afflicted by catastrophic illnesses. More appropriations are asked for medical schools and for scholarships to aid medical students. These bills all call for Federal spending at a national level for problems that could be more economically and efficiently handled at a local level.

Six Regional Conferences on Legislation have been held by the A.M.A. at strategic points over the United States in the past two months. These conferences were sponsored by the Chicago office to study current legislation and to discuss these important subjects so that a general consensus of opinion could be obtained by the Legislative Committee. These conferences were well attended and were extremely enlightning, both to the delegates and to members of the National Legislative Committee. It made possible a more intelligent and democratic viewpoint of our program. It behooves us to keep informed in regard to the progress of this legislation so that we may furnish convincing answers to the public and to consult with our members of Congress in their thinking on these important bills of health and legislation.

Sincerely yours,

John E McDonald M.D.

President

Clinical Results* with Banthīne® Bromide

(Brand of Methantheline Bromide)

22 Published Reports Covering Treatment of 1443 Peptic Ulcer Patients with Banthine

Comprising the reports published in the literature to date which give specific facts and figures of the results of treatment

AUTHORS	No. of Patients	Chronic Resistant to Other Therapy	TYPES OF ULCERS				RELIEF OF SYMPTOMS (Chiefly Pain)				Surgery or Complications	Side Effects Requiring Discontinuance of Drug	EVIDENCE OF HEALING			
			Duodenal	Jejunal	Stomal	Gastric	Good	Fair	Poor	No Report			Complete	Moderate	None	No Report
Grimson, Lyons, Reeves	100	100	93	7			80	11	4		5		42		19	29
Friedman	15	15	14			1	5		4	6¹			2			13
Bachgaard, Nielsen, Bang, Gravlund, Tobiassen	26	26	21			5	16	4	6				8	6	12	
McHardy, Browne, Edwards, March, Ward	162		162				136	12	11		1	1	14	9	7	129
Segal, Friedman, Watson	34	34	34				14	13			7	2	5		8	14
Brown, Collins	117	99	117				97	7	8		5	8	55	9	8	40
Asher	77		65		7	5	52	9	16			16		9	21	47
Rodriguez de la Vega, Reyes Diaz	5	2	5				4		1					3	2	
Winkelstein	116	116	102	8		6	102		14				53		18	45
Hall, Hornisher, Weeks	18	18	18				11		1	6¹			18			
Maier, Meili	38	38	24			14¹	27	7	4¹				10	2	5	21
Meyer, Jarman	25	18	25				21		4							25
Poth, Fromm	37	37	37				33	3	1				33	3	1	
Plummer, Burke, Williams	41	41	41				36		5				36		3	
McDonough, O'Neil	104	100	104				63	10	31			11	4		11	89
Broders	60	60	56		1	1	35	19	6				10	1	49	
Leggerton, Texter, Ruffin	11		11				11									11
Holouben, Hulzubeh, Langford	76	69	76				35	27	10		4	10	26		10	36
Ogburn	42		39	2		1	42									42
Shapiro	48	48	48				33	10	3		2		33	10	3	
Johnston	145	145	145				143		2			2	143		2	
Rosoll, Knox, Stephenson	146		141			5	146						53			93
TOTALS	1443	968	1380	17	8	38	1142	132	131	12	26	54	552	52	179	634
PERCENTAGES		67.8	95.6	1.2	0.6	2.6	81.3	9.4	9.3			3.7	70.5	6.6	22.9	

1. Not included in totals/figures.
2. Included in "Relief of Symptoms" as "Poor" and in "Evidence of Healing" as "None."
3. Four had no symptoms when Banthine therapy was begun.
4. Of which seven were penetrating lesions and five partially obstructive.
5. No symptoms were present in four.
6. Two with symptoms only; no demonstrable ulcer.
7. Three were psychopathic patients and one had a ventricular ulcer of the lesser curvature.
8. Roentgen findings after treatment period of two weeks; forty-seven had duodenal deformity.
9. All returned to work within a week.
10. In three four, after relief of symptoms, Banthine was discontinued because of urinary retention.

During the past three years, more than 250 references to Banthine therapy in peptic ulcer and other parasympathotonic conditions have appeared in medical literature. Of these reports, 22 have presented specific facts and figures on the results of treatment in a total of 1,443 peptic ulcer patients, 67.8 per cent of whom were reported as chronic or resistant to other therapy. These results are tabulated above and show:

"Good" relief of symptoms was obtained in 81.3 per cent of the 1,405 patients on whom reports were available.

"Complete" evidence of healing was obtained in 70.5 per cent of the 783 patients on whom reports were available.

In all but 9.3 per cent, relief of pain was "good" or "fair." In all but 22.9 per cent, evidence of healing was "complete" or "moderate."

During treatment, 26 patients required surgery or developed complications other than ulcer which required discontinuance of the drug before results could be evaluated.

Of the remaining 1,417 patients, only 3.7 per cent experienced side effects sufficiently annoying to require discontinuance of the drug.

*Volume containing complete references, with abstracts of 39 additional reports, will be furnished on request by

G. D. SEARLE & Co.
P. O. Box 5110, Chicago 80, Illinois

Medical News and Events

A. M. A. Trustees Issue Statement On Health Plan

After an all day meeting held in Chicago January 24, the A. M. A. Board of Trustees issued the following statement concerning the implications of the proposed Eisenhower health plan:

"The Board of Trustees of the American Medical Association has given careful study to the President's Message on Health delivered to Congress on January 18. The Board is pleased to find in this message so many of the ideas and principles for which the American Medical Association has striven for so many years.

"The Board endorses the general objectives of the President to extend needed facilities, to promote further research, to increase coverage under voluntary health insurance and to rehabilitate the disabled.

"There are certain basic principles which the American Medical Association feels are essential in the consideration of any voluntary health insurance program: there must be free choice of physicians and hospitals: the program must be founded on sound actuarial data and there must be no direct or indirect control of the program by the government.

"The Administration's federal reinsurance proposal is indefinite. It is not clear whether this is true reinsurance or another form of government subsidy. This whole subject needs careful study and until the plan is spelled out in detail the American Medical Association can make no further comment.

"The American Medical Association feels that there may be other approaches to the problem of the extension of health coverage than that of federal reinsurance. For example, the A.M.A. has strongly supported legislation to permit deduction from income for tax purposes of medical and hospital bills and premiums paid for voluntary health insurance."

First Industrial Conference Slated

The University of Oklahoma School of Medicine will hold its first postgraduate Industrial Medicine symposium on May 20 and 21 at the School of Medicine auditorium in Oklahoma City.

This program is one of several activities spearheading the inclusion of industrial medicine in the curriculum of the school. The meeting represents an effort toward bringing together industry, medicine, law, safety engineering and industrial relations for joint discussions of topics pertinent to these groups.

Subjects to be covered include: Recent Advances in Traumatic Surgery, Industrial Challenge to the Medical Profession, Aspects of Occupational Diseases of Interest to the General Practitioner, Fundamentals of Industrial Medical Practice, Mental Health in Industry, The Role of the Physician in Labor Relations, Industrial Problems of the Painful Back, Workmen's Compensation in Oklahoma, Current Psychosomatic Understandings, Rehabilitation of the Industrially Injured, Injury Case Handling, Current Industrial Hygiene Methods, Industrial Safety and Disability Evaluation.

Among the speakers are: Dr. Earl D. McBride, Oklahoma City; Mr. W. H. Seymour, vice president of the Liberty Mutual Insurance Company, Boston; Dr. Stewart G. Wolf Jr., Oklahoma City; Dr. Kieffer Davis, Bartlesville, Okla., and Dr. Jean S. Felton, Oklahoma City.

The symposium is sponsored jointly by the School of Medicine through its Office of Postgraduate Instruction, the Liberty Mutual Insurance Company, and the Oklahoma Academy of General Practice.

Credit is given for attendance to the members of the Oklahoma Academy of General Practice and the registration fee will be $10. Those who are interested should register in advance with the Office of Postgraduate Instruction, University of Oklahoma School of Medicine, 800 N. E. 13th Street, Oklahoma City 4, Okla.

Physiological test
compares Kent's
"Micronite" Filter with other cigarette filters

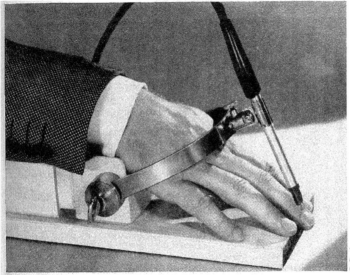

To compare the efficiency of various filters as they affect physiological responses in the cigarette smoker, drop in surface skin temperature at the last phalanx was measured.

Using well-established procedures, the subject smoked conventional filter cigarettes and the new KENT with the exclusive Micronite Filter.

For every other filter cigarette, the drop in temperature averaged over 6 degrees. For KENT's Micronite Filter, there was no appreciable drop.

These findings confirm the results of other scientific measurements that show these facts: 1) KENT's Micronite Filter takes out *far more* nicotine and tars than any other cigarette, *old or new*. 2) Ordinary cotton, cellulose or crepe paper filters remove a small but ineffective amount of nicotine and tars.

Thus KENT, with the first filter that really works, gives the one smoker out of every three who is susceptible to nicotine and tars the protection he needs . . . while offering the satisfaction he expects of fine tobacco.

For these reasons, smokers have made the new KENT the most popular new brand of cigarette to be introduced in the last 20 years.

If you have yet to try the new KENT with the exclusive Micronite Filter, may we suggest you do so soon?

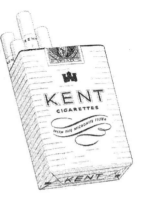

Course on Pulmonary Disease

Listed below is the initial program for the Pulmonary Disease Postgraduate course to be offered at the University of Oklahoma School of Medicine April 9 and 10.

Friday Morning—April 9

Chairman: Dr. L. J. Moorman

9:00-9:45—Dr. J. Burns Amberson (New York University, Bellevue Hospital) The Early Tuberculosis Lesion and Its Treatment.

10:00-10:45—Dr. Thomas Burford (Washington University, Barnes Hospital) Indications for Surgery in Pulmonary Tuberculosis

11:00-12:30—Panel Discussion — Treatment of the Complications of Tuberculosis. Moderator: Dr. P. M. McNeill

Panel Members: Dr. J. Burns Amberson, Dr. Thomas Burford, Dr. Samuel M. Glasser.

12:45-1:45—Lunch—University Cafeteria

Friday Afternoon

Chairman: Dr. Floyd Moorman

2:00-2:45—Dr. Richard V. Ebert. Mechanics of Pulmonary Ventilation and Tests of Pulmonary Function.

3:00-4:00—Panel Discussion—Case Presentation—Pulmonary Emphysema. Moderator: Dr. Stewart Wolf

Panel Members: Dr. Richard V. Ebert (Northwestern University, Veteran Research Hospital), Dr. R. H. Furman, Dr. A. E. Greer, and Dr. Simon Dolin.

4:15-4:45—Dr. Allen E. Greer. Management of Empyema.

5:00-5:30—Dr. James F. Hammarsten. Hypertrophic Osteoarthropathy.

(Continued on page 78)

ANNOUNCEMENTS

Oklahoma State Medical Association
May 10-11-12, 1954, Municipal Auditorium, Oklahoma City. House of Delegates, Sunday, May 9.

Rural Health Conference
Ninth National conference on rural health sponsored by the Council on Rural Heatlh of the American Medical Association, March 4-6, Baker Hotel, Dallas, Texas. Pre-conference session *for doctors only* will be held Thursday morning, March 4, beginning at 10:00 a.m.

Chicago Medical Society
Annual clinical conference, Palmer House, Chicago, Ill., March 2, 3, 4, 5, 1954.

Doctors in Alcoholics Anonymous
Fifth annual international group, Mayflower Hotel, Akron, Ohio, May 14, 15 and 16. For information and reservation address: Mayflower Hotel, Akron, Ohio.

American Medical Association
June 21-25, San Francisco, Calif.

Industrial Medicine Symposium
May 20 and 21. University of Oklahoma School of Medicine, Oklahoma City. Registration Fee $10.00. Those interested should register in advance with the Office of Postgraduate Instruction, University of Oklahoma School of Medicine, 800 N. E. 13th St., Oklahoma City.

Pan-Pacific Surgical Association
Sixth Congress will be held in Honolulu in October, 1954. For further information write F. J. Pinkerton, M. D., Director General, Pan-Pacific Surgical Association, Suite Seven, Young Bldg., Honolulu, Hawaii.

American Goiter Association
Annual meeting will be held April 29, 30 and May 1, Somerset Hotel, Boston, Mass.

The President's Health Message To Congress

In a special message to Congress on the nation's health problems, President Eisenhower proposes the following:

Medical Care — Reinsurance. "Better health insurance protection for more people can be provided. . . The government can and should work with them (private and non-profit organizations) to study and devise better insurance protection to meet the public need. . . I recommend the establishment of a *limited federal reinsurance service* to encourage broader health protection to more families. This service would reinsure the special additional risks involved in such broader protection. It can be launched with a capital fund of $25 million provided by the government, to be retired from reinsurance fees."

(An administration spokesman said the program would not involve "subsidies." The Department of Health, Education, and Welfare expects to send its specific recommendations to Congress within the next two or three weeks.)

Rehabilitation. "There are 2,000,000 disabled persons who could be rehabilitated and thus returned to productive work. Only 60,-00 now are being returned each year. Our goal should be 70,000 in 1955 . . . For 1956, 100,000. . . In 1956 states should begin to contribute to the cost of rehabilitating these additional persons. . . By 1959, with. . . states. . . sharing with the federal government, we should reach the goal of 200,000 . . . We must extend greater assistance to the states (for). . . specialized training of personnel. . . research, clinical facilities for rehabilitative services. . . the development of community centers and special workshops." Details of cost to be set forth in budget message.

Construction of Medical Facilities. "New hospital construction continues to lag behind the need. . . (but). . . hospital construction meets only part of the urgent need for facilities. . . I. . . propose added assistance or assistance in the construction of (a) non-profit hospitals for care of chronically ill, (b) non-profit medically supervised nursing and convalescent homes, (c) non-profit rehabilitation facilities for the disabled, (d) non-profit diagnostic or treatment centers for ambulatory patients. . . I (also) recommended. . . special funds be made available to the states to help pay for surveys of their needs."

(Legislation already introduced in both houses provides for grants of $20 million for diagnostic or treatment centers, a like amount for chronic disease centers, and $10 million each for rehabilitation facilities and nursing homes. These sums would be in addition to the appropriation under the regular Hill-Burton Act, which this year is $65 million.)

Union Leaders Insist on National Health Insurance at Hearings. Spokesmen for the AFL and the CIO have informed the House Interstate and Foreign Commerce Committee they still favor a compulsory national health plan as "the only adequate answer to the need of our people." Not all labor witnesses took the all-or-nothing position. *A. J. Hayes,* president of the International Association of Machinists and former member of the Truman Health Commission, testified: "Since it appears that the chances of achieving the ultimate solution are fairly remote, we will cooperate in any program which is a step in the right direction."

Jerry Voorhis, executive secretary, Cooperative Health Federation of America, and former California Congressman, advocated more emphasis by physicians on group practice. He said state and county medical societies have been carrying on a "running attack" against such practice and he hoped there would be "spontaneous action by the AMA and its constituent organizations" against such "discrimination."

Dr. Dean A. Clark, general director, Massachusettes General Hospital, who also served ed on the Truman Health Commission, testified in favor of matching funds to states to encourage development of comprehensive prepayment plans

Relegation of Army SG Proposed: A proposed Army reorganization would relegate the Surgeon General on the administrative scale. The proposal is to create a Supply Command, responsible for the Technical Services, including the Medical Department. The recommendations are from an advisory committee under the chairmanship of Paul L. Davies, San Jose, Calif. industrialist.

1953 Interns Are
Potential State Doctors

For the benefit of physicians and communities desiring information about physicians seeking locations, the following list is published of the 1953 University of Oklahoma Medical School class and their internship appointments. It is pointed out, however, that some of the group will be going into military service while others will be taking additional postgraduate work. It is hoped that the list will be of some value because a number of the group will be going into private practice upon completion of their internships.

Adams, Jerome M., Wm. Beaumont Army Hosp., El Paso, Texas; Allen, Rollie E., Brackenridge Hosp., Austin, Texas; Allison, Robert L., Brackenridge Hosp., Austin, Texas; Amdall, Robert O., University — 2 year, Oklahoma City, Oklahoma; Athey, Clanton R. Jr., Wichita St. Joseph's Hosp., Wichita, Kansas.

Bailey, Harry K., University — 2 year, Oklahoma City, Oklahoma; Ballinger, Thomas I., St. Joseph's Hosp., Fort Worth, Texas; Beasley, Gerald L. Jr., V. A. Hosp., Oklahoma City, Oklahoma; Bennett, Wayne E., U. S. Navy Hosp., San Diego, California; Boles, Robert D., Army-Navy Gen. Hosp., Hot Springs, Arkansas; Bricker, Earl M. Jr., St. Anthony Hosp., Oklahoma City, Oklahoma; Brooks, Quentin T., Wesley Hosp., Oklahoma City, Oklahoma; Brown, Claude H. B., University — 2 year, Oklahoma City, Oklahoma;

Carey, Philip O., Brooke Army Hosp., San Antonio, Texas; Castle, Eugene A., University — 1 year, Oklahoma City, Oklahoma; Cathey, Charles W., Denver Gen. Hosp., Denver, Colorado; Collins, William R., Kansas city Gen. Hosp. #1 Kansas City, Missouri; Cox, Walter M., St. Anthony Hosp., Oklahoma City, Oklahoma; Crawford, Perry F., St. Luke's Hosp., Chicago, Illinois.

Davenport, Charles D., Wichita St. Joseph's Hosp., Wichita, Kansas; Denny, William F., George Wash. Univ. Hosp., Washington, D. C.; Devine, J. C., Univ. of Texas Hosps., Galveston, Texas; Dietrich, Bailey L., V. A. Hosp., Oklahoma City, Oklahoma; Dowdy, Gerald S. Jr., V. A. Hosp., Oklahoma City, Oklahoma; Duffy, Mary L., University—1 year, Oklahoma City, Oklahoma.

Eddington, Allen B., University — 1 year, Oklahoma City, Oklahoma; Engles, Raymond L., V. A. Hosp., Oklahoma City, Oklahoma; Ewing, William F. Jr., Salt Lake Gen. Hosp., Salt Lake City, Utah.

Finn, Thomas C. Jr., University — 1 year, Oklahoma City, Oklahoma; Floyd, John H. University — 1 year, Oklahoma City, Oklahoma.

Harris, Jack A., East Tenn. Baptist Hosp., Knoxville, Tennessee; Harrison, William S., University Hosp., Ann Arbor, Michigan; Harvey, William G. Jr., University — 2 year, Oklahoma City, Oklahoma; Honaker, Jack D., Providence Hosp., Waco, Texas; Honick, Gerald L., University — 1 year, Oklahoma City, Oklahoma.

Jacobs, Luster I. Jr., Fitzsimons Army Hosp., Denver, Colorado; Jeter, Wiley P. Jr., University — 1 year, Oklahoma City, Oklahoma.

Lair, Burke, Providence Hosp., Seattle, Washington; Lively, Gerald A., St. Joseph's Hosp., Fort Worth, Texas; Lowell, James R., Good Samaritan Hosp., Dayton, Ohio; Lumpkin, Lee Roy, Tripler Army Hosp., Moanalua, Honolulu, T. H.

Mahan, Frank L., Letterman Army Hosp., San Francisco, California; Masters, Paul L., Wichita St. Joseph's Hosp., Wichita, Kansas; Mauldin, Howard P., Wichita St. Joseph's Hosp., Wichita, Kansas; McCabe, Jack M., Fitzsimons Army Hosp., Denver, Colorado; McCabe, William R., University — 1 year, Oklahoma City, Oklahoma; McFarland, James R., University — 1 year, Oklahoma City, Oklahoma; McGovern, Joseph D. Jr., Wesley Hosp., Oklahoma City, Oklahoma; Moore, Benjamin H. Jr., University — 2 year, Oklahoma City, Oklahoma; Moore, Robert, Wichita St. Joseph's Hosp., Wichita, Kansas; Moore, William R., Hillcrest Memorial Hosp., Tulsa, Oklahoma; Morgan, Robert F., University — 2 year, Oklahoma City, Oklahoma; Morgan, William L., Hillcrest Memorial Hosp., Tulsa, Oklahoma; Morse, James O., Los Angeles County Hosp., Los Angeles, California; Morton, Donald G., Mercy Hosp., Oklahoma City, Oklahoma; Moseley, Jack E., Wichita St. Joseph's Hosp., Wichita, Kansas.

(Continued on page 78)

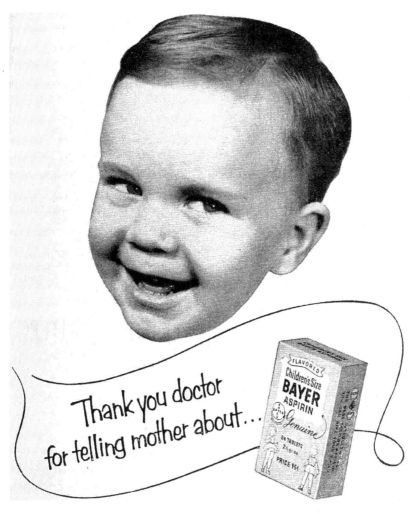

Thank you doctor for telling mother about...

FLAVORED
Children's Size
BAYER
ASPIRIN
Genuine
24 TABLETS
2½ grs.
PRICE 15¢

The Best Tasting Aspirin you can prescribe   The Flavor Remains Stable down to the last tablet   Bottle of 24 tablets 15¢ (2½ grs. each)

We will be pleased to send samples on request
THE BAYER COMPANY DIVISION of Sterling Drug Inc., 1450 Broadway, New York 18, N.Y.

Deaths

J. E. HARBISON, M. D., 1878-1954

J. E. Harbison, M. D., founder of Oklahoma City General Hospital (now Mercy Hospital), Oklahoma City, died January 5 of coronary thrombosis.

Doctor Harbison had retired in 1951 after more than 50 years in the medical profession. He was born in Benton, Tenn. and was graduated from Baylor University in 1901. He moved to Indian Territory near Duncan in 1905 and practiced there until moving to Oklahoma City in 1911.

(Continued from page 76)

Nunnery, Arthur W., Strong Mem. & Roch. Mun., Rochester, New York.

Overstreet, Robert J., St. Luke's Hosp., Chicago, Illinois.

Parrish, Jack W., Hillcrest Memorial Hosp., Tulsa, Oklahoma; Peffly, Elmer D., Wesley Hosp., Wichita, Kansas; Petrie, Robert B., Wesley Hosp., Oklahoma City, Oklahoma; Pinkerton, Clarence B., University — 2 year, Oklahoma City, Oklahoma; Power, Robert E., Henry Ford Hosp., Detroit, Michigan.

Rahhal, Lindbergh J., Kansas City Gen. Hosp. #1, Kansas City, Missouri; Rhine, John R., Hillcrest Memorial Hosp., Tulsa, Oklahoma.

Seelig, Darrell A., V. A. Hosp., Oklahoma City, Oklahoma; Sheffel, Donald J., U. S. Navy Hosp., San Diego, California; Smith, carl W. Jr., Barnes Hosp., St. Louis, Missouri; Standifer, John J., U. S. Navy Hosp., Bremerton, Washington; Stover, Robert M. University — 2 year, Oklahoma City, Oklahoma; Svoboda, Catherine A., Wesley Hosp., Oklahoma City, Oklahoma.

Taylor, Thomas W., Hillcrest Memorial Hosp., Tulsa, Oklahoma.

Wall, Henry L., University — 2 year, Oklahoma City, Oklahoma; Webb, James A., Army-Navy Gen. Hosp., Hot Springs, Arkansas; Whitcomb, Walter H., Salt Lake Gen. Hosp., Salt Lake City, Utah; Williams Richard G., Hillcrest Memorial Hosp., Tulsa, Oklahoma; Winters, Richard L., Denver Gen. Hosp., Denver, Colorado.

Zumwalt, Robert B., Kansas City Gen. Hosp. #1, Kansas City, Missouri.

(Continued from page 74)
Friday Evening

6:30-7:30—Buffet Supper . . . for Registrants and Participants. Oklahoma Medical Research Foundation.

8:00—Open Lecture. All physicians, medical students, nurses and medical personnel invited.

Dr. J. Burns Amberson. Pathogenesis of Unresolved Pneumonia. Introduction by Dr. L. J. Moorman.

Saturday Morning—April 10

Chairman: Dr. C. E. Bates

9:00-9:45—Dr. Thomas Burford. Diagnosis and Management of Chest Tumors.

10:00-10:45—Dr. Richard V. Ebert. Differential Diagnosis of Cardiac and Pulmonary Dyspnea.

11:00-11:30—Dr. Peter E. Russo. Recent Advances in X-ray Diagnosis of Diseases of the Chest.

11:30-12:30—Panel Discussion — Case Presentation—Bronchiectasis.

Moderator: Dr. James E. Hammarsten.

Panel Members: Dr. J. Burns Amberson, Dr. Thomas Burford, Dr. Richard V. Ebert, and Dr. Peter E. Russo.

Neo-Synephrine®
hydrochloride

Running noses, sneezing, watery eyes, clogged-up nasal passages quickly yield to administration of Neo-Synephrine hydrochloride — a nasal decongestant of proved clinical value. Ciliary activity is nearly untouched, sting and congestive rebound are practically absent, and effectiveness is undiminished on repeated use throughout the cold season.

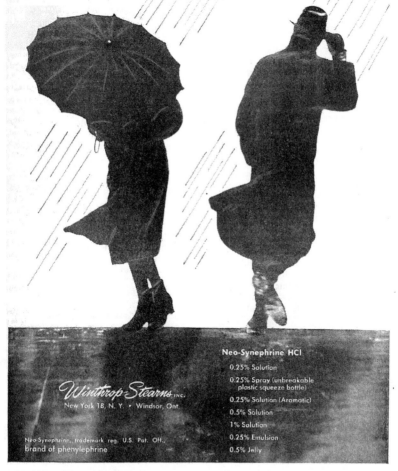

Winthrop-Stearns INC.
New York 18, N. Y. • Windsor, Ont.

Neo-Synephrine, trademark reg. U.S. Pat. Off.,
brand of phenylephrine

Neo-Synephrine HCl

0.25% Solution

0.25% Spray (unbreakable plastic squeeze bottle)

0.25% Solution (Aromatic)

0.5% Solution

1% Solution

0.25% Emulsion

0.5% Jelly

Book Reviews

DIET MANUAL. Compiled by Special Committees of the Oklahoma Dietetic Association and the Oklahoma State Medical Association. 1953.

This 33 page loose leaf manual is compiled by a special committee of the Oklahoma Dietetic Association and a committee from the Oklahoma State Medical Association and is just off the press. It is well printed on legible, heavy paper. It contains a normal diet, three variations of a liquid diet, a soft diet, a bland diet with three variations, a low residue diet, a food allergy detection regime, low sodium diet with 500 mgs and a low sodium diet with four gms in a 24 hour allowance as well as directions for varying the caloric content of the low sodium regime. There is a complete diet for pregnancy, supplemental schedule for infants, diets for pre-school and school children, seven variations of the A.D.A. diabetic meal plan with the complete A.D.A. food exchange lists, tables of of desirable weights and measures for both men and women, tables of percentiles for height and weight from birth to 16 years and a table of recommended dietary allowances for men, women during pregnancy, children and infants for various degrees of activity. There is a rather complete chart of food constitutents and their common sources and directions for making bread without salt for a low sodium diet. There are two blank pages and a food comparison table for the short method of dietary analysis followed by an index of the material contained in the manual.

The purpose of getting out this manual was to answer the demand for such a manual in small hospitals where a dietitian is not in attendance and for use by the general practitioner in his office and I feel that this manual answers the purpose quite well and probably answers the general purposes for most cases which are seen by the general practitioner or in small hospital practice. However, it appears to this reviewer that there are three rather blatant omis-sions in the manual. Since it seems that a weight reducing regimen or a 1000 calorie diet could have well been included in this manual. Since disturbances of purine metabolism, likewise, are far more common than is recognized at present in general practice and since we feel that gout is a very frequently overlooked cause of rheumatic complaints a low purine diet could have well been included in this manual and since so much recent work has shown the importance of a low cholesterol regimen in cardiovascular disorders it would seem to this reviewer that a book which does not include any of these three diets is rather incomplete.

There is included with each manual an order blank for any of the individual diets outlined in the manual (numbering 29 separate diets) and these diets may be ordered by anyone in lots of 50 or 100 for dispensing to patients at a very reasonable price for the quality and grade of printing and paper on which they are presented.

I feel that by and large the project has been well inaugurated and with a few additions in the future with some possible deletions as, for instance, in the diet for pregnancy I know of no particular difference from the diet for pregnancy and a normal diet or a normal bland diet. Therefore, the inclusion of this diet seems rather superfluous.

I also question the necessity of so many diabetic diet plans included in a brief manual of this sort.

However, I feel that the diet manual published at this reasonable price of $1.25 is well worth the investment for anyone who has small institution where dieticians are not available in which case this is an easily followed regimen for most of the commonly encountered disorders.

—Turner Bynum, M.D.

GIFFORD'S TEXTBOOK OF OPHTHAL-MOLOGY. Francis Heed Adler, M. D. W. B. Saunders Company, Philadelphia and London, Fifth Edition. 1953.

in arthritis

and allied disorders

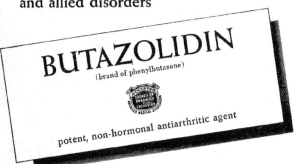

BUTAZOLIDIN
(brand of phenylbutazone)

potent, non-hormonal antiarthritic agent

Its therapeutic effectiveness substantiated by more than fifty
published reports, BUTAZOLIDIN has recently received
the Seal of Acceptance of the Council on Pharmacy and Chemistry
of the American Medical Association.

In the treatment of arthritis BUTAZOLIDIN produces prompt relief
of pain. In many instances relief of pain is accompanied
by diminution of swelling, resolution of inflammation and increased
freedom and range of motion of the affected joints.

BUTAZOLIDIN is indicated in:

Gouty Arthritis	Rheumatoid Arthritis
Psoriatic Arthritis	Rheumatoid Spondylitis

Painful Shoulder (including peritendinitis, capsulitis, bursitis, and acute arthritis)

Since BUTAZOLIDIN is a potent agent, patients for therapy should
be selected with care; dosage should be judiciously controlled;
and the patient should be regularly observed so that treatment may be
discontinued at the first sign of toxic reaction.

Physicians unfamiliar with the use of BUTAZOLIDIN are urged to send
for complete descriptive literature before employing it.

BUTAZOLIDIN® (brand of phenylbutazone), coated tablets of 100 mg.

 GEIGY PHARMACEUTICALS
Division of Geigy Chemical Corporation
220 Church Street, New York 13, N.Y.
In Canada: Geigy Pharmaceuticals, Montreal   360

This book is directed to medical students who will be expected to practice general medicine and as such the author has wisely attempted to concentrate on those eye diseases which the general practitioner can be expected to see most frequently. Accordingly the sections on the hypertensive diseases and diabetes are both thorough and detailed, whereas, the section dealing with surgery of the eye is limited only to the general indications for operative procedures. The book will provide a valuable reference for the general practitioner since it contains much about "ocular manifestations of general diseases". There is much in these sections which is not even mentioned in the better known textbooks of internal medicine.

The sections dealing with the various layers and media of the eye as well as the extra ocular apparatus are presented in clear and lucid fashion in the classical textbook style. The illustrations are excellent although full color photographs of retinoscopic findings are all too infrequent. It seems a shame that there are so many black and white pencil drawings and that these cannot be replaced with the much easier to understand full color illustrations, either sketches or actual Kodachrome reproductions such as are employed for delineating the external appearance of the eye. This is, nevertheless, a fine text which any general physician or internist might well own.

—John P. Colmore, M. D.

THE NURSING MOTHER, Frank Howard Richardson, M. D., Prentice-Hall, Inc., New York. 1953.

This is a very readable and well organized book which answers most questions in the minds of pregnant women who are contemplating the dilemma whether or not to nurse their baby. The answers are forcefully stated but frankly biased. The author's contention that natural breast feeding is healthiest for all babies is based more on exhortation than evidence and is a bit long winded. On the other hand the sections dealing with supposed dangers of breast feeding are well handled and the fear in the expectant mother's mind is swept out with clearly stated recourse to the facts.

Obstetricians who favor breast feeding will find persuasive backing in this book which is intelligible to almost any patient who is able to read.

—Stewart Wolf, M. D.

AN ATLAS OF PELVIC OPERATIONS. Langdon Parsons, M. D. and Howard Ulfelder, M. D. Illustrated by Mildred B. Codding, A. B., M. A. W. B. Saunders Company, Philadelphia. 1953. Price $18.00.

"One picture is worth a thousand words" — an old Chinese proverb.

If one accedes to this view then Doctors Parsons and Ulfelder with the very apparent capable surgical artist have written a tome of enormous dimensions.

This reviewer has always held to the idea that if one wishes to learn technique of surgical procedures nothing helps like drawing it. Throughout the years this has been recommended to medical students and doctors. Graphic instruction is actually paramount.

The addition of certain procedures usually classified as General Surgery has been a happy inclusion. Bowel resection, henial repair and abdomino-perineal resection of the rectum come to mind.

From "Biopsy of the Cervix" to "Repair of Vesico-Vaginal Fistula," this Atlas is of great importance and value, not alone to gynecologists, but to the general surgeon as well.

—L. J. Starry, M. D.

broad-spectrum therapy

Terramycin®

BRAND OF OXYTETRACYCLINE

established

an agent of choice

in the treatment of a wide range of infections due to gram-positive and gram-negative bacteria, spirochetes, rickettsiae, certain large viruses and protozoa.

clinical advantages *known*

rapid absorption

wide distribution

prompt response

excellent toleration

Within an hour after oral administration in fasting or non-fasting state, effective serum concentrations of Terramycin may be attained.[1] It is widely distributed in body fluids, organs and tissues and diffuses readily through the placental membrane.[2,3] Immediate evidence of Terramycin's efficacy is often obtained by the rapid return of temperature to normal.[4] Widely used among patients of all ages, this tested broad-spectrum antibiotic is well tolerated.[5,6]

1. Sayer, R. J., et al.: Am. J. M. Sc. 221:256 (Mar.) 1951.
2. Welch, H.: Ann. New York Acad. Sc. 53:253 (Sept.) 1950.
3. Werner, C. A., et al.: Proc. Soc. Exper. Biol. & Med. 74:261 (June) 1950.
4. Wolman, B., et al.: Brit. M. J. 1:419 (Feb. 23) 1952.
5. Potterfield, T. G., et al.: J. Philadelphia Gen. Hosp. 2:6 (Jan.) 1951.
6. King, E. Q., et al.: J.A.M.A. 143:1 (May 6) 1950.

Available in convenient oral, parenteral and ophthalmic preparations.

PFIZER LABORATORIES, *Brooklyn 6, N. Y.*
Division, Chas. Pfizer & Co., Inc.

GLYNAZAN

(Brand of Theophylline-Sodium Glycinate)

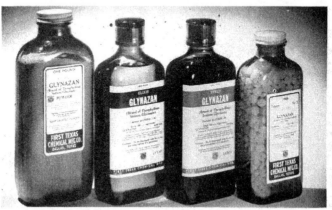

POWDER	ELIXIR	SYRUP	TABLETS
(Equivalent to Theophylline, U.S.P. 50%)	(Glynazan 1 grain per c.c.)	(Glynazan ½ grain per c.c.)	(2½ and 5 grains)

COUNCIL ACCEPTED GLYNAZAN PRODUCTS AVAILABLE FOR PRESCRIPTION USE.

ADVANCING

THEOPHYLLINE THERAPY

A Theophylline Compound exhibiting maximal solubility with minimal gastric iritation. Permits intensive Theophylline therapy in bronchial and circulatory disturbances.

FIRST TEXAS
CHEMICAL MANUFACTURING CO.

1903 - 1954: Celebrating 51 Years of Making FINE PHARMACEUTICALS

1810 N. Lamar   Dallas

Editorials

The Sixty-First Annual Meeting

More than 50 years ago my Indian ponies and I traveled down from Jet to Oklahoma City for an early meeting of the State Medical Association. They needed new belly bands and I needed a brain dusting. Although the trip was hard and time consuming, we couldn't afford to miss it.

The scientific program was simple, brief, and fairly adequate considering the time and place. There was no fanfare, no loudspeaker, no radio, no television and no fancy touches, but the program was loaded with the experiences of plain country doctors, practical reports by aspiring town surgeons, and other methods of treatment. It seemed fairly adequate for that day.

Medical practice had added impiricism to magic and it had become at least impirico-rational. The meetings of these hard, early days prepared the way for organized medicine and modern medical science.

The 61st meeting will convene in Oklahoma City May 10-11-12. Time, conditions, and people have changed. There'll be no ponies; no belly bands, unless for some members of the profession. The need for brain dusting may be just as real but less obvious because of the superficial gloss that comes through improved, but time consuming, communications. The needs of physicians are much greater now than when I came down so many years ago. But the knowledge required to meet current needs is more nearly adequate and more readily available than ever before. Every physician in the state should be here to receive it.

Fifty years ago transportation was slow and difficult. Now it is easy and swift. Then the people were satisfied with their doctors and thankful for medical care. There were no grievance committees and malprac-

tice suits were rare. Today many of the people are restless, exacting, and often distrustful. Some of them mistake *Reader's Digest*, medical indigestion for medical knowledge and often became unduly concerned and reach false conclusions. They need more guidance than ever before. Although "a little learning is a dangerous thing," they are well enough informed to know that physicians must attend medical meetings if they are to be professionally competent and thus worthy of individual and community confidence.

It is obvious that the physician of today cannot afford to miss the Annual Meeting of his State Medical Association. In contrast to the meeting of 50 years ago, the approaching session in Oklahoma City offers two and one-half days of intensive scientific presentations and discussions. Communications will be facilitated by the most approved methods. Each day television will bring surgical and clinical procedures within reach of all in attendance.

Ten carefully picked guest speakers from all points of the compass will bring up to the minute applied medical knowledge from various schools of thought and different sections of the country.

The sessions should be most stimulating and provocative of much original thought and the individual take for home consumption should amply compensate for loss of time and money.

This year the Council and the House of Delegates have much important business on their respective agendas. Those entrusted with official duties must come early and be prepared for serious deliberations.

This should be the most significant and the best attended meeting in 60 years.

Association Activities

PRESIDENT'S LETTER

May 9, 10, 11, 12 are the dates for the 61st Annual Meeting of the Oklahoma State Medical Association.

From the beginning, 61 years ago, the strides made by Oklahoma medicine have bordered on the miraculous. The pioneers of Oklahoma medicine, many of whom are still with us, should be justly proud of the heritage they have created for those of the profession yet to come along, to keep alive.

The advancements of medicine in these 61 years have been not only in the field of scientific medicine, but medical education and, of more recent years, scientific research.

While it would be difficult to pin point any one thing that has brought about these advancements, it is extremely unlikely that any single activity has been more important than the Annual Meeting. This meeting, which brings together for four days the medical profession of the State not only for scientific advancement but for a discussion of the economic ills, together with professional fraternalism, should be attended by every physician who can possibly attend. The Annual Meeting, a time when East may meet West and North consult with South, when old acquaintances can be renewed and new friendships made, is well worth any physician's time.

Any physician who has been accorded the privilege of being President fully realizes how his horizon broadens as he travels the State of Oklahoma and learns and enjoys the profession he finds everywhere. Each of you can have the same enjoyment attending the Annual Meeting.

With these few words of general comment, but firmly and honestly believed, I hope and urge that all of you will make every effort to be in Oklahoma City for part or all of the 61st Annual Meeting of your Association.

John E McDonald M.D.

President

Officers and Councilors

OKLAHOMA STATE MEDICAL ASSOCIATION

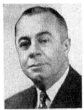

John E. McDonald, M.D.
Tulsa
President

Lewis J. Moorman, M.D.
Oklahoma City
*Secretary-Treasurer
Editor*

Sixty-First Annual Meeting

Zebra Room—Municipal Auditorium
Oklahoma City, Oklahoma

May 9-10-11-12, 1954

COUNCIL MEETING—Saturday, May 8—
7:00 p.m., Oriental Room, Biltmore Hotel

HOUSE OF DELEGATES—Sunday, May 9
—1:00 p.m., Hall of Mirrors, Municipal
Auditorium

District No. 1: Craig, Delaware, Mayes, Nowata, Ottawa, Rogers, Washington.
Councilor (1956)_____F. S. Etter, M. D., Bartlesville
Vice-Councilor (1956)____J. E. Highland, M. D., Miami

District No. 2: Kay, Noble, Osage, Pawnee, Payne.
Councilor (1964)____Clifford Bassett, M. D., Cushing
Vice-Councilor (1954)__E. C. Mohler, M. D., Ponca City

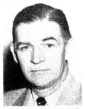

Bruce R. Hinson, M.D.
Enid
President-Elect

District No. 3: Garfield, Grant, Kingfisher, Logan.
Councilor (1955)____C. M. Hodgson, M. D., Kingfisher
Vice-Councilor (1955)____Wm. P. Neilson, M. D., Enid

District No. 4: Alfalfa, Beaver, Cimarron, Ellis, Harper, Major, Texas, Woods, Woodward.
Councilor (1956)_____L. R. Kirby, M. D., Cherokee
Vice-Councilor (1956)__Joe L. Duer, M. D., Woodward

District No. 5: Beckham, Blaine, Canadian, Custer, Dewey, Roger Mills.
Councilor (1954)_____A. L. Johnson, M. D., El Reno
Vice-Councilor (1954)____Ross Deputy, M. D., Clinton

District No. 6: Oklahoma.
Councilor (1955) R. Q. Goodwin, M. D., Oklahoma City
Vice-Councilor (1955)_____
_____Elmer Ridgeway, Jr., M. D., Oklahoma City

District No. 7: Cleveland, Creek, Lincoln, Okfuskee, Pottawatomie, Seminole.
Councilor (1956)_____Paul Gallaher, M. D., Shawnee
Vice-Councilor (1956)_____
_____Charles A. Smith, M. D., Norman

District No. 8: Tulsa.
Councilor (1954)_____Wilkie Hoover, M. D., Tulsa
Vice-Councilor (1954)__W. A. Showman, M. D., Tulsa

District No. 9: Adair, Cherokee, McIntosh, Muskogee, Okmulgee, Sequoyah, Wagoner.
Councilor (1955)_____F. R. First, Jr., M. D., Checotah
Vice-Councilor (1955)_____
_____I. W. Bollinger, M. D., Henryetta

District No. 10: Haskell, Hughes, Latimer, LeFlore, Pittsburg.
Councilor (1956)_____E. H. Shuller, M. D., McAlester
Vice-Councilor (1956) Paul Kernek, M. D., Holdenville

District No. 11: Atoka, Bryan, Choctaw, Coal, McCurtain, Pushmataha.
Councilor (1954)_____A. T. Baker, M. D., Durant
Vice-Councilor (1954)_____T. E. Rhea, M. D., Idabel

District No. 12: Carter, Garvin, Johnston, Love, Marshall, McClain, Murray, Pontotoc.
Councilor (1955)_____J. H. Veazey, M. D., Ardmore
Vice-Councilor (1955)_____W. T. Gill, M. D., Ada

Dsitrict No. 13: Caddo, Comanche, Cotton, Grady, Jefferson, Stephens.
Councilor (1956)____H. M. McClure, M. D., Chickasha
Vice-Councilor (1956)____J. B. Miles, M. D., Anadarko

District No. 14: Greer, Harmon, Jackson, Kiowa, Tillman, Washita.
Councilor (1954)___ L. G. Livingston, M. D., Cordell
Vice-Councilor (1954)____J. B. Hollis, M. D., Mangum

General Information

HOTEL ACCOMMODATIONS

Physicians planning to attend the Annual Meeting are asked to return the hotel reservation form in this issue as soon as possible. Make reservations with the Hotels Committee, Oklahoma State Medical Association, 1227 Classen Drive, Oklahoma City 3, Okla. *Do not write hotels direct.* State date of arrival and departure, approximate time of arrival, type of accomodations desired (single, double, twin bedroom suite, etc.) There is no headquarters hotel.

REGISTRATION

Registration will open Monday, May 10, at 8:30 a.m. in the Zebra Room of the Municipal Auditorium. Delegates may register Sunday, May 9, on the Mezzanine of the Municipal Auditorium immediately preceding the House of Delegates session. Physicians may register until 5:00 p.m. every day until Wednesday when the meeting closes at noon.

HOUSE OF DELEGATES

Members of the Association who are not Delegates or Alternates are invited to attend the session of the House as spectators. The House will convene at 1:00 p.m., Sunday, May 9, in the Hall of Mirrors, Municipal Auditorium. A special section will be reserved for those who are not Delegates.

ROUNDTABLE LUNCHEONS

Roundtable luncheons will be held at 12:15 p.m. Monday and Tuesday, May 10 and 11 at the YWCA Auditorium. The YWCA is two and one-half blocks east of the Municipal Auditorium located on the south side of the street at 320 N. W. First St.

GOLF TOURNAMENT

A golf tournament sponsored jointly by the Association and Pfizer Laboratories will be held at Twin Hills Country Club Wednesday afternoon, May 12. Entries may register at Twin Hills from noon until 1:00 p.m. Prizes will be awarded and a social hour and dinner will be held at Twin Hills following the tournament, compliments of Pfizer.

CHEST-X-RAYS

The Scientific Exhibits Committee, in cooperation with the Oklahoma State Health Department, has arranged for a booth at the Annual Meeting in which all members and guests in attendance are urged to have miniature chest x-ray films made. The equipment used in this project will be the same type that is being recommended for use by hospitals throughout the state for the screening of all patients.

Interpretation and the film will be forwarded to the physicians having x-rays made. Guests having films made will give the name of the physician to whom they desire their film to be sent.

RELATED MEDICAL MEETINGS

Several allied organizations are planning conventions to coincide with the O.S.M.A. Annual Meeting. Meeting schedules of these groups may be found elsewhere in this issue.

PAST PRESIDENTS' BREAKFAST

The annual breakfast honoring Past Presidents of the Association will be held Monday morning, May 10, at 8:00 a.m. in the Blue Room, Mezzanine, Skirvin Hotel. All past presidents are urged to attend.

PRESIDENT'S ANNUAL DINNER-DANCE

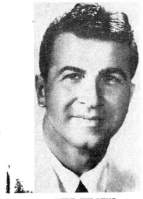

DICK JURGENS

Tuesday, May 11, 1954

Persian Room

Skirvin Tower Hotel

6:00 p.m. SOCIAL HOUR, Balinese and Crystal Rooms, Mezzanine, Skirvin Hotel

7:00 p.m. DINNER, Persian Room, Skirvin Tower Hotel
Introduction of guests and officers
Inaugural of Bruce R. Hinson, M.D., as President

9:00 p.m. DANCING, Persian Room, Skirvin Tower

Dick Jurgens . . .

Dick Jurgens and his Orchestra featuring Al Galante, vocalist, and Paul Allen, vocalist

As a composer of popular tunes, Dick Jurgens rates among the best. Among his triumphs are his theme song, "Day Dreams Come True at Night," "Careless," written with bandleader Eddy Howard when he was a vocalist with the J u r g e n s crew, "One Dozen Roses," dedicated to his brother-in-law who is a florist, "Elmer's Tune," "A Million Dreams Ago," "I Do, Do You," "If I Knew Then," "It's a Hundred to One I'm In Love," and "I Won't Be Home Anymore When You Call."

Reservations . . .

Tickets to the President's Annual Dinner Dance are limited to the capacity of the Persian Room. Price is $7.50 per person and includes the social hour, dinner, inaugural program, and the Dick Jurgens dance. Members may purchase tickets in advance by sending their checks, payable to the Oklahoma State Medical Association to the Association at 1227 Classen Drive, Oklahoma City 3, Oklahoma. Tickets will be available at the Registration Desk as long as they last.

Distinguished Guest Speakers

C. ALLEN GOOD, M.D.
Rochester, Minnesota

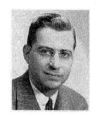

Associate Professor of Radiology, Mayo Foundation, University of Minnesota (Rochester); Consultant, Section on Diagnostic Roentgenology, Mayo Clinic; M.D., Washington University (St. Louis); A.B., Williams College; M.S. in Radiology, University of Minnesota; Diplomate, American Board of Radiology; President, Minnesota Radiological Society; Fellow, American College of Radiology; Member, American Roentgen Ray Society, Radiological Society of North America.

Sponsor—Edmond H. Kalmon, M.D., Oklahoma City

JOHN B. HAZARD, M.D.
Cleveland, Ohio

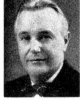

Head of Department of Pathology, Cleveland Clinic; Graduate of Harvard Medical School, 1930; Assistant Professor of Pathology and Bacteriology, Tufts College Medical School; hospital affiliations, the Faulkner Hospital and Robert B. Brigham Hospital, Boston, Massachusetts; Army Service: Chief of Laboratory, Harvard Unit; Command, Central Laboratory in Europe; Command, United Kingdom Base Laboratory; Diplomate of American Board of Pathology; Specialty Societies: American Society of Clinical Pathologists; College of American Pathologists; American Association of Pathologists and Bacteriologists; Councilor, International Association of Medical Museums; President-elect, Ohio Society of Pathologists.

Sponsor—Allen E. Greer, M.D., Oklahoma City

J. RODERICK KITCHELL, M.D.
Philadelphia, Pennsylvania

B.A., Rice Institute, 1928; M. D., University of Texas, 1932; F.A.C.P., 1941, Life Member, 1944; Fellow, American College of Cardiology, 1953; Certified by American Board of Internal Medicine in Internal Medicine, 1945 and Cardiovascular Disease, 1947; Associate in Medicine, University of Pennsylvania, School of Medicine; Associate Professor of Cardiology, University of Pennsylvania, Graduate School of Medicine; Chief, Department of Cardiovascular Disease, Presbyterian Hospital, Philadelphia; Staff and Member, Board of Directors, Childrens Heart Hospital of Philadelphia; Chairman of Rheumatic and Congenital Heart Disease Committee, Pennsylvania Heart Association; Member, Founders Group of the Scientific Council, American Heart Association.

Sponsor—F. Redding Hood, M.D., Oklahoma City

H. RELTON, McCARROLL, M.D.
St. Louis, Missouri

A.B. Degree, Ouachita College, Arkadelphia, Arkansas, 1927; M.D. Degree, Washington University School of Medicine, 1931; Certified by the American Board of Orthopedic Surgery; Assistant Professor of Clinical Orthopedic Surgery, Washington University School of Medicine, St. Louis, Missouri; Member of the Staffs of Barnes, St. Louis Children's, St. Luke's, Deaconness, Jewish, and Shriners Hospitals, St. Louis, Missouri; Member of the Clinical Orthopedic Society, The American Academy of Orthopedic Surgeons, and the American Orthopedic Association; Treasurer of the American Academy of Orthopedic Surgeons, 1948-1954; Chairman of Orthopedic Section of the American Medical Association, 1952-1953; Positions on Editorial Boards: Member of Board of Associate Editors, The Journal of Bone and Joint Surgery; Member of Board of Associate Editors, Quarterly Review of Surgery.

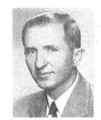

Sponsor—Don H. O'Donoghue, M.D., Oklahoma City

EARL D. OSBORNE, MD..
Buffalo, New York

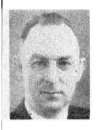

B.S. Degree, 1917; M.D., 1919, University of Michigan; Internship and Fellowship, Mayo Clinic, 1919-1923; M.S. University of Minnesota, 1924; Professor of Dermatology and Syphilology, University of Buffalo, School of Medicine and chief attending Dermatologist and Syphilologist at Buffalo General Hospital, Meyer Memorial Hospital and Children's Hospital; Founder, American Academy of Dermatology and Syphilology, 1937; Secretary-Treasurer, 1937-1949, President, 1950, Chairman of Committee on Education. Recognized by the Academy for efforts in its organization by establishment, Earl D. Osborne Fellowship in Dermal Pathology at the Armed Forces Institute of Pathology in Washington, 1949; President, American Dermatological Association, 1952; Author of more than fifty scientific publications.

Sponsor—John H. Lamb, M.D., Oklahoma City

E. H. PARSONS, M.D.
St. Louis, Missouri

M.D., Vanderbilt University, 1930; Postgraduate, Colorado General Hospital, Denver and St. Elizabeth Hospital, Washington, D.C.; Psychiatric consultant in Orient before war; Combat Psychiatry, European Theater three years during World War II as Head of 101st Neuropsychiatric General Hospital; now associate clinical professor Neuropsychiatry, Washington University and Member of Staff of Barnes, Baptist, St. Vincent, and other hospitals, St. Louis; Publications deal with Research in Experimental Embryology, Fever Therapy, Clinical Psychiatry, and Neurology.

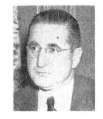

Sponsor—Moorman P. Prosser, M.D., Oklahoma City

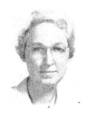

VIRGINIA APGAR, M.D.
New York, New York

B.A., Mt. Holyoke College, 1929; M.D., Columbia University College of Physicians and Surgeons, 1933; Internship in Surgery, Presbyterial Hospital, 1933-1935; Resident in Anesthesiology, Presbyterian Hospital, Wisconsin General Hospital, Bellevue Hospital, 1935-1937; Clinical Director, Anesthesia Service, Columbia Presbyterian Medical Center; Professor of Anesthesiology Columbia University.

Sponsor—Grace C. Hassler, M.D., Oklahoma City

PHILIP B. PRICE, M.D.
Salt Lake City, Utah

A.B., Davidson College; M.D., Johns Hopkins Medical School, 1921; Internship and Surgical Residency, Union Memorial Hospital, Baltimore; Medical Missionary Work, 1925-1938; Assistant and Associate Professor of Surgery, Cheeloo University (China), 1928-1938; Associate Surgeon, Johns Hopkins Medical School and Hospital, 1938-1943; Professor and Head of the Department of Surgery, University of Utah; Surgeon-in-Chief, Salt Lake General Hospital; Senior Surgical Consultant, Salt Lake VA Hospital and Grand Junction (Colorado) VA Hospital; Fellow, American College of Surgeons, American Surgical Association, Western Surgical Association, Society of University Surgeons; President, Southwestern Surgical Congress.

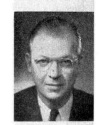

Sponsor—C. R. Rountree, M.D., Oklahoma City

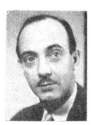

FRED M. TAYLOR, M.D.
Houston, Texas

M.D., Stanford University School of Medicine, 1943; Internship and Pediatric Residency, Colorado General Hospital and Children's Hosptial, Denver; Diplomate, American Board of Pediatrics; Fellow, American Academy of Pediatrics; Associate Professor of Pediatrics, Baylor University College of Medicine, Houston.

Sponsor—C. M. Bielstein, M.D., Oklahoma City

J. ROBERT WILLSON, M.D.
Philadelphia, Pennsylvania

M.D., University of Michigan, 1937; M.S., (Obstetrics and Gynecology) University of Michigan, 1942; Internship, University of Michigan Hospital, 1937-1938; Residency, Obstetrics and Gynecology, University of Michigan Hospital, 1938-1941; Assistant Professor, Obstetrics and Gynecology, University of Chicago, Attending Obstetrician and Gynecologist, Chicago Lying-in Hospital, 1943-1946; Professor and Chairman of Department of Obstetrics and Gynecology, Temple University School of Medicine and Temple University Hospital. Societies: American Association for Advancement of Science; Society for Experimental Biology and Medicine, American Board of Obstetrics and Gynecology, American Association of Obstetricians, Gynecologists and Abdominal Surgeons, American Gynecological Society, American Academy of Obstetricians and Gynecologists.

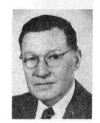

Sponsor—Robert D. Anspaugh, M.D., Oklahoma City

Scientific Program

MONDAY MORNING, *May 10, 1954*

Zebra Room, Municipal Auditorium

TELEVISION

9:00 - 9:20 SURGERY
Cancer of the Breast—Demonstration of Cases
Philip B. Price, M.D., Salt Lake City, Utah

9:20 - 9:40 ORTHOPEDICS
Insertion of Hip Prosthesis
H. Relton McCarroll, M.D., St. Louis, Missouri

9:40 - 10:00 GYNECOLOGY
Abdominal Hysterectomy
J. Robert Willson, M. D., Philadelphia, Pennsylvania

GENERAL SESSION

10:00 - 10:20 MEDICINE
The Evaluation of the Surgical Cardiac
William Best Thompson, M.D., Oklahoma City

10:20 - 10:40 OPHTHALMOLOGY
Funduscopic Findings of Some Common Internal Diseases
Robert P. Dennis, M. D., Lawton, Oklahoma

10:40 - 11:00 RADIOLOGY
Operative Cholangiography
Bruce H. Brown, M.D. and George M. Brown, Jr., M.D., McAlester, Oklahoma

11:00 - 11:20 PEDIATRICS
Erythroblastosis
Robert D. Shuttee, M.D., Enid, Oklahoma

11:20 - 12:00 RADIOLOGY
The Roentgenologic Contribution to the Diagnosis of Bronchogenic Carcinoma
C. Allen Good, M.D., Rochester, Minnesota

12:15 - 1:45 ROUNDTABLE LUNCHEON
YWCA AUDITORIUM

MONDAY AFTERNOON, *May 10, 1954*

Zebra Room, Municipal Auditorium

GENERAL SESSION

2:00 - 2:40 DERMATOLOGY

The Treatment of Skin Infections
Earl D. Osborne, M.D., Buffalo, New York

2:40 - 3:20 ANESTHESIOLOGY

Obstetric Anethesia in General Practice
Virginia Apgar, M.D., New York, New York

3:20 - 4:00 PEDIATRICS

Obscure Fever in Infants and Children
Fred M. Taylor, M.D., Houston, Texas

4:00 - 4:20 THORACIC SURGERY

Emergency Treatment of Chest Injuries
Allen E. Greer, M.D., Oklahoma City

4:20 - 5:00 ORTHOPEDICS

Practical Points in the Management of Common Fractures
H. Relton McCarroll, M.D., St. Louis, Missouri

MONDAY NIGHT

The Arrangements Committee has planned no activity for Monday
evening in the belief that those in attendance would prefer to have one
evening open for their own individual planning.

TUESDAY MORNING, *May 11, 1954*

Zebra Room, Municipal Auditorium

TELEVISION

9:00 - 9:20 MEDICINE

Rheumatic Heart Disease with Mitral Valvulitis-Indications and Contra-indications for Surgery
J. Roderick Kitchell, M.D., Philadelphia, Pennsylvania

9:20 - 9:40 PEDIATRICS

A Case of Focal Motor Convulsive Seizures
Fred M. Taylor, M.D., Houston, Texas

9:40 - 10:00 RADIOLOGY

Roentgenologic Demonstration of Gastric Lesions
C. Allen Good, M.D., Rochester, Minnesota

GENERAL SESSION

10:00 - 10:40 ANESTHESIOLOGY

Infant Resuscitation
Virginia Apgar, M.D., New York, New York

10:40 - 11:20 PATHOLOGY
The Solitary Thyroid Nodule
John B. Hazard, M.D., Cleveland, Ohio

11:20 - 12:00 OBSTETRICS

The Management of the Third Stage of Labor and Prevention of Postpartum Hemorrhage
J. Robert Willson, M.D., Philadelphia, Pennsylvania

12:15 - 1:45 ROUNDTABLE LUNCHEON

YWCA AUDITORIUM

TUESDAY AFTERNOON, *May 11, 1954*

Zebra Room, Municipal Auditorium

GENERAL SESSION

2:00 - 2:40 DERMATOLOGY

A Therapeutic Armamentarium for General Practitioners
Earl D. Osborne, M.D., Buffalo, New York

2:40 - 3:20 SURGERY

Suture Materials and General Principles of Suturing Wounds
Philip B. Price, M.D., Salt Lake City, Utah

3:20 - 4:00 PSYCHIATRY

Cinderella is a Growing Child
E. H. Parsons, M.D., St. Louis, Missouri

4:00 - 4:20 GYNECOLOGY

Endometriosis, Cause and Effect
Eugene S. Cohen, M.D., Tulsa, Oklahoma

4:20 - 4:40 MOTION PICTURE

The Well Child Examination
Presented by the School Health Committee in cooperation with the Oklahoma State Health Department

4:40 - 5:00 MEDICINE

A Critical Appraisal of Therapy for Duodenal Ulcer
Stewart G. Wolf, Jr., M.D., Oklahoma City

PRESIDENT'S ANNUAL DINNER DANCE

Featuring Dick Jurgens Orchestra

Social Hour, 6:00 P.M.
Balinese and Crystal Rooms
Skirvin Hotel

Dinner, 7:00 P.M.
Persian Room
Skirvin Tower

WEDNESDAY MORNING, *May 12, 1954*

Zebra Room, Municipal Auditorium

GENERAL SESSION

9:00 - 9:40 PATHOLOGY

Pulmonary Disease as Reflected in Lung Biopsy
John B. Hazard, M.D., Cleveland, Ohio

9:40 - 10:20 MEDICINE

Management of the Patient with Coronary Atherosclerosis
J. Roderick Kitchell, M.D., Philadelphia, Pennsylvania

10:20 - 11:00 PSYCHIATRY

Medicine Is Also An Art
E. H. Parsons, M.D., St. Louis, Missouri

11:00 - 12:30 CLINICAL PATHOLOGIC CONFERENCE

John B. Hazard, M.D., Cleveland, Ohio
J. Roderick Kitchell, M.D., Philadelphia, Pennsylvania
Robert H. Bayley, M.D., Oklahoma City

Annual Meeting Committees

Arrangements Committee:

Richard A. Clay, M.D., Chairman
Wm. H. Reiff, M. D.
E. E. Cooke, M. D.
Harold Binder, M. D.

Roundtable Luncheon Chairmen:

Lynn H. Harrison, M. D.
James J. Gable, Jr., M. D.

Commercial Exhibits Committee:

T. C. Points, M. D., Chairman
I. O. Pollock, M. D.
W. L. Waldrop, M. D.

Scientific Exhibits Committee:

John D. Ingle, M. D., Chairman
Allen D. Greer, M. D.
P. E. Russo, M. D.

Golf Chairman:
P. E. Russo, M. D.

Housing Chairman:
J. P. Luton, M. D.

Television Committees:
A. H. Bungardt, M. D.
Frank E. Darrow, M. D.
Robert D. Anspaugh, M. D.
Simon Dolin, M. D.
John P. Colmore, M. D.
Charles E. Delhotal, Jr., M. D.

Scientific Work Committees:
James C. Amspacher, M. D., Chairman
Joe M. Parker, M. D.
Henry G. Bennett, Jr., M. D.
John R. Danstrom, M. D.
W. T. McCollum, M. D.
Charles W. Freeman, M. D.

Woman's Auxiliary

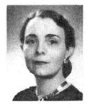

Mrs. Millard L. Henry
McAlester

*President, Woman's
Auxiliary to the O.S.M.A.*

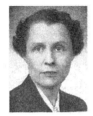

Mrs. W. R. Cheatwood
Duncan

*President-Elect, Woman's
Auxiliary to the O.S.M.A.*

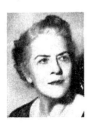

Mrs. George Turner
El Paso

*President-Elect, Woman's
Auxiliary to the A.M.A.*

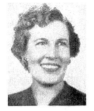

Mrs. George Feldner
New Orleans

*President, Woman's
Auxiliary to the Southern
Medical Association*

Skirvin Hotel   Oklahoma City, Okla.

MAY 9-12, 1954

CONVENTION COMMITTEES

Convention Chairman . . . . . Mrs. Elias Margo
Headquarters and Registration . Mrs. J. H. Robinson
Credentials . . . . Mrs. P. K. Graening
Hospitality . . . . Mrs. P. B. Rice
Tickets . . . . Mrs. Harold Binder
Transportation . . . . Mrs. Richard E. Carpenter
Luncheon . . . . Mrs. George S. Bozalis
Style Show . . . . . . Mrs. Carroll M. Pounders
Publicity . . . . Mrs. John Lamb
Past Presidents . . . . . . Mrs. James McMurry

SUNDAY, MAY 9, 1954

THEME: *Together We Progress*

1:00 p.m. to 3:00 p.m.—REGISTRATION—Mezzanine
Floor, Skirvin Hotel

3:00 p.m. to 5:00 p.m.—TEA—Honoring Mrs. George
Turner, El Paso, Texas, President-Elect of Woman's Auxiliary to the American Medical Association; Mrs. George Feldner, New Orleans, President of Woman's Auxiliary to the Southern Medical Association; State Officers and Visiting
Wives of members of the Oklahoma State Medical Association and wives of Guest Speakers.
Home of Mrs. W. K. Ishmael, 1500 Glenwood.
Courtesy of the Woman's Auxiliary to the Oklahoma County Medical Society.

8:00 p.m.—EXECUTIVE BOARD MEETING—Hospitality Room, Skirvin Hotel, Mrs. Millard L.
Henry, Presiding

MONDAY, MAY 10, 1954

THEME: *Together We Progress*

8:30 a.m.—PAST PRESIDENT'S BREAKFAST—Empire Room, Skirvin Hotel, Mrs. W. K. West, hostess

9:00 a.m. to 4:00 p.m.—REGISTRATION—Mezzanine Floor, Skirvin Hotel
INFORMATION — Mezzanine Floor, Skirvin Hotel

9:00 a.m. to 5:00 p.m.—HOSPITALITY ROOM HOSTESS COUNTIES

10:00 a.m. GENERAL MEETING—Mrs. Millard L. Henry, Presiding. Continental Room, Skirvin Hotel. All members and visiting physicians' wives welcome.

CALL TO ORDER—Mrs. Millard L. Henry, President of the Woman's Auxiliary to the Oklahoma State Medical Association.

INVOCATION—Mrs. Elbert H. Shuller, McAlester

PLEDGE OF LOYALTY—Mrs. Logan Spann, Tulsa

"I pledge my loyalty and devotion to the Woman's Auxiliary to the American Medical Association. I will support its reputation, and ever sustain its high ideals."

WELCOME—Mrs. Howard B. Shorbe, President, Oklahoma County Auxiliary.

GREETINGS—Bruce Hinson, M.D., Enid, President-Elect of the Oklahoma State Medical Association.

ROLL CALL BY COUNTIES—Mrs. John Cunningham, Oklahoma City, Secretary-Treasurer of the Woman's Auxiliary to the Oklahoma State Medical Association.

READING AND ADOPTION OF THE MINUTES—Mrs. Cunningham

PRESENTATION OF PAGES—Mrs. Floyd T. Bartheld, McAlester; Mrs. Hartzell Schaff, Holdenville.

INTRODUCTIONS—State Officers, Committee Chairmen, County Presidents and Guests.

PRESENTATION OF REPORTS OF ALL OFFICERS—Mrs. Henry

GUEST SPEAKER—Mrs. George Feldner, New Orleans, President of the Woman's Auxiliary to the Southern Medical Association. ADDRESS—*Southern's Star Shines Brightly*

REPORT OF REVISIONS AND RESOLUTIONS CHAIRMAN—Mrs. John F. Kuhn, Jr., Oklahoma City.

REPORT OF NOMINATING COMMITTEE—Mrs. W. R. Cheatwood, President-Elect of the Woman's Auxiliary to the Oklahoma State Medical Association.

MEMORIAL SERVICE—Mrs. George H. Garrison, Oklahoma City. Music—Mrs. Gerald Bednar, Oklahoma City, Okla.

ANNOUNCEMENTS—Mrs. Elias Margo, Convention Chairman.

1:00 p.m.—LUNCHEON—Style Show by Al Rosenthal's, Crystal and Balinese Rooms, Skirvin Hotel. Mrs. Howard B. Shorbe, President, Woman's Auxiliary to the Oklahoma County Medical Society, presiding.

INVOCATION—Mrs. James McMurry, Oklahoma City, Okla.

TUESDAY, MAY 11, 1954

THEME: *Together We Progress*

9:00 a.m. to 1:00 p.m.—REGISTRATION—Mezzanine Floor, Skirvin Hotel

INFORMATION—Mezzanine Floor, Skirvin Hotel

10:00 a.m.—GENERAL MEETING—Mrs. Millard L. Henry, Presiding. Continental Room, Skirvin Hotel

CALL TO ORDER—by President

INVOCATION—Mrs. I. F. Stevenson, Alva

REPORT OF CREDENTIALS—Mrs. P. K. Graening, Oklahoma City

ROLL CALL OF VOTING DELEGATES—Mrs. John A. Cunningham

GUEST SPEAKER—Mrs. George Turner, El Paso, President-Elect of Woman's Auxiliary to the American Medical Association. ADDRESS—

RESOLUTIONS—Mrs. John F. Kuhn, Jr., Oklahoma City

UNFINISHED BUSINESS

NEW BUSINESS

GUEST SPEAKER—John E. McDonald, M.D., Tulsa, President of the Oklahoma State Medical Association. ADDRESS—*Veterans Medical Care* ELECTION OF OFFICERS AND DELEGATES REPORT OF FINANCE AND BUDGET CHAIRMAN—Mrs. George Bozalis, Oklahoma City

INSTALLATION OF OFFICERS—Mrs. Clinton Gallaher, Shawnee

1:00 p.m.—LUNCHEON—Regency Room, Skirvin Hotel

BOARD MEETING—Mrs. W. R. Cheatwood, President, Presiding. Post Convention School of Instruction including all State Officers, Chairmen of Committees, Council Women, County Presidents, Presidents-Elect, Members and Guests.

6:00 p.m. to 1:00 a.m.—ANNUAL PRESIDENT'S INAUGURAL DINNER-DANCE — Social Hour, Dinner and Dance, Persian Room, Skirvin Tower Hotel. Dick Jurgen's Orchestra will play for the dance.

Scientific Exhibits

The following Scientific Exhibits will be on display in the Zebra Room of the Municipal Auditorium Monday and Tuesday, May 10 and 11, from 9:00 a.m. to 5:00 p.m. and until noon Wednesday, May 12.

AMERICAN CANCER SOCIETY, OKLAHOMA DIVISION
Oklahoma City

"Recent Advances in the Treatment of Lung Cancer"

This exhibit, which was produced by the American Cancer Society and the Memorial Cancer Center, graphically outlines some of the newer diagnostic methods including exfoliative cytology, as well as indicating various types of treatment which are now in use in many institutions — surgery, radiotherapy, including the betatron and million volt x-ray machine, chemotherapy, etc. It also includes a number of investigative trends which are currently under study as a solution to this problem.

AMERICAN COLLEGE OF APOTHECARIES
Oklahoma City

An exhibit depicting pharmacy's part in the defense of pain, disease and death.

SIMON DOLIN, M. D. AND PETER E. RUSSO, M. D.
Oklahoma City

"Angiocardiography in Congential Malformations of the Heart and Great Vessels Amenable to Surgical Correction"

Serial Roentgenograms of congenital malformations of the heart amenable to surgical correction with brief clinical histories and drawings, as well as explanation of the radiographic features will be presented. All cases have been proved and operated. Some of the cases also have cardiac cathertization findings.

S. M. GLASSER, M. D.
Oklahoma City

"Uncommon Lesions of the G. I. Tract"

Exhibit is a collection of several of the more uncommon conditions which involve the esophagus, stomach, small and large bowel as demonstrated in the roentgenograms of patients admitted to the general medical and surgical services of the V. A. Hospital.

HOWARD C. HOPPS, M. D., HARRY WILKINS, M. D. AND WALTER JOEL, M. D.
Oklahoma City

'Pathology of Central Nervous System Disease Including Brain Tumors"

Selected gross specimens illustrating pathologic processes in the brain will be arranged in specially designed cases. This will be supplemented by descriptive data which will include history, physical findings, pertinent laboratory information, and, in some-instances, a brief description of the histopathology. In addition, arranged on special transilluminated panels there will be presented large (macro) sections of selected central nervous system lesions which can be viewed to advantage with hand lenses, which will be part of the exhibit.

JAMES W. KELLEY, M. D.
Tulsa

"Nasal Deformities"

Preoperative and postoperative photographs of cases illustrating different types of nasal deformities with short accompanying legends explaining the correction will be shown.

GEORGE H. KIMBALL, M. D.

"Plastic and Reconstructive Surgery"

Photographs and colored slides will be shown.

GILBERT HYROOP, M. D.
Oklahoma City

"Plastic Surgery and Hand Surgery"

Photographs before and after surgery will be exhibited.

LAWRENCE McHENRY AND MARY ELLEN HARPER

"Great Men in the History of Medicine, an Exhibit of Sculpturing by Doris Appel"

This is an exhibit of busts and plaques of great physicians throughout the ages from Imhotep to Osler created by the medical sculptress, Doris Appel of Lynn, Mass.

NATIONAL FOUNDATION FOR INFANTILE PARALYSIS
New York City

"Definitive and Differential Diagnosis of Poliomyelitis"

The exhibit presents pertinent data on the symptomology, muscles and nerves most frequently involved, traumatizing factors, the physical examination and clinical laboratory findings which contribute to making a diagnosis of poliomyelitis.

OKLAHOMA ASSOCIATION FOR MENTAL HEALTH, INC.
Oklahoma City
"The Nation's Number 1 Health Problem"

A large, colorful exhibit with flashing lights created to attract persons to read the facts about mental illness and the answer such as more guidance services, hospital treatment, education, etc.

OKLAHOMA SOCIETY OF ANESTHESIOLOGISTS
Oklahoma City
"Airway Management of the Unconscious Patient"

Management of the airway of the unconscious patient will be discussed and a demonstration of techniques used will be illustrated.

OKLAHOMA SOCIETY OF MEDICAL TECHNOLOGISTS
Oklahoma City
"Medical Technology"

Exhibit will consist of material in printed form containing information concerning requirements and training of medical technologists as well as information on various phases of work done by medical technologists. A registered medical technologist will be at the booth at all times to answer questions.

OKLAHOMA STATE HEART ASSOCIATION
Oklahoma City
"Heart Research and Diagnostic Procedures"

An exhibit of the use of the Ultracentrifuge in various phases of lipid metabolism and showing the use of cardiac catherization in diagnosis and congential cardiac disorders will be presented.

AVERILL STOWELL, M. D.
Tulsa
"Whip-lash Injuries of the Neck"

Exhibit will consist of x-rays and posters.

HENRY H. TURNER, M. D.
Oklahoma City
"Endrocrine Disorders of Growth and Development"

This exhibit is composed of photographs of patients with various types of endocrine disorders affecting growth and development. All have adequate legends and many illustrate results of therapy.

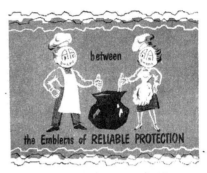
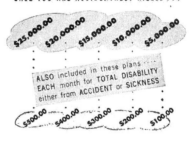

Related Meetings

Technologists To Meet

Miss Wanda Echols, University of Oklahoma, 1950, will speak at the annual convention of the Oklahoma Society of Medical Technologists. She will talk on microchemistry technics in clinical laboratory work. The convention will be held May 1 and 2 in Oklahoma City.

State Diabetes Association

A meeting of the Oklahoma State Diabetes Association will be held during the O. S. M. A. Annual Meeting. A social hour, dinner and panel discussion on "What's New in the Treatment of Diabetes" is planned for Monday night, May 10 at the Biltmore Hotel. The social hour is scheduled for 6:30 with the dinner to begin at 7:15. Advance reservations may be made with R. C. Lawson, M. D., Secretary, 301 N. W. 12th St., Oklahoma City; or Kelly West, M. D., Program Chairman, 1200 N. Walker, Oklahoma City. All physicians interested in diabetes are invited to attend whether they are members of the Diabetes Association or not.

Reunion For Class of '44

The University of Oklahoma School of Medicine graduating class of 1944 will hold its 10 year reunion Monday night, May 10, at Twin Hills Country Club.

A social hour, dinner, dance, and old class movies are planned for those who attend. Price is $10.00 per person. Transportation will be arranged for all who need it.

Reservations can be made with Robert J. Morgan, M. D., 216 Pasteur Building, 1111 North Lee, Oklahoma City. When making reservations, it is requested that the following information be given: permanent address (home and office), names of spouse and children.

Oklahoma Arthritis and Rheumatism Foundation

Complete program has been announced for the Oklahoma Arthritis and Rheumatism Foundation which will meet Sunday, May 9 at the Biltmore Hotel. Advance reservations may be made by writing J. N. Owens, Jr., M. D., Secretary, 605 N. W. 10th, Oklahoma City. Program is as follows:

8:30 a.m. Registration — North Lounge, Biltmore Hotel

9:30 a.m. Business Meeting

10:00 a.m. Movie on the Use of Compound F in Joints

10:15 a.m. Symposium on Hip Disease
Medical Aspects — W. K. Ishmael, M. D., Oklahoma City
Surgical Aspects—Earl D. McBride, M. D., Oklahoma City
Physical Medicine — John W. Deyton, M. D., Okmulgee

11:20 a.m. "Non-Articular Rheumatism" Richard Smith, M. D., Philadelphia

12:15 p.m. Luncheon with Question and Answer Period—Doctor Smith

1:30 p.m. "Rehabilitation of the Hand" S. Y. Andelman, M. D., Tulsa

2:00 "Lupus Erythematosus"
Medical Aspects — Richard W. Payne, M. D., Oklahoma City
Pathology—J. N. Owens, Jr., M. D., Oklahoma City

2:30 p.m. Roundtable Discussion on Current Treatment of Fiber Collagen Disease"
Richard Payne, M. D., Moderator
Participants — Richard Smith, M. D.
A. A. Hellbaum, M. D.
E. Goldfain, M. D.
S. Y. Andelman, M. D.
W. K. Ishmael, M. D.

Oklahoma State Dermatological Association Announce Meeting

Dermatologists from Oklahoma, Texas and Kansas are invited to attend the meeting of the Oklahoma State Dermatological Association scheduled for 10:00 a. m., Sunday, May 9 at University Hospital, Oklahoma City.

The clinical session will feature presentation and discussion of cases. There will be a luncheon following the clinical session. Earl D. Osborn, M. D., Buffalo, N. Y., O. S. M. A. guest speaker, will be a guest and participate in the discussions. For further information contact William G. McCreight, M. D., 525 N. W. 11th, Oklahoma City, Secretary of the group.

Society of Anesthesiologists

The Oklahoma Society of Anesthesiologists will meet Sunday, May 9, at the Oklahoma Club. Reservations may be made by writing the secretary, Betty Bamforth, M. D., University Hospital, 800 N. E. 13th St., Oklahoma City. The scientific program will begin at 10:00 a.m. and a luncheon is planned for 12:30.

Guest speaker will be Virginia Apgar, M. D., New York, who will discuss "'Management of Anesthetic Emergencies" and "Anesthetic Aspects of Cardiac Surgery."

State Radiological Society

The Oklahoma State Radiological Society will meet Sunday, May 9, at 2:30 p.m. at Wesley Hospital, 300 N. W. 12th St., Oklahoma City. C. Allen Good, M. D., an OSMA guest speaker, will be the speaker. Election of officers will be held and a dinner and social hour will be held in the evening with the time and place to be announced later. John R. Danstrom, M. D., Medical Arts Building, Oklahoma City, is Secretary of the group.

Society of Neurologists And Psychiatrists

The annual meeting for the election of officers and scientific program of the Society of Neurologists and Psychiatrists will be held Sunday, May 9, at the Oklahoma Club, Oklahoma City, beginning at 2:00 p.m. The busi-

ness meeting will be held in the afternoon and a dinner with guest speaker will be held Sunday night. For further information, please contact A. A. Hellams, M.D., President, 1200 N. Walker, Oklahoma City; or Charles A. Smith, M.D., Secretary, Lockett Hotel, Norman.

Special Memberships

LIFE MEMBERSHIP

Petition for Life Membership have been filed in the Executive Office for the following and the Council recommends their approval by the House of Delegates:

Lin Alexander, M. D._____Okmulgee
H. A. Angus, M. D._____Lawton
E. R. Barker, M. D._____Healdton
Charles E. Calhoun, M. D.____Sand Springs
Roy F. Cannon, M. D._____Miami
Samuel C. Dean, M. D._____Howe
Paul Grosshart, M. D._____Tulsa
Edgar Frank Harbison, M. D.____Okla. City
Bunn Harris, M. D._____Jenks
John Evans Heatley, M. D._____Okla. City
A. E. Hennings, M. D._____Tuttle
Clarence C. Hoke, M. D._____Tulsa
E. F. Hurlbut, M. D._____Meeker
H. L. Johnson, M. D._____Woodward
Powell K. Lewis, M. D._____Stillwater
W. T. Mayfield, M. D._____Norman
James W. Rogers, M. D._____Tulsa
R. E. Sawyer, M. D._____Durant
Harry A. Stalker, M. D._____Pond Creek
William J. Trainor, M. D._____Tulsa
I. D. Walker, M. D._____Tonkawa
J. Clay Williams, M. D._____Durant
Divonis Worten, M. D._____Pawhuska

HONORARY MEMBERSHIP

Petition for Honorary Membership has been filed in the Executive Office for the following and the Council recommends its approval by the House of Delegates:

George H. Niemann, M. D., Ponca City

ASSOCIATE MEMBERSHIP

Petitions for Associate Membership have been filed in the Executive Office for the following and the Council recommends their approval by the House of Delegates:

Louis Lipnick_____Muskogee
Thomas Worobec_____Shawnee

OKLAHOMA STATE MEDICAL ASSISTANTS SOCIETY

Biltmore Hotel, Oklahoma City

Friday Evening, May 7

7:00 p.m. Board of Directors Meeting

8:00 p.m. Reception honoring out of town guests

Saturday Morning, May 8

9:00 a.m. Registration—South Alcove, Lobby

10:00 a.m. Call to Order—East Room—Bobbie Antrim, State President

10:10 a.m. Official Welcome—Mr. Dick Graham, Executive Secretary, Oklahoma State Medical Association

10:20 a.m. Response

10:30 a.m. Personality Improvements for the Medical Assistant—Nelleta Cooper, Personal Relations Counselor

11:15 a.m. Business Session—Minutes, Treasurer's Report, Officers and Committee Chairmen Reports, Registration Report, and Announcements

12:00 Noon Luncheon — President's Room, Oklahoma Club, 202 West Grand

Saturday Afternoon, May 8

1:30 p.m. Call to Order—East Room, Roll Call by Counties, Minutes of Previous Session, Jeanne O'Dell, Bartlesville, Okla.

2:15 p.m. Election of Officers—Nell Pulver, Oklahoma City, Parliamentarian
County Reports
Business Session

3:00 p.m. Barco Uniform Style Show—John A. Brown Co., Sponsor

Saturday Evening, May 8

6:00 p.m. Convivial Hour

7:00 p.m. Dinner—Civic Room

7:30 p.m. Invocation—W e l c o m e, Introduction of Guests, Officers; Ruby Kemp, Guthrie, Convention Chairman

7:40 p.m. Response — S. Fulton Tompkins, M.D., Oklahoma County Medical Advisor

8:00 p.m. Guest Speaker—Mr. Steven T. Donohue, Assistant Director Public Relations, American Medical Association, Chicago

8:30 p.m. Eccentric Operations—"Dr. Wizard and His Musical Assistant"

9:00 p.m. to 12:30 a.m. Dancing—Wynn Myers, and the Stardusters, Civic Room

Sunday Morning, May 9

9:00 a.m. Coffee Hour—Biltmore Hotel

9:45 a.m. Call to Order, Invocation—West Lounge, Katherine Kroeger, Guthrie

10:15 a.m. Presentation of State Project Contribution to Medical Research Foundation—Florence Witt, Stillwater, State Project Chairman

10:20 a.m. Acceptance—Mr. Gene White, Coordinator Public Relations, Oklahoma Medical Research Foundation

10:40 a.m. "Christ the Physician"—Msgr. John Mason Connor, Cathedral of Our Lady of Perpetual Help, Oklahoma City

11:30 a.m. Installation of Officers — Bobbie Antrim, President

12:00 noon—Buffet, Civic Room

12:30 p.m. Blue Cross Highlights—Miss Velma Neely

Sunday Afternoon, May 9

1:15 p.m. Call to Order—Invocation, West Lounge
Address and Appointments, New President

1:30 p.m. "The Inside Story" or "You and Your Ulcer" —Turner Bynum, M.D., Oklahoma City

2:15 p.m. Final Business Session
Invitation of 1955 Convention
Adjourn

For information regarding reservations, fees, etc., please contact Convention Co-Chairmen: Bobbie Antrim, 437 N.W. 12, Oklahoma City or Ruby Kemp, 523 E. Warner, Guthrie.

Registration fee $6.00. Not limited to members—guests welcome.

Telephone Call Center At Annual Meeting

A complete message center service will be provided for your convenience at the State Medical Association Annual Meeting May 9-12. This service will handle your incoming calls and every effort will be made to locate you as rapidly as possible upon receipt of a call. This service will also assist you in locating other registered members and guests.

Soon you will receive a fold card for use in your office giving the telephone numbers of the message center. This message center is a service of the Oklahoma City Chapter of the Medical Service Society.

Commercial Exhibits

A. S. ALOE COMPANY
St. Louis, Misouri
Booth 13

Visit Booth 13 where the Aloe representatives will show you a cross section of the complete line of physicians' equipment and supplies carried by the A. S. Aloe Company. Highlighted will be New Model Steeline — tomorrow's treatment room furniture today — featuring the body contour table top, magnetic door catches, and advanced design, all in new decorators' colors. Our representatives will be William R. Jones and William L. Edelen.

AMES COMPANY, INC.
Elkhart, Indiana
Booth 30

CLINITEST, for urine sugar, is standardized. This assures uniformly reliable results whenever and wherever a test is performed — office, ward, clinic or patient's home. Standardization not only curtails error, but saves personnel's time by elimination of preparing and mixing of reagents.

ACETEST for Acetonuria, BUMINTEST for Albuminaturia, HEMATEST for occult blood, and ICTOTEST for Bilirubin will also be on display. Representatives at our booth will be Robert W. Dafforn, Edwin J. Rohan, and William N. Sallee.

AYERST LABORATORIES
New York, New York
Booth 61

Physicians attending the Oklahoma State Medical Association meeting are cordially invited to visit the Ayerst Laboratories booth where you will receive a warm welcome. Our representatives, V. Van Franklin Jr., Charles R. Dinehart, and Elmer C. Trueblood, will be present to answer any questions you may have relative to 'Premarin", Trilene", Mediatric" or any other product in our line of prescription specialties.

THE BAKER COMPANY—
AUDOGRAPH DISTRIBUTORS
Oklahoma City, Oklahoma
Booth 60

Showing three complete systems for office dictation. The Audograph individual units, the automatic PhonAudograph for remote dictation by special built telephone sets and the automatic PhonAudograph for remote dictation by special built telephone sets and offices using telephone in the same manner, as the automatic PhonAudograph. You owe yourself the finest — Gray Audograph. Representatives at the booth will be C. E. Barrett, W. G. Dinsmore, H. H. Hill, Delbert Cooper, and J. Roy.

BELTONE HEARING SERVICE
Oklahoma City, Oklahoma
Booth 26

The BELTONE HEARING SERVICE exhibits a complete range of Beltone Hearing Aids designed to fit almost every need for better hearing. The new, all-transistor aid — the Concerto, climax of BELTONE'S quality aids — is demonstrated to the medical profession. With the increased interest of many physicians in the problems of the hard of hearing, BELTONE is proud to demonstrate the physician's choice of hearing test instruments — ADC Diagnostic Audiometer. With the ADC Audiometer, a complete hearing analysis of your patient can be easily and quickly made by you or your staff. Our representatives will be Walter L. Metcalfe and Robert L. Millier.

BLUE CROSS AND BLUE SHIELD
Tulsa, Oklahoma
Booth 59

Our exhibit will illustrate the functions and activities of Blue Cross and Blue Shield in the State of Oklahoma with particular emphasis on physician relations. Representatives in charge of our booth will be Velma Neely and Jim Dennis.

GEORGE A. BREON & COMPANY
New York, New York
Booth 41

George A. Brown & Co., distributors of Lanteen products, invites convention members to their exhibit of reproductions of well-known paintings by famous European artists at Booth 41 Lithographic prints of these beautiful paintings are available upon request. Representatives will also be happy to discuss Lanteen products with visiting members. Bob McKanna and Ken Shaw will be our representatives.

CARNATION COMPANY
Los Angeles, California
Booth 55

You are invited to visit Booth No. 55 where you will see an attractive display on Carnation Evaporated Milk — 'The Milk Every Doctor Knows.' Some valuable information on the use of this milk for infant feeding, child feeding and general diet will be explained and the reasons why Carnation Milk deserves consideration as your first choice for infant formulas. Interesting and valuable literature will also be available for you. Our representatives will be D. C. Earnest, W. J. Miller, W. R. Wooten, and C. M. Dietz.

CARROL DUNHAM SMITH PHARMACAL COMPANY
New Brunswick, New Jersey
Booth 22

Our exhibit will feature Lipotriad (Smith) a new unusually potent lipotropic and oxytropic product, in both liquid and capsule form for the treatment of many conditions associated with faulty fat metabolism. Our representatives, T. R. Mafit and George W. Griffin, will also welcome the oportunity to discuss Calferbee, Hemo-Vitol, Neo-Sedaphen and other specialties.

CIBA PHARMACEUTICAL PRODUCTS, INC.
Summit, New Jersey
Booth 64

The Ciba exhibit will feature SERPASIL, a pure crystalline alkaloid of Rauwolfia which usually produces mild, gradual sustained lowering of blood pressure with a slowing of the pulse rate. Representatives in charge, W. L. Williams, C. J. Wise, and J. C. Dorsey, will be pleased to discuss the role of SERPASIL in the treatment of hypertension and to furnish literature on this new drug.

OKLAHOMA COCA-COLA BOTTLING CO.
Oklahoma City, Oklahoma
Booth 19

The exhibit will consist of a bamboo type back-bar and counter with a Coca-Cola trademark and the phrase "Drink Coca-Cola with our compliments". There will be attendants present to serve free Coca-Cola to all delegates. Our representatives will be Tom Bogart, Kerney Tunnell and Mel Rathert.

CONNIE'S PRESCRIPTION SHOP, INC.
Oklahoma City, Oklahoma
Booth 36

Our booth will be a goodwill booth. We shall have some special items and merchandise on display, and shall have matches, pencils, emery boards, etc., for the doctors and visitors. Our representatives will be C. J. 'Connie" Masterson, Juanita Mosley, and Wanda Burford.

CREDIT SERVICE
Oklahoma City, Oklahoma
Booth 48

Credit Service is an organization designed to furnish credit information and collection assistance to the professional men and commercial interests of the state. The management of this organization is giving to our clientele, thirty-seven years of credit and collection experience. We are members of the national association of Medical-Dental Bureaus, and we are bonded through our membership in the American Collectors Association, Incorporated; a world wide service. Collections are made as quickly as possible and remittances are mailed from our office before the end of each month. Each employee is personally trained and supervised in the handling of professional accounts. Our organization is the oldest and largest of its kind in the Southwest. Representatives at the booth will be Robert R. Sesline, Robert F. Hughes, and Harold Fudge.

DICTAPHONE CORPORATION
Oklahoma City, Oklahoma
Booth 43

Office Dictating and Transcribing Machines. Revolutionary new Dictaphone Time-Master Models. Telecord Network dictation system. Combination machines especially designed for busy doctors. Our representatives will be Bob Simpson, Carl Fairchild, Don Hagan, and M. P. Garner.

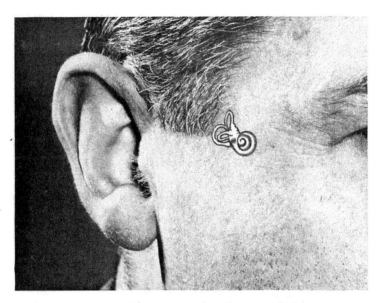

Through its probable action on the labyrinth,
dependable control of vertigo and nausea has made
Dramamine the most widely-prescribed product in its field.

Vertigo: The Labyrinthine Structure and Dramamine®

Dramamine's remarkable therapeutic efficiency is believed to be the result of suppression of the over-stimulated labyrinth. Thus it prevents the resulting symptom complex of vertigo, nausea and, finally, vomiting.

First known for its value in motion sickness, Dramamine is widely prescribed for nausea and vomiting of pregnancy, electroshock therapy, certain drugs and narcotization. It relieves vertigo of Ménière's syndrome, fenestration procedures, labyrinthitis, hypertensive disease and that accompanying radiation and antibiotic therapy.

A most impressive number of clinical studies shows that Dramamine has a high therapeutic index and minimal side actions. Drowsiness is possible in some patients but in many instances this side action is not undesirable.

Dramamine (brand of dimenhydrinate) is available in tablets of 50 mg. each; liquid containing 12.5 mg. per 4 cc. Dramamine is accepted by the Council on Pharmacy and Chemistry of the American Medical Association. G. D. Searle & Co., Research in the Service of Medicine.

DOHO CHEMICAL CORPORATION
Franklin Park, Illinois
Booth 24

Doho Chemical Corporation is pleased to exhibit: AURALGAN, the ear medication for the relief of pain in Otitis Media and removal of Cerumen; NEW OTOSMOSAN, the effective, non-toxic ear medication which is Fungicidal and Bactericidal (gram negative-gram positive) in the suppurative and aural dermatomycotic ears; RHINALGAN, the nasal decongestant which is free from systemic or circulatory effect and equally safe to use on infants as well as the aged. Mallon Chemical Corporation, Subsidiary of the Doho Chemical Corporation, is also featuring: RECTALGAN, the liquid topical anesthesia, also for relief of pain and discomfort in hemorrhoids, pruritus and perineal suturing. Louis C. Cassell will be the DOHO representative.

H. G. FISCHER & COMPANY
Franklin Park, Illinois
Booth 24

Latest models of Modern X-ray, F.C.C. approved Physical Medicine and Rehabilitation Equipment all of highest quality materials and construction, will be on display. Representatives in attendance will welcome an opportunity to give demonstrations and quote todays low prices. Your visit will be appreciated.

L. A. Melanson will be in charge of our booth.

FLINT, EATON & COMPANY
Decatur, Illinois
Booth 45

Ferrolip — a new organic choline complex of iron is on display. This new iron complex will not precipitate protein, is not astringent, and thus avoids gastrointestinal irritation. This new iron complex is soluble in acid and alkaline media and available for absorption through the entire pH range of the gastrointestinal tract. Representatives of the company who will be at the booth are Richard Carruthers, and John Hale.

GENERAL ELECTRIC COMPANY, X-RAY DEPARTMENT
Oklahoma City, Oklahoma
Booth 49

Displaying the new type DWB CARDIOSCRIBE and the new improved type IN-

DUCTOTHERM, together with a complete line of X-Ray supplies and Accessories. Our representatives will be C. A. Bohan, J. O. Jones, V. R. Troop, E. R. Rector, and G. L. Shirk.

GREB X-RAY COMPANY
Oklahoma City, Oklahoma
Booth 32

Exclusive Picker X-Ray Accessory Items. Representatives of the company who will be in the booth are Rodney D. Smith, John M. Miller, Glenn F. Conger, and Robert E. Miller.

HOLLAND-RANTOS COMPANY, INC.
New York, New York
Booth 42

Physicians interested in Medical Contraception are cordially invited to discuss with H-R convention representatives, Charles S. Donahue and James M. Zipen, the latest information on new clinical and laboratory data concerning the efficacy of KOROMEX products.

R. P. KINCHELOE COMPANY
Oklahoma City, Oklahoma
Booth 27

The R. P. Kincheloe Company of Oklahoma, Louisiana and Texas will display Keleket X-ray Apparatus, Liebel-Flarsheime Diathermy Units, and Cambridge Eletrocardiograph. Our representatives will be H. H. Kirby, F. W. Kirbey and R. P. Kincheloe, Jr.

ELI LILLY AND COMPANY
Indianapolis, Indiana
Booth 62

You are cordially invited to visit the Lilly exhibit located in space number 62. The display will contain information on recent therapeutic developments and will feature the story of the Lilly Junior Taste Panel. Lilly sales people, W. N. Burks, Bert Tunnell, and E. W. Griffith, will be in attendance. They welcome your questions about 'Ilotycin' (Erythromycin, Lilly) and other Lilly products.

J. B. LIPPINCOTT COMPANY
Philadelphia, Pennsylvania
Booth 15

J. B. Lippincott Company presents, for your approval, a display of professional books and journals geared to the latest and

most important trends in current medicine and surgery. These publications, written and edited by men active in clinical fields and teaching, are a continuation of more than 100 years of traditionally significant publishing. J. L. Rosencrants will represent the company at our booth.

J. A. MAJORS COMPANY
(W. B. SAUNDERS COMPANY)
New Orleans, Louisiana
Booth 53

The W. B. SAUNDERS COMPANY, Medical Publishers of Philadelphia, represented by their Southern Agents, J. A. MAJORS COMPANY, will occupy Space No. 53 at the State Meeting. The doctors attending the meeting will find many new works on display, namely Conn's "Current Therapy 1954"; Mayo Clinic Volume 1953; Gross' "Surgery of Infancy and Childhood"; Bakwin & Bakwin "Clinical Management of Behavior Disorders in Children"; Haymaker's "Peripheral Nerve Injuries"; Sweet's "Thoracic Surgery", 2nd edition; Conant and others "Clinical Mycology", 2nd edition, and many others. Representatives at the booth will be J. Speight and B. J. McClendon.

THE S. E. MASSENGILL COMPANY
Bristol, Tennessee
Booth 10

You are invited to visit the S. E. Massengill Company booth. Adrenosem, the new Massengill systemic hemostatic, is featured. Adrenosem is a specific in treating those conditions characterized by increased capillary permeability. Our representatives, J. L. Hedges, Casey O'Dell and R. N. Ross, will be glad to discuss with you the latest information and clinical evaluation of this product.

MEAD JOHNSON AND COMPANY
Evansville, Indiana
Booth 34

Mead Johnson & Company Booth No. 34 will feature Lactum, Mead's liquid formula for infant feeding; Poly-Vi-Sol and Tri-Vi-Sol, superior vitamin supplements for infants; Panalins and Panalins-T, new vitamin capsule based on the new National Research Council's recommendations for vitamin maintenance and therapy. Natalins, the smaller, complete prenatal capsules and Mul-

cin, the new orange flavored vitamin liquid, will also be shown. In charge of the booth will be J. D. Parks.

MEDCO PRODUCTS COMPANY
Tulsa, Oklahoma
Booth 52

The MEDCOLATOR Stimulatorm for the stimulation of innervated muscle or muscle groups ancillary to treatment by massage, is a low volt generator that will generate plenty of your interest. Electrical muscle stimulation is a valuable form of rehabilitation therapy. Be sure to visit our booth for a personal demonstration. Mark E. DeGroff will be in charge of our booth.

MEDICAL AIDS, INC.
Chicago, Illinois
Booth 44

Medical Aids, Incorporated will feature a complete line of pressure bandages, including the well-known Dalzoflex and Primer Combination, recommended in the treatment of Varicose Ulcers, Phlebitis, etc. The Nulast elastic crepe bandage, constructed of Viscolax Rubber Threads, Dalmas Elastic Strapping, which is waterproof, oil and grease resistant and Dalmaplast Plastic Adhesive Strapping. Our representatives will be S. V. Bentley, and D. C. McLintock.

MELTON COMPANY, INC.
Oklahoma City, Oklahoma
Booth 25 & B

MELTON COMPANY will exhibit the new popular priced ABCO line, Welch Allyn Headlight, Burdick EKG, Cardiall EKG, Raytheon Microtherm and many more popular and new items that will be interesting to the doctors visiting this Oklahoma State Medical Association Meeting. Representatives at the booth will be J. B. Dixon, Tom Brennan, Bill Hughes, Joe Snider, B. B. Benson, and Bill Jones.

MIDWESTERN ADJUSTMENT CO., INC.
Oklahoma City, Oklahoma
Booth 3

Our exhibit will consist of photostatic copies of out statements and checks. We will also have a small man who is supposed to be casting a fishing line to not let the delinquent accounts get away from him. We will have literature to pass out to the doctors who attend the meeting. C. Bill Davis will be in charge of our booth.

NATIONAL DRUG COMPANY
Philadelphia, Pennsylvania
Booth 37

The National Drug Company cordially invites you to visit their booth. Dimethylane and Rau-Vertin, two products recently developed by the Company's Research Laboratories, will be featured. Displayed along with these new products will be Resion, AVC Improved, Hesperidin-C and Protinal Powder. Dimethylane is a new nontoxic relaxant which gives prompt relief from anxiety tension states. Rau-Vertin provides effective oral therapy for hypertension, capable of producing a significant lowering of high blood pressure and of maintaining it at the lowered level. Our representatives, C. M. Kelly and Jeff W. Chalmers will attend at our booth.

OKLAHOMA PHYSICIANS SUPPLY, INC.
Oklahoma City, Oklahoma
Booth 31

The Oklahoma Physicians Supply will display in its booth at the Oklahoma State Medical Association's Annual Meeting many of the routine items used in the physicians office. It also intends to show the new Ultrasonic machine developed by the Birtcher Manufacturing Company. Another piece of equipment which should be of special interest to the doctors that will be shown is the Vibrabath which we feel is the latest thing in inexpensive hydro-therapy massage. Those in charge of the booth will be Ray W. Broadfoot, Fulsom Scott, L. A. Wamsley, O. B. Bradshaw, Fred Schrandt, and Clifford Arney.

ORTHO PHARMACEUTICAL CORP.
Raritan, New Jersey
Booth 58

ORTHO cordially invites you to booth 58. Featured will be their product for conception control, PRECEPTIN℞ vaginal gel, designed for use without a vaginal diaphragm. Preceptin vaginal gel has achieved an outstanding record of clinical effectiveness and has been widely acclaimed by the medical profession. Your inquiries on Preception vaginal gel are invited. Our representatives will be Noble S. Birkett, and Jesse C. Mayfield.

PARKE, DAVIS & COMPANY
Detroit, Michigan
Booth 65

Medical service members of our staff will be in attendance at our exhibit for consultation and discussion of various products of particular interest to members of the Association. Important specialties, such as Milontin, Amphedase, Benadryl, Penicillin S-R, Ambodryl, Dilantin Suspension, Vitamins, Oxycel, Thrombin Topical, etc., will be featured. You are cordially invited to visit our exhibit. Representatives at our booth will be S. N. Downs and D. L. Porter.

PET MILK COMPANY
St. Louis, Missouri
Booth 29

Specially trained representatives will be in attendance to discuss the use of Pet Evaporated Milk in infant feeding and Pet Nonfat Dry Milk for high protein diets. A variety of services that are time-savers for busy physicians will be furnished on request. Miniature Pet Milk cans will be given to visitors at the exhibit. In charge of the both will be A. E. Besch, Jr., and R. L. Miller.

PFIZER LABORATORIES
Brooklyn, New York
Booth 50

Bothered by motion-sickness? Stop by for your homeward-bound supply of new Bonamine. Our exhibit includes Cortril, the anti-inflammatory hormone, and other Pfizer-Syntex steroids; Terramycin in a variety of practical dosage forms; and many other items from the world's largest producers of antibiotics. Our representatives will be George Lane, Arnold Belding and Murl Nance.

R. J. REYNOLDS TOBACCO COMPANY
Winston-Salem, North Carolina
Booth 16

Welcome to the CAMEL-CAVALIER Exhibit! You are cordially invited to receive a cigarette case (monogrammed with your initials) containing your choice of CAMELS, America's most popular cigarette, or CAVALIERS the king size cigarette of extra mildness and distinctive flavor.

Representatives at the CAMEL-CAVALIER booth will be J. W. McDowell and J. W. White.

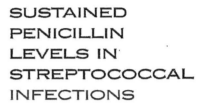

SUSTAINED PENICILLIN LEVELS IN STREPTOCOCCAL INFECTIONS

"... it has been shown that the treatment of streptococcic infections by adequate amounts of penicillin will prevent rheumatic fever ... On the basis of our experience, we feel that BICILLIN for injection more nearly supplies the need than any other product available at present."[1]

"Following the injection of 600,000 units of this drug in aqueous suspension, 100 per cent of ambulatory adult males show blood concentrations of 0.105 to approximately 0.03 unit per ml. for 10 days, and about 50 per cent of these subjects maintain demonstrable concentrations for 14 days ... The development of BICILLIN is one of the important milestones in antibiotic therapy."[2]

"The demonstration of detectable amounts of penicillin in the serum of most patients for four weeks following the administration of 1,250,000 units of BICILLIN suggests the feasibility of maintaining continuous drug prophylaxis against recurrences [of rheumatic fever] by administration of single monthly intramuscular injections."[3]

BICILLIN *is available in oral suspension, tablet, and injectable forms*

1. Breese, B. B.: J.A.M.A. *152*:10 (May 2) 1953
2. Welch, H.: Antibiot. & Chemo. *3*:347 (April) 1953
3. Stollerman, G. H., and Rusoff, J. H.: J.A.M.A. *150*:1571 (Dec. 20) 1952

BICILLIN ®

Benzathine Penicillin G
Dibenzylethylenediamine Dipenicillin G

Streptococcus haemolyticus.
Right: *Electron micrograph (from Mudd, S., and Lackman, D. B.: J. Bacteriol., Williams & Wilkins Co.).* Above: *Blood-agar plate, showing hemolysis.*

Philadelphia 2, Pa.

PIED PIPER SHOE COMPANY
Wausau, Wisconsin
Booth 47

Shoes and lasts (corrective and regular) from Pied Piper will be on display. Our representatives will be Jake Owen, Della M. Harrold, Cinnie Bell Oldfield, and Frances Wiggins.

A. H. ROBINS COMPANY, INC.
Richmond, Virginia
Booth 51

ENTOZYME, comprehensive digestant; ROBALATE, antacid-demulcent; and DONNALATE, combining Robalate with Donnatal formula; are featured at the A. H. Robins exhibit. Also shown are PABALATE, PABALATE-SODIUM FREE AND ALL-BEE with C. Robins' representatives welcome the opportunity to discuss with physicians the therapeutic advantages of these and other Robins prescription specialties. Our representatives will be Ellsworth Draper and C. D. Wheeler.

J. B. ROERIG & COMPANY
Chicago, Illinois
Booth 20

Attending physicians are cordially invited to visit the J. B. Roerig and Company exhibit booth No. 20 where information is available on Tetracyn the newest broad spectrum antibiotic. Professional Service Representatives will be glad to supply samples, literature and clinical data on the efficacy of this basic antibiotic which can make your patient afebrile in hours, in the great variety of infections caused by a wide range of microbial invaders. Information, samples and literature will also be available on our well known nutritional products, such as Viterra, Viterra Therapeutic, Heptuna Plus, Amplus, Obron, Obron Hematinic, etc. Our representatives will be Jim Southerland, C. K. Dougherty, C. E. Seitz, and Bob Riley.

LESTER J. SABOLICH ORTHOPEDIC APPLIANCE COMPANY
Oklahoma City, Oklahoma
Booth 46

Artificial limbs, Back Braces, Leg Braces and Corsets. Our representatives will be Lester J. Sabolich, B. Ray Buddin, T. H. Wengert, and Ella Brinson.

SANDOZ CHEMICAL WORKS, INC.
New York, New York
Booth 23

Sandoz Pharmaceuticals cordially invites you to visit our display at the Oklahoma State Medical Meeting — Booth 23. FIORINAL, A new approach to therapy of tension headaches and other head pain due to sinusitis and myalgia. CAFERGOT, Available in oral and rectal form for effective control of head pain in migraine and other vascular headaches. HYDERGINE, A vasorelaxant with central and peripheral action useful in hypertension and peripheral vascular disorders and geriatric conditions. BELLERGAL, Valuable as an autonomic inhibitor in a variety of functional ills — the volume of favorable clinical reports is constantly increasing. Any of our representatives in attendance, will gladly answer questions about these and other Sandoz products. In charge of our booth will be W. Mack Doyle.

SCHERING CORPORATION
Bloomfield, New Jersey
Booth 12

Members of the Oklahoma State Medical Association and their guests are cordially invited to visit the Schering exhibit where new therapeutic developments will be featured. Schering representatives, Ralph Couch and Joseph Ingola, will be present to welcome you and to discuss with you these products of our manufacture.

G. D. SEARLE AND COMPANY
Chicago, Illinois
Booth 63

You are cordially invited to visit the Searle booth where our representatives, Frank R. Cotten and T. R. Sellers, will be happy to answer any questions regarding Searle Products of Research. Featured will be Vallestril, the new synthetic estrogen with extremely low incidence of side reactions; Banthine, and Pro-Banthine. the standards in anti-cholinergic therapy; and Dramamine, for the prevention and treatment of motion sickness and other nauseas.

E. R. SQUIBB AND SONS
New York, New York
Booth 33

At Booth No. 33, E. R. Squibb & Sons features Raudixin, the safe hypotensive agent. Raudixin contains the whole root of Rauwolfia serpentina accurately standardiz-

in arthritis
and allied disorders

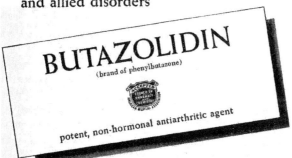

BUTAZOLIDIN
(brand of phenylbutazone)

potent, non-hormonal antiarthritic agent

Its therapeutic effectiveness substantiated by more than fifty
published reports, BUTAZOLIDIN has recently received
the Seal of Acceptance of the Council on Pharmacy and Chemistry
of the American Medical Association.

In the treatment of arthritis BUTAZOLIDIN produces prompt relief
of pain. In many instances relief of pain is accompanied
by diminution of swelling, resolution of inflammation and increased
freedom and range of motion of the affected joints.

BUTAZOLIDIN is indicated in:

Gouty Arthritis	Rheumatoid Arthritis
Psoriatic Arthritis	Rheumatoid Spondylitis

Painful Shoulder (including peritendinitis, capsulitis, bursitis, and acute arthritis)

Since BUTAZOLIDIN is a potent agent, patients for therapy should
be selected with care; dosage should be judiciously controlled;
and the patient should be regularly observed so that treatment may be
discontinued at the first sign of toxic reaction.

Physicians unfamiliar with the use of BUTAZOLIDIN are urged to send
for complete descriptive literature before employing it.

BUTAZOLIDIN® (brand of phenylbutazone), coated tablets of 100 mg.

GEIGY PHARMACEUTICALS
Division of Geigy Chemical Corporation
220 Church Street, New York 13, N.Y.
In Canada: Geigy Pharmaceuticals, Montreal   260

ed for uniform hypotensive and sedative effect. Our representatives, M. A. Fortner, S. E. Wilson, R. A. Grantham, and K. E. Lisle, will be glad to discuss with you the advantages of Raudixin used alone or in combination with other drugs.

U. S. VITAMIN CORPORATION
New York, New York
Booth 35

Exhibit features original, complete lipotropic therapy. . . METHISCHOL. . . the combination of five proven lipotropic agents: B_{12}, choline, methionine, inositol and liver extract. Also NEW GERIATRONE ELIXIR . . . a new kind of geriatric nutritive-metabolic tonic which furnishes the important digestive enzymes pepsin and pancreatin together with lipotropic factors, B-Complex and calcium and manganese glycerophosphate. You are invited to stop at the booth and sample this very palatable new preparation. John Wilbourn and Guy W. Anderson will be in charge of the booth.

THE UPJOHN COMPANY
Kalamazoo, Michigan
Booth 56

The Upjohn exhibit will feature CORTEF, brand of hydrocortisone. Reports from clinicians and practitioners reveal dramatic results in the use of CORTEF where cortisone is indicated. CORTEF is available in tablet or ointment form for oral or topical use. Upjohn representatives will welcome the opportunity to furnish additional information to the profession.

WARNER-CHILCOTT LABORATORIES
New York, New York
Booth 38

Two important cardiovascular agents will be featured at the Warner-Chilcott booth: Methium — to lower blood pressure and relieve hypertensive symptoms and Peritrate — to prevent attacks in angina pectoris. A new drug, Parisdol — for the efficient management of Parkinson's disease will also be exhibited. Represenatives and research personnel will welcome an opportunity to discuss these drugs with you. In charge of the booth will be William J. Havey and Theron F. Spigener.

THE WARREN-TEED PRODUCTS CO.
Columbus, Ohio
Booth 28

The Warren-Teed Products Company cordially invites all members of the Oklahoma State Medical Association and their guests to visit our new exhibit at booth No. 28. This exhibit will feature our new product, Glu-Sal Tablets, a combination of Glucuronolactone and Salicylamide, indicated for the relief of pain and corrective therapy of rheumatic conditions, arthritis, gout, sciatica, neuritis and neuralgia, by reversal of degenerative changes without side effects. Other products of interest to the medical profession will also be displayed. Our representatives, Robert E. Loftus, W. Allen Davis, and James M. Hamilton, will be in attendance to discuss these products and assist registrants in any way possible.

WINTHROP-STEARNS, INC.
New York, New York
Booth 66

WINTHROP-STERNS, INC., New York, invite you to visit booth No. 66, where the following products will be featured — LEVOPHED bitartrate, the most powerful pressor antidote for shock due to myocardial infarction, surgical and nonsurgical trauma, hemorrhage and other causes. Levophed is noted for its prompt, predictable, reliable, and easily controlled action. Administer diluted in 5 per cent dextrose or dextrose in saline infusion; APOLAMINE, synergistic compound for more efficient control of nausea and vomiting due to pregnancy, radiation sickness, and other causes. Our representatives will be G. W. Shilling, P. R Kirk, and V. C. Moreland.

WYETH LABORATORIES
Philadelphia, Pennsylvania
Booth 40

The display of Wyeth Laboratories will feature BICILLIN[R] — the new long-acting penicillin compound — in various forms: BICILLIN Injection (several strengths) for treatment of infections caused by penicillin-sensitive organisms and for prevention of rheumatic fever: BICILLIN C-R, for use in general practice; BICILLIN All-Purpose, for prophylaxis and treatment in surgical infections; widely prescribed BICILLIN Oral Suspension, effective, stable delightfully palatable and BICILLIN Tablets, useful, convenient oral form — unaffected by gastric juice, hence can be given without regard to meals. Also featured will be PHEN-ERGAN[R], powerful antihistamine for the treatment of all allergic manifestations, and WYDASE[R], the purified, "spreading factor" hyaluronidase with a wide range of clinical applications. The Wyeth representatives will be H. A. Dicken, W. W. Bush, Harold Green, R. L. Woods, I. J. Vaughn, and J. A. Parker.

AUDIO-DIGEST FOUNDATION
Glendale, California
Booth 57

AUDIO-DIGEST FOUNDATION gives a busy physician an effortless tour through the best of current medical literature each week. This medical "newscast"—compiled and reviewed by a professional Board of Editors—may be heard in the physician's automobile, home, or office. The Foundation— whose profits are distributed among the nation's medical schools—also offers tape-recorded medical lectures by nationally-recognized authorities. Representatives for the Foundation booth will be H. O. McCumber, Ph.D. and Harold Heller.

ST. PAUL INDEMNITY COMPANY
Oklahoma City, Oklahoma
Booth 14

THE ST. PAUL MERCURY INDEMNITY COMPANY will offer an opportunity at its booth No. 14 for the members of the Association to discuss with their experts the problems in regard to malpractice insurance. They are prepared to offer complete information in regard to policies, coverage, and the handling of claims. The company representatives in attendance at the St. Paul booth will be Don Hawkins, Forrest Cress, Roger Bainbridge, Gordon Fransen, Gordon Gorney, Gordon Estes, and M. J. Herod.

Please return your Dinner Dance and Hotel Reservation Forms on page 116 as soon as possible.

CLASSIFIED ADS

DINNER-DANCE TICKET ORDER BLANK

Enclosed is my check in the amount of $_____for_____ tickets to the annual Dinner-Dance. (Tickets are $7.50 each and include the social hour, dinner, inaugural program and Dick Jurgens dance.) Checks should be made payable to the Oklahoma State Medical Association and mailed to 1227 Classen **Drive,** Oklahoma City 3, Oklahoma.

Name_____, M.D.
(please print or type)

- -

HOTEL RESERVATION FORM

Please make reservations for_____persons at the_____

Hotel (give first and second choice of hotels) for a single room_____,

double room_____, twin bedroom_____, suite_____, other_____

(check one). Arrival date and time_____

Departure date and time_____. Leading Oklahoma City hotels are the Biltmore, Black, Huckins, Roberts, Skirvin and Skirvin Tower.

Name _____
(please print or type)

Address_____

City and State_____

Oklahoma State Medical Association

INCOME AND EXPENSE STATEMENT

January 1, 1953—December 31, 1953

INCOME

Dues		$58,021.75
United States Bond Interest		167.50
Annual Meeting'		11,248.25
Journal		15,177.36
History of Medicine Appropriation		1,500.00
Directory Advertising		974.40
Rural Health Luncheon		575.30
Miscellaneous		1,068.75
		88,733.31

EXPENDITURES

Office Expense	$34,209.55	
Annual Meeting	9,997.26	
Journal	21,179.38	
Public Policy Committee	3,956.50	
Public Health Committee	1,607.87	
Legal Expense	1,421.52	
Travel—In and Out of State	7,006.49	
History of Medicine—University of Oklahoma	3,000.00	
Retirement Insurance Program	3,991.91	
Miscellaneous	1,056.20	87,426.68
INCOME OVER EXPENSE		$ 1,306.63

BALANCE SHEET

December 31, 1953

ASSETS

CURRENT ASSETS

Petty Cash	$ 6.00	
Cash in Bank	40,813.39	$40,819.39
FIXED ASSETS		
Furniture and Fixtures	10,537.36	
Less Reserve for Depreciation	2,784.14	7,753.22
INVESTMENTS		
U. S. Government Bonds		12,398.88
TOTAL ASSETS		$60,971.49

LIABILITIES AND NET WORTH

ACCRUALS

Withholding Tax	1,095.02	
Social Security	52.09	
Retirement Fund	425.95	1,573.06
Operating Reserve		59,398.43
TOTAL LIABILITIES AND NET WORTH		60,971.49

Respectfully Submitted,
H. E. COLE COMPANY, Public Accountants

Editorials

Lay Publicity in Action

Perrin H. Long's address in Tulsa February 15 before the Oklahoma Academy of General Practice promptly made news. The February 16 *Daily Oklahoman* headline reads, "Doctor Warns Miracle Drugs Can Be Deadly". Space will not permit a full discussion. Suffice it to say that while the *Journal* finds no fault with the reporter and her reporting, the fact remains that the unqualified statements leave the public with only half the truth.

The explanation appears in an editorial appearing in the *Journal* of March, 1954, titled "The Matter of Lay Medical Publicity".

The justifiable caution should have been accompanied by the significant fact that largely on account of these same new drugs in the past 15 years, morbidity and mortality have been greatly reduced. To cite only one example, pneumonia, one of the greatest killers of the past, is now practically non-existent as a cause of death.

Before Doctor Long spoke in Tulsa, the editorial "Drug Addicts" referring to the fact that physicians may become addicted to overprescribing in the presence of miracle drugs, was in the February *Journal*.

Though the unwarranted and promiscuous prescribing cannot be condoned, we must insist that it is unfortunate that the publicity was not accompanied by the full truth showing that any damage resulting from over-prescribing cannot compare with the good accomplished by the new drugs. The number of lives lost is insignificant compared with the number saved.

Maryland Indebted to Oklahoma

The University of Oklahoma Medical School's Robert H. Riley, who graduated in the class of 1913 has been cited for unusually meritorious service in public health.

At the November 5, 1953, convention in Washington, D. C. the Association of State and Territorial Health Officers "honored Dr. Robert H. Riley, Director of the Maryland State Department of Health, with the 1953 Arthur T. McCormack Award. . . Dr. Riley has been Director of the Maryland State Department of Health for the past twenty-five years. He has been instrumental in successfully guiding the course of public health in Maryland during this period which has seen some of the greatest changes in the field of health administration. Prior to this time Dr. Riley served as Assistant State Health Officer of Oklahoma."[1]

Oklahoma is proud of Robert H. Riley. Through his service in public health his influence in the cause of human weal will live long after he hands over "the lamp of life".

[1]Baltimore Health News. Published monthly by the Baltimore City Health Department. Vol. XXX, No. 12, December, 1953.

Needle Biopsy of the Liver

In the August *Journal* (1952) there is an editorial under the above title. Briefly it discussed indications, diagnostic efficacy, dangers and the importance of standard technique.

In the *New England Medical Journal* Norman Zamcheck and Richard L. Sidman[1] under "Medical Progress" discuss the procedure in two issues of the Journal: 1. Its use in clinical and investigative medicine and 2. The Risk of Needle Biopsy.

Those who read and heeded the principles set forth in the previous editorial are in line with progress as reported. For the benefit of our readers we lift the author's conclusions from *New England Medical Journal* and recommend this report with its long list of references to all who are interested in this important diagnostic method:

"A review of 20,016 needle biopsies of the liver indicates clearly that at present this is the most useful adjunct available for the diagnosis of clinical liver disease. In the hands of unqualified persons, misled by its apparent simplicity, the procedure is hazardous, but, when performed by experienced personnel, it is remarkably safe, having a true mortality of less than 1:1000. The proper use of needle biopsy can save many lives by permitting early diagnosis and prompt institution of correct medical or surgical therapy."

New England Journal of Medicine. Vol. 249, Nos. 25-26 (December 17 and 24) 1953. Pages 1020-29; 1062-69. Norman Zamcheck, M.D., Richard L. Sidman, M.D. and Oscar Klausenstock, M D.

Hospitals in the Practice of Medicine

The following contribution by P. E. Russo, M.D., opens an old wound. Since the subject is a controversial one, it deserves editorial notice. Any member desiring to comment on the statement presented by Doctor Russo should address the Editor or any member of the Editorial Board:

"I am submitting for your consideration the following statement with reference to the new Health Insurance contract for the meat packing industry. The health insurance contracts for the meat packing industry do not permit *'free choice of physician and fee for service.'* The contract distinctly restricts professional services in radiology, pathology, anesthesiology and physiatry to services 'when rendered by a salaried employee of a hospital.' This excludes such professional service when rendered by a physician in his office or by a physician conducting a private practice of these specialties in a hospital on a fee for service basis. Such restrictions of professional services to those rendered by an employee of a hospital are sinister influences undermining a private practice of medicine and promoting the progressive institutionalization of medical practice in hospitals.

"The restriction of benefits for professional services to 'when rendered by a salaried employee of a hospital' and the implication that these represent hospital care rather than medical practice are being encountered more and more frequently in the health insurance contracts of insurance carriers. It is particularly difficult to correct the policies of such private insurance companies in which our profession has no representation or voice. The Oklahoma Blue Cross accepted the 'Swift Contract' which contains such restrictions and was put into effect December 6, 1953.

"It is recommended that our Medical Association go on record as definitely opposed to the restriction of any Blue Shield or private insurance benefits for professional services to those 'rendered by a salaried employee of a hospital' and to insurance contracts which by implication tend to define radiology, pathology, anesthesiology or physiatry as 'ancillary hospital service'."

Coronary Disease

In the *British Medical Journal* of January 9, 1954, there is an editorial on "Coronary Disease and Work". The long considered riddles connected with this condition are still unsolved. Nobody knows why coronary disease is more common in professional groups than in other classes. On the whole current studies present insoluble paradoxes. Dr. J. N. Morris and co-workers in Britain find this is true. Their investigations of drivers, conductors and guards, aged 35 to 64, employed by the London Transport show that conductors have less coronary disease than the other groups, all in virtually the same social strata. This leads them to believe that lack of physical activity is a contributing factor. This doesn't explain the higher incidence in general practitioners than in consultants.

Admittedly the disease etiologically arises through both genetic and environmental influences. We would like to know about genetics. Before it is too late, the students of cardiovascular disease should tell us whether to be poor or rich, whether to be sedentary or physically active, whether to smoke and drink, what to eat and how much, whether to worry or not to worry and if it is within their power to be so merciful how to develop a rapidly fatal coronary thrombosis just before obvious senility sets in.

British Medical Journal. Coronary Disease and Work. January 9, 1954. Pages 86-87.

CERVICO-FACIAL ACTINOMYCOSIS

DAN E. BRANNIN, D.D.S., Tulsa

THE AUTHOR

Dan E. Brannin, D.D.S., M.S.D., Tulsa oral surgeon, has a paper on "Cervico-Facial Actinomycosis" in this issue. Doctor Brannin received his B.S. degree from Oklahoma A. and M. in 1946 and his D.D.S. from the University of Kansas City in 1950. In 1952 he was granted his M.S.D. from the University of Minnesota with a major in oral surgery and a minor in oral pathology.

Actinomycosis is a disease which occurs with relative infrequency in man. Clinically, it is characterized by suppuration, the formation of granulation tissue, fistulas, sinuses, and by the presence in the pus of yellow granules, the so-called "sulfur granules."[1] Three areas of the body are most commonly affected in approximately the following percentages: thoracic 14 per cent, abdominal 8-18 per cent, and cervico-facial 60 per cent.[1] In reference to the last, Burket[3] states that the submaxillary region is the most frequent site of involvement in cervico-facial actinomycosis. There is characteristically a slowly progressive swelling of the cheek or neck which is indurated in nature. As the disease progresses, foci of suppuration develop which tend to form chronic sinuses through which pus containing sulfur granules escapes. The skin in the area about the drainage sites is described as possessing a characteristic bluish or violaceous color.[4] Actinomycosis of the submaxillary area is easily confused with osteomyelitis. In osteomyelitis, however, the pain is more severe, there is greater destruction of bone, and suppuration occurs more quickly.[3] In addition to osteomyelitis, one must differentiate from many diseases such as syphilis, tuberculosis, and malignancy.

The infective organisms are anaerobic fungi belonging to the group, Actinomyces. They are gram-positive, filamentous organisms which are probably strict parasites.[2] Most workers believe that there are two pathogenic types of Actinomyces: Actinomyces israeli, which causes most infections in man; and Actinomyces bovis, which is the etiological agent in bovine infections but may be the insulting organism in man. Until recently it had been thought that human infections arose from contact with infected animals or contaminated plants. Hall states

that at the present time there is little reason to cling to such a belief.[2] The organisms commonly reside in the human mouth in carious teeth, periodontal pockets, and tonsillar crypts. The mechanism whereby these harmless Actinomyces of the mouth invade tissues and lead to disease is not known. Thoma[6] states that they may enter through root canals, periodontal pockets, and oral wounds.

The positive diagnosis of actinomycosis can only be made from isolation of anaerobic Actinomyces from infected tissue or pus by curvature.[2] The presence of "sulfur granules" while helpful is not diagnostic. Other microorganisms may cause the formation of such structures by forming a matrix about which lime salts are deposite. In actinomycosis these granules are actually colonies of the fungus.[1] The demonstration of mycelial fibers within a granule is highly suggestive but not conclusive. Nocardia, for example, also presents such a picture. Biopsies of the wound frequently reveal only granulomas and suppuration. Most laboratories, however, are willing to make a presumptive diagnosis of actinomycosis if sulfur granules are present and if gram-positive mycelia can be demonstrated in these granules.

The treatment of actinomycosis in recent years has been revolutionized. Iodides, x-ray therapy and the sulfa drugs, combined with radical surgery were employed but

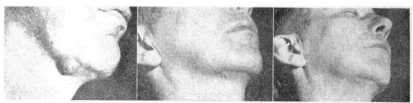

FIG. 1. Preoperative appearance of patient. The right submandibular swelling is plainly visible.

FIG. 2. The right submandibular area 30 days postoperatively.

FIG. 3. The right submandibular area three months after initiation of treatment.

these yielded little success. However, the antibiotics penicillin and more recently, aureomycin and terramycin, have demonstrated effectiveness in the treatment of the disease. Incision and drainage followed by curettage in combination with large doses of penicillin for three to six weeks is the treatment most universally employed at the present time. Cervico-facial actinomycosis has demonstrated itself to be responsive to this therapy and numerous cures have been reported.

Report of a Case

Mr. A. M., a 43-year-old postal clerk, was admitted to the hospital, September 2, 1952, complaining of a painful swelling just inferior to the right lower jaw.

History: Approximately two and one-half months prior to admission the mandibular right molars were extracted. Following these extractions, the "lower jaw swelled" and incision and drainage was done. Two injections of penicillin and twelve oral tablets of penicillin were given. His condition improved until 10 days later when a "hard swelling like a hard rubber ball" developed in the right upper neck just below the mandible. He was admitted to a hospital and remained there for eight days during which time he received four injections of penicillin a day and application of warm moist packs externally to the swelling. His condition improved considerably but the swelling did not completely resolve. He was discharged, however, from the hospital and informed that he could expect the swelling to disappear completely within a few days.

A further medical history revealed no additional contributory information and was essentially negative except for a stated intolerance to fatty or fried foods.

Examination: The patient was a well developed, well nourished 43-year-old postal clerk in no distress. Physical examination demonstrated no abnormality except for that associated with the right lower face and upper neck. A reddish-blue, raised, fluctuant mass approximately two centimeters in diameter was present in the right submandibular area. (Fig. 1) It was movable, apparently unattached to the mandible, non-painful, and non-tender to palpation. Palpation of the cervical lymph nodes revealed no deviations from normality. Intraorally, the examination was negative except for some slight increased tenderness in the right mandibular muco-buccafold. The previous extraction sites were almost completely healed.

Repeated blood studies were done but the results of all performed were well within normal limits as was examination of the urine. Serology and heterophile antibody studies were likewise negative.

Treatment: The patient was given crystalline penicillin intramuscularly 100,000 units every four hours beginning immediately after admission to the hospital. On the day following admission, aspiration of the mass followed by incision and drainage was performed in the operating room under trichlorethylene analgesia. A 20 gauge needle was inserted into the mass and approximately one milliliter of sero-purulent material aspirated. This material was submitted for bacteriologic study. An incision approximately one inch in length was made directly over the point of greatest fluctuation and parallel to the inferior border of the mandible. Five to 10 milliliters of sero-purulent fluid was evacuated. Jelly-like granulation tissue was curetted from the area and portions submitted for microscopic study. The inferior

122

border of the mandible was visualized, but no defects in this structure seen. A Penrose drain was inserted into the wound and fixed in place with one 000 silk suture.

Close examination of the aspirated material revealed the presence of peculiar yellowish specks, presumably "sulphur granules." Examination of these granules under the microscope demonstrated them to be formed masses of gram positive mycelial fibers. A presumptive diagnosis of actinomycosis was made. Cultures later showed the organisms to be Actinomyces bovis.

Microscopic study of the tissue curetted from the wound revealed, "massive inflammatory infiltrate."

The postoperative course was uneventful. Continuous hot moist packs were applied for three days at the end of which time drainage had ceased. The drain was removed and the patient transferred to the medical service for completion of treatment. Penicillin was continued and given in increments of 300,000 units every 12 hours. The wound healed without further incident and the patient discharged 30 days after admission, apparently cured. (Fig. 2) He was seen three months later and no evidence of recurrence was found. (Fig. 3)

REFERENCES

1. Jordan, E. O., Burrows, W.: Textbook of Bacteriology, 14th. Ed., pp 599-615, W. B. Saunders Co., Philadelphia, 1945.
2. Hall, W. H.: Actinomycosis in Man, Surgical Staff Seminars, Minneapolis Veterans Hospital, 9:84-91, Sept. 5, 1950.
3. Burket, L. W.: Oral Medicine, pp. 498-501, J. B. Lippincott Co., Philadelphia, 1946.
4. Blair, V. P., and Ivy, R. H.: Essentials of Oral Surgery, 4th. ed., pp. 102-106, C. V. Mosby Co., St. Louis, 1951.
5. Miller, S. C.: Oral Diagnosis and Treatment, 2nd ed., pp. 154-155, Blakiston Co., Philadelphia, 1946.
6. Thoma, K. H.: Oral Pathology, 2nd. ed., pp. 848-851, C. V. Mosby Co., St. Louis, 1944.

DEVELOPMENT of CLINICAL AUDIOLOGY

JOHN W. KEYS, Ph. D., Oklahoma City

Audiology is the science of hearing. The scope and subject matter of this field, including as it does certain aspects of many academic disciplines, physiology, anatomy, medicine, psychology, electrical engineering, and speech, is so broad, that it is almost an impossibility today for one person to be an expert in every and all phases of the subject. It would be somewhat unusual to find an otologist, who normally is concerned with the pathological and medical aspects of hearing, to be also a trained teacher of the deaf, a specialist in speech reading, and a psychophysicist. Neither would one expect to find as a usual circumstance, a teacher of the deaf who had completed four years of medical school, a year of internship, and one or two years of residency in otology. However, in spite of the fact that it is very unlikely that any one person can become proficient in the entire field of audiology, it is possible for him to become a specialist in one and possibly two aspects of that field

Presented before the Rocky Mountain Speech Conference in Denver February, 1953.

THE AUTHOR

John W. Keys, Ph.D. wrote "The Development of Clinical Audiology" in this issue. Doctor Keys is director of the speech and hearing clinic, Crippled Children's Hospital, Oklahoma City. Doctor Keys had a previous article appearing in the December, 1953, issue of the Journal.

with at least a general acquaintance with the others.

In this paper for purposes of discussion and since it will best serve our needs, we shall divide the field of audiology into three broad areas: otology, the medical science of hearing; clinical audiology, the measurement and evaluation of hearing; education of the deaf and/or the hard of hearing. Additional divisions and subdivisions could, perhaps, be made, but our principal concern here is with the growth and development of clinical audiology, so that additional classification does not seem to be necessary.

Each of the fields just mentioned, notwithstanding the fact that there is a certain amount of subject matter common to all these areas has its own sphere of responsibility and each has professional integrity in its own right

As a matter of fact, it is only through the proper cooperation and careful integration of the medical, clinical, and educational services represented in these areas that the greatest benefits to the hearing handicapped can be achieved.

Causes for the Growth of Audiology

The development in the whole field of audiology in the past two decades has been a rapid one. There are certain basic causes for this development and perhaps it is important, at least historically, to review some of these causes which made possible, and in fact constitute, the foundation for the advancements in clinical audiology, the topic with which this paper will be primarily concerned.

The first great impetus to the field came with the development of the vacuum tube and its subsequent adaptation for use in various types of hearing testing equipment and somewhat later, in the hearing aid. We shall have more to say later about hearing testing equipment, but I should like to point out here that the vacuum tube hearing aid gave thousands of people a new lease on life. It provided the opportunity for countless numbers of hard of hearing children, who otherwise would have dropped out of school, to continue their education in a normal manner, and to take their place in a hearing society.

By the same token, thousands of adults were able to hold their jobs, maintain their self respect and carry on a normal life who might have been relegated to the sidelines to lead a life of non-productivity and misery. The hearing aid was truly a god-send to the hard of hearing and it awakened a general interest in the potentialities and possibilities of the use of amplification to aid those who have hearing losses — an interest which is still very much alive. In fact, the 14 or 15 years which have passed since the first vacuum tube hearing aid became a reality to the development of the new transistor aid now coming on the market, marks an era of progress that can scarcely be duplicated anywhere.

A second great contributing factor to the advancement of audiology came with the discovery of the anti-biotics. For the first time medicine had a really effective means of combatting middle ear infections. Their discovery did a great deal to stimulate the awareness of the scientist and the public that preventive measures were possible that could, to a large extent, eliminate otitis media as a prime cause of hearing loss in children.

The third development which proved to be a much needed stimulus for the field of otology as well as a new source of help for persons with otosclerosis (a disease in which there is an osseous growth in the middle ear which may impede, or in the advanced stage, prevent the movement of the ossicular chain) was the fenestration operation. Although the operation holds no benefit for those whose hearing loss results from other causes, the fact that operative procedures are now available for even one type of hearing loss gave tremendous encouragement to all.

It is hardly possible to evaluate the tremendous contributions of the aural rehabilitation programs of World War II toward the advancement of audiology. Thousands of soldiers were returned to normal life through the training received in centers at Deson, Borden, Hoff, and Philadelphia Naval Hospitals. The tremendous progress made by these men during their concentrated programs of speech reading, auditory training, and hearing aid instruction surprised even those who were intimately involved in the training procedures. The whole program drove home the point to everyone that the hard of hearing can and must be rehabilitated.

From an analysis of the records of the thousands of soldiers tested came valuable research contributions to the field. Concomitantly, programs of investigation were carried on at Harvard Psycho-Acoustic laboratory, Central Institute for the Deaf, and other places which developed more effective tools for testing hearing in the form of new tests, new equipment, and new procedures.

The advancements made in the area of psychological testing have also had a profound effect in audiology, as well of course, as in the entire educational field. Particularly important has been the standardization of certain performance or non-verbal tests on deaf children. It is no secret to any of us that many acoustically handicapped children have been relegated to the ranks of the feeble-minded when careful examination by a competent psychologist could have demonstrated their normalcy in everything but hearing. Other tests, diagnostic in nature, have been devised which have aided greatly in improving our insight into the actual causes operating to interrupt the development of a child's communicative processes. Achievement and other types of tests are now available which allow a comparison of these children with their normal hearing playmates. All of this has given purpose, direction and validation to the educatiohal training of these youngsters.

The last great influence in the field of audiology in recent years which I shall mention was the awakened interest on local, state, and national levels in the deaf and the hard of hearing. The Federal Government set up a program providing hearing aids for Veterans and also contributed funds through various agencies such as the Children's Bureau and the Commission for Crippled Children for special projects in speech and hearing. Universities and colleges by the dozens established speech and hearing programs; states passed measures which provided special education, or if you prefer, education for special children in the public schools. Speech and hearing surveys were conducted on a state wide basis; and special social or philanthropic groups set up day schools for the deaf in various large cities throughout the country or in some other way contributed to the program. The country has become "hearing" conscious as never before.

In fact, there has been such an effective job done in selling the program that we are now in a position of having created the demand and interest, but do not have trained personnel to fill the need. If we can do as good a job in selling competent seniors in high school on becoming teachers of the deaf, audiologists, and speech therapists, some day we may be able to supply the demand.

The Development of Clinical Audiology

We have reviewed what we conceive to be the major contributing factors to the growth of audiology in general. It now becomes pertinent to talk more specifically in terms of the advancement of the youngest member of the hearing field, academically speaking at least, clinical audiology.

We have previously mentioned the development of the vacuum tube and its effect on the field of audiology. One piece of equipment made possible by this development was, of course, the pure tone audiometer. Previous to this time, the tuning fork had been the principal instrument used by the otologist in differentiating between conductive and perceptive hearing loss.

It had been known for years, that loss by air conduction with relatively normal bone conduction is characteristic of conductive type hearing loss while a loss by both bone and air is a strong indication of perceptive involvement. The Rinné tuning fork test, in fact, was designed to demonstrate the bone-air relationship, clinically.

The tuning fork tests, however, had certain weaknesses. In the first place, the intensity of the fork tone could not be determined accurately, nor could a constant intensity level be maintained for the exploration and measurement of threshold. There was simply no way of knowing the exact amount of hearing loss of the patient.

As a result of these deficiencies, no accurate records of a patient's hearing loss could be kept from year to year as it was most difficult for the otologist to determine, except within gross limits, that a Rinné was more negative or more positive than it had been six months previously or that, as in the Weber, a tone was more lateralized or less lateralized than it had been the last time the individual was tested. Further, if a child were to move to another community there could be no accompanying chart which would convey to his new teacher or doctor just what the child's hearing picture was.

Although it cannot be said that the audiometer solved all of the problems connected with hearing testing, it certainly has helped with many of them. Today the fact that we can send an audiogram across the nation and know that it will have the same meaning to the doctor, clinician, or teacher that it had to us has proved to be an invaluable asset. Further, as was previously mentioned, a statistical analysis of a large number of these records from the files of hearing centers has yielded valuable clinical information.

Manufacturers of audiometers must meet certain specific and rather rigid requirements relative to the physical properties of the instrument. Such matters as distortion, air threshold calibrations, frequency range and accuracy, hum level, and maximum allowable error in attenuation are carefully regulated. There are problems yet to be solved in relation to certain variables encountered in bone conduction testing, not the least of which is the accurate calibration of the bone conduction receiver. These difficulties notwithstanding, the audiometer today has become an essential instrument for hearing testing and some, if not all, the problems connected with the testing of hearing by bone conduction may be eliminated in the future.

The Audiometer as an Aid in Diagnosis

Not only is the audiometer important in hearing testing, but it has also become one of the primary tools in diagnosis, i. e., in differentiating one type of hearing loss from another. Perhaps at the risk of boring those who are thoroughly familiar with the use of the audiometer, it might be well to review briefly some of the things we can learn from the audiogram. Before doing so, however, I should like to offer some precautionary remarks to the beginning audiologist.

First, although it is the obligation of every clinical audiologist worthy of the name to be completely familiar with and to be able to administer and interpret the various kinds of clinical diagnostic tests, the diagnosis of the individual's hearing loss must be made by the medical doctor.

I conceive it to be the responsibility of the audiologist to make complete reports of the results of his tests to the doctor and it is permissible to include a general summary of what those results seem to indicate if the doctor requests it. On the other hand, the audiologist's report to the patient should be in terms only of the severity of his loss, in what frequency range he has the greatest deficiency; what his loss means in terms of his ability to communicate with others; and his possibilities for receiving satisfaction from a hearing aid.

It is the responsibility of the otologist to keep abreast of the clinical developments in the field that he may properly utilize the information which the audiologist can furnish him.

Further it should also be stated catergorically that no diagnosis should be, or in fact, can be made from an audiogram alone. The case history, the medical examination, and other clinical tests to be mentioned later are all necessary to complete the diagnostic picture.

It must also be remembered that any review of diagnostic interpretations from an audiogram must be in terms of generalities and as such are subject to exceptions. With these precautions in mind suppose we proceed with our review by simply listing diagnostic indications of conductive loss which may be attained from the audiogram or from the testing procedure itself.

Conductive loss may be suspected when the following conditions exist: (1) When there is a loss of air conduction with relatively normal bone conduction. (2) When there is a greater loss of hearing in the low frequencies than in the high frequencies or the loss is straight across the audiogram. (3) When the patient shows no unusual sharpness or accuracy in the determination of threshold. (4) When there is no evidence of recruitment in testing particularly in the higher frequencies.* (5) When there is no evidence of a lowered pain threshold.** (6) A pure conductive hearing loss will never exceed 65 db.

*Recruitment may be defined as a more rapid increase in the sensation of loudness for a given increase in intensity than that experienced by normal ear.

**Although the audiometer is not usually employed as a test of recruitment, many times the phenomenon becomes apparent in the testing situation. If the patient demonstrates unusual accuracy in selecting threshold or complains that the test tone presented at above threshold levels for identification by the patient is uncomfortably loud, recruitment may be suspected.

Indications of perceptive loss are, in general, opposite to those just mentioned. We expect a loss by bone conduction as well as air; recruitment; a greater loss in the high than in the low frequencies; a particular sharpness and accuracy in the observation of thresholds; and in some cases a lowered pain threshold. Perceptive hearing loss can, of course, be of any degree.

Close observation of the patient's responses during the testing procedure as well as a careful examination of the audiogram—should point up some of the differences between conductive and perceptive loss. The picture may be somewhat confusing in cases of mixed deafness. It must again be noted that exceptions to these rules are common. Cases suffering from blocked eustachian tubes or blocked external canals, for instance, often produce a hearing deficiency in the high frequencies which may be mistaken for perceptive loss. Also, the bone conduction test may yield spurious results. In general, however, the above observations can be regarded as true. Careful consideration of the facts revealed by the case history in addition to the test results will further clarify the hearing picture.

The problem is still further complicated from the diagnostic standpoint because it is essential not only to be able to differentiate conductive from perceptive loss, but also to be able to diagnose a conductive loss caused by otosclerosis from one caused by otitis media or a perceptive loss in which there is damage to the hair cells and nerve endings of the cochlea from a perceptive loss where a lesion has occurred on the eighth cranial nerve itself. Although time will not permit a complete discussion of all the clinical developments which may be used in arriving at a differential diagnosis, I should like to mention a few of the most promising ones which may add greatly to our confidence in the final decision.

Carhart's Notch

It has not been many years ago that a prominent otologist is reported to have made the statement that, without instituting operative procedures, there was no sure way to diagnose otosclerosis except by post mortem examination. Such a diagnosis was obviously a little tardy to benefit the patient.

Clinical audiology has come a long way since then and today such a diagnosis is possible with more than considerable accuracy.

Carhart at Northwestern University was the first to note that the pre-operative bone conduction curves in cases who later underwent operations for otosclerosis took a particular and characteristic form. He found that such a curve usually showed a loss of 5 db. at 500 cycles; 10 db. at 1000 cycles; 15 db. at 2000 cycles; and 5 db. at 4000 cycles.* This characteristic curve has been named the Carhart Notch. Such a curve becomes apparent in routine bone conduction audiometry and therefore a careful study of the audiogram on the part of the clinician and the doctor becomes increasingly significant. Previous to this time such a loss in the middle frequencies probably would have been interpreted as perceptive involvement.

It is thought that this loss by bone conduction has been brought about by the change in the mechanical system of the middle ear through otosclerotic involvement. A similar loss by bone does not occur in cases of otitis media.

The Luscher Test

The term recruitment has been previously mentioned. It was pointed out that this abnormal acceleration in the sensation of loudness which we have called recruitment does not occur in conductive hearing loss. Therefore any test which can accurately and consistently determine whether recruitment is present will automatically be valuable in differentiating conductive from perceptive loss. Bruine-Altes and Dix, Hallpike, and Hood[2] demonstrated that recruitment occurs in perceptive loss cases of the cochlear type, that is, where the damage occurs in the organ of Corti. Cases of perceptive loss in which lesions occur beyond the cochlea usually do not exhibit this phenomenon, or if so, only partially.[3]

Thus a sure fire test for recruitment also would be highly valuable in differentiating retrolabyrinthine from cochlear perceptive loss. There have, of course, been such tests

*Bruine-Altes as cited in Jerger, J. F.: "A Difference Lumen Recruitment Test and Its Diagnostic Significance," *The Laryngoscope*, Vol. LXII, Dec. 1952, No. 12.
*These values have since been refined. See McConnell and Carhart, "Fenestration Surgery," Laryngoscope, Vol. LXII, Dec. 1952, p. 1267.

devised previously, among them the equal loudness balance test. There are, however, clinical difficulties in the presentation of this test which limit its usefulness. One test which seems to show considerable promise for clinical use is the Luscher test which may be easily and quickly administered and seems to have great validity.

Since recruitment is an acceleration in the sensation of loudness, it is reasonable to suppose that the recruited ear should also be capable of recognizing more and therefore smaller intensity changes, or DLs (difference limens) within a given increase in intensity above threshold than does the normal ear. Doerfler has demonstrated that this is true.[5] Because such an ear can detect smaller DLs, it would follow that it should also detect the increment (or decrement) in the intensity of a tone before the normal ear is able to do so.

This is the basic principle upon which the Luscher test operates. The Luscher equipment may be attached to the conventional audiometer which furnishes the signal source.* The equipment itself allows the operator to modulate the signal tone from 0 db. in small but ever increasing intensity steps up to 6 db. or 50 per cent maximum modulation. At some point, as the degree of modulation is increased from its zero value, the ear will begin to hear the test signal as a warble tone. This, of course marks the difference limen or the point at which the ear has recognized a just noticeable increase in intensity. The intensity of the test tone may be varied as can the rate at which the modulation is increased.

Luscher recommended that the test tone be presented at the 40 db. level above threshold. Jerger,[4] however, in a recent study at Northwestern University presented the tone at 15 db. level since Doerfler found that the size of the DLs in perceptive loss cases is reduced in greater degree in the 15-30 db. range above threshold than at higher levels where the DLs tend more nearly to approach normal values.

*The Luscher apparatus comes as standard equipment on the Sonotone Model 23—Advanced Clinical Audiometer.

**The difference in the level at which the test tones were presented has just been mentioned. Luscher presented the test tone with maximum modulation gradually diminishing it until the loudness beat disappeared. Jerger reversed the procedure, using the ascending method of stimulus presentation in which he proceeds from no modulation to full modulation. Luscher had also employed an interrupter switch in the presentation of the modulation tone which Jerger eliminated.

Although the procedure for administering the test differed somewhat in the Luscher and Jerger studies,** the results were similar. In general, these results may be summarized in the following statements:

1. In certain types of perceptive loss, notably those in which the etiology was indicative of cochlear damage such as acoustic trauma and Menieres disease, the DLs were abnormally small.

2. The DLs in conductive loss were normal in size.

3. In certain types of perceptive loss where retrolabyrinthine damage was present the DLs were of normal size.

Two other tentative conclusions made in these studies should be mentioned although further investigation seems necessary for verification.

1. Both Luscher's and Jerger's results indicated that in psychogenic hearing losses, the DLs are abnormally large.

2. Jerger also discovered that the DLs for people suffering from presbycusis (senile deafness) in the majority of cases were normal in size. In fact only two out of ten individuals tested exhibited reduced DLs.

It seems probable, therefore as Jerger points out, that senile deafness may not be strictly a cochlear type deafness as had been supposed previously.

Although further research is necessary, the Luscher test seems to have possibilities as a diagnostic tool and will undoubtedly be added as a routine procedure to the implementaria already employed in hearing testing.

Békésy Audiometer

Other types of hearing testing equipment and procedures also hold promise of diagnostic value. Recently Békésy[1] designed an audiometer which allows the patient to conduct his own hearing test. The instrument presents a tone which automatically but gradually increases in a sweep frequency manner through the usual testing range. The equipment is so constructed that the patient may increase or decrease the intensity alternately.

When the intensity of the tone decreases below the threshold level the patient immediately presses a button which reverses the direction of the attenuator and the intensity increases until the tone is again just audible. This procedure is repeated throughout the test frequency range, the signal at one moment being just audible, and the next just inaudible. The result which is automatically recorded by the up and down excursion of a stylus on an audiogram form is therefore a continuous frequency audiogram showing the patient's observation of the stimulus between perceptibility and imperceptibility.

In cases of perceptive hearing loss, the variability in the length of the excursion of the stylus between the just perceptible and just imperceptible tone is considerably less than in the normal ear, particularly in the high frequences. The audiogram therefore graphically points out the reduced size of the DLs found only in perceptive loss, and the test becomes another important means of arriving at a correct diagnosis.

Speech Test

Although the use of speech as a means of testing hearing is not new, it is only in recent years, in fact since World War II, that standardized and objectively measured speech tests have assumed a prominent place in routine clinical examinations. It has long been recognized that the audiometer, as important as it is in testing hearing, has one great deficiency — it reveals what the patient cannot hear, but it fails to tell what the patient can hear, that is, how well the patient can use the hearing that remains to him.

Research done at the Harvard Psycho-Acoustic Laboratory during the war provided the means for obtaining this information in the form of certain speech tests, two of which are familiarly known as the Spondee and PB word lists. The former test consists of lists of two syllable words such as "earthquake" and "outlaw" which also have equal accent on both syllables. The PB test is composed of monosyllabic words in which the frequency of occurrence of speech sounds is in approximately the same ratio as the same sounds occur in spoken English.

It is evident that accurate and objective measurements of hearing by speech neces-

sitate well calibrated, high fidelity electro-acoustic systems. Speech testing to be meaningful requires that in test-retest situations, scores can be duplicated within the limits of observational error. Furthermore, to be practical, a speech score in one clinic must have meaning in a similar clinic elsewhere. In addition to the specially designed equipment which is necessary to make these ends possible, acoustically treated rooms in which to perform the testing are highly desirable if not essential.

Two measurable aspects of speech testing are significant — speech intelligibility and speech discrimination. The speech intelligibility score, commonly referred to as the speech reception score, marks that level at which the Spondee words must be presented in order that 50 per cent of the words will be correctly understood. The discrimination score is determined by the number of words repeated correctly by the patient from the PB list when the test is presented at a predetermined level above the speech reception threshold.*

The speech threshold obtained on the Spondee test yields important information to the clinician in several ways. It not only marks the patient's loss of hearing for speech in decibels, but at the same time it reveals the amount of hearing which remains to the individual in which to hear speech. Further, some tentative judgment of the amplification which may be necessary to raise the person's level of hearing within normal range can be made by observing the degree of speech loss. In some instances a wide discrepancy between speech loss and average pure tone loss on the audiogram may have valuable diagnostic implications.

The PB scores are of particular diagnostic significance. It has long been known that the ear afflicted with perceptive loss has difficulty in discriminating between speech sounds. One of the common complaints of persons suffering from this type of loss is, "I can hear you, but I can't understand you." In this situation, unlike that in conductive loss cases, the problem is not one of simply over-riding the hearing

*The PB word list is usually presented at 25 db. above the speech reception score when the words are presented by live voice, i.e., through a microphone, and at 35 db. when phonograph records are used. In obtaining the Social Adequacy index score the list is presented at 110 db. re. 0002 dynes² cm.

loss by increasing the intensity until the ear hears in a normal fashion.

We expect discrimination to be affected in cases of perceptive loss and regardless of the amount of intensity added above the threshold level, the individual's ability to discriminate will not improve beyond a certain degree, that degree being determined by the amount and place of damage in the cochlea. To state it another way, discrimination is a function of intensity only up to a certain point in perceptive loss. Any intensity increment beyond that point may prove actually detrimental to hearing rather than beneficial.

We can thus conclude that the perceptive ear is characterized not only by a reduced ability to discriminate speech sounds, but that it may also have a relatively narrow comfortable loudness range. Sounds below a given level are too loud. The "in between" range in which the ear may hear fairly well may be only a relatively few decibels.

The ear with conductive loss behaves in a different fashion. Its ability to discriminate will improve as the intensity is increased until it understands all or nearly all the test words. The behavior of the conductive loss ear is similar to that of the normal ear once the hearing loss has been overcome by sufficient intensity increment.

Thus the PB test is a valuable diagnostic aid in differentiating conductive from perceptive involvement. There are other ways in which speech testing may be employed advantageously, particularly in testing for malingerers and in discovering those suffering from psychogenic hearing loss, but they cannot be discussed here. Suffice it to say that the development and use of the speech tests have marked a great step forward in the development of clinical audiology.

In this paper an attempt has been made to present the reasons for the rapid growth of the whole field of audiology and to mention at least the significant developments and advancements in diagnostic testing in clinical audiology. The future undoubtedly holds additional and perhaps even more startling discoveries than has the past. No one can deny, however, that the developments thus far have contributed much to the betterment of that large group of individuals who suffer from loss of hearing.

REFERENCES

1. Bekesy, G.: A New Audiometer. *Acta Otolaryngol.,* 35:411-422, 1947.
2. Dix, M. R.; Hallpike, C. S.; and Hood, J. D.: Observations Upon the Loudness Recruitment Phenomenon with Especial Reference to the Differential Diagnosis of Disorders of the Internal Ear and VIIIth Nerve. *Jour. Laryngol. and Otol.,* 62:671-686, Nov., 1948.
3. Doerfler, L. G.: Differential Sensitivity to Intensity in the Perceptively Deafened Ear. Doctoral Dissertation, Northwestern University, 16:75-79, 1948.
4. Jerger, J. G.: "A Difference Limen Recruitment Test and Its Diagnostic Significance," *The Laryngoscope,* Vol. LXII, Dec. 1953, No. 12.
5. Luscher, E., and Zwislocki, J.: A Simple Method of Monaural Determination of the Recruitment Phenomenon. *Prac. Oto-Rhine-Laryngol.,* 10:521-522, 1948.
6. McConnell, F. and Carhart, R.: "Fenestration Surgery," *The Laryngoscope,* Vol. LXII, Dec. 1953.

Oklahoma Has Twenty-four Accredited Hospitals

Twenty-four Oklahoma hospitals have been included in the list of accredited hospitals recently released by the Joint Commission on Accreditation of Hospitals.

The list is the first published by the Joint Commission since it took over the actual hospital surveyal work from the American College of Surgeons January 1, 1953. The Commission is supported by the American College of Physicians, the American College of Surgeons, the American Hospital Association, the American Medical Association and the Canadian Medical Association. Oklahoma hospitals meeting the requirements are:

Valley View Hospital, Ada; Hardy Sanitarium, A r d m o r e ; Chickasha Hospital, Chickasha; Western Oklahoma State Hospital and Western Oklahoma Tuberculosis Sanatorium, Clinton; Enid General Hospital and St. Mary's Hospital Annex, Enid; Benedictine H e i g h t s Hospital, Guthrie; St. Mary's Hospital, McAlester; Muskogee General and Oklahoma Baptist Hospital, Muskogee; Ellison Infirmary and Norman Municipal Hospital, Norman;

Bone and Joint Hospital, Mercy Hospital, St. Anthony Hospital, University Hospital and Oklahoma Hospital for Crippled Children, and Wesley Hospital, all of Oklahoma City; Ponca City Hospital, Ponca City; A.C.H. Hospital, Shawnee; Stillwater Municipal Hospital, Stillwater; Hillcrest Memorial Hospital and St. John's Hospital, Tulsa.

Case Report

Benign Inoculation Lymphoreticulosis

CATSCRATCH DISEASE

J. NEILL LYSAUGHT, M.D.

THE AUTHOR

J. Neill Lysaught, M.D., author of the Case Report on Cat Scratch Disease is an Oklahoma City pediatrician. He was graduated from the University of Kansas School of Medicine in 1944. Certified by the American Board of Pediatrics, and a member of the American Academy of Pediatrics, he was director of the pediatric outpatient department at Johns Hopkins and instructor in pediatrics at Johns Hopkins before coming to Oklahoma.

Although only four years have elapsed since Debré first described catscratch disease, cases have now been reported in all European countries, Canada, and over the entire United States. Since the entity must be considered in the differential diagnosis of any regional lymphadentis, it is felt that a description of the disease and some illustrative case reports may be of value.

Typically, there is a history of contact with and/or a scratch by a cat. In a few days, a papule or pustule forms at the site of the scratch. Following this by from four days to three weeks there is enlargement of the lymph nodes draining the area involved. The nodes are moderately tender and the skin overlying them exhibits increased local heat. Fever may or may not be present, although sometimes it is a very prominent symptom. Occasionally transient rashes resembling erythema multiforme or erythema nodosum appear.

Laboratory examination of the blood shows only slight or no leukocytic response. The only proof of diagnosis is the demonstration of a positive skin test to an antigen made from pus aspirated from a suppurating node of a patient with the disease. This material is prepared just as is a Frei antigen. A positive test is denoted by a wheal with erythema and induration starting in 24 to 36 hours and persisting for days. Occasionally, vesiculation and even superficial sloughing occur at the site of skin testing. Positive skin tests generally persist over periods of years.

The course of the disease as mentioned is one of slow indolent enlargement of the areal lymph nodes over a period of three to 12 weeks. These nodes may eventually suppurate and require drainage or excision.

Nodes removed surgically show an epithelioid cell type of chronic inflammatory reaction. There is no histologic specificity to the appearance of the nodes that will allow microscopic diagnosis.

Recently Mollaret and his co-workers have proved the viral origin of the disease and have been able to transmit it to monkeys and to humans.

Case I: L. B., a four-year-old white male had been given a cat 18 days before, which on the first day had scratched him on the upper lip and on each cheek. Four days later, swelling of the anterior cervical and submaxillary glands on the right was noted, with the appearance of a red pustule at the site of the original scratch on the right cheek. The nodes had enlarged progressively and almost painlessly to a mat two and one half by one and one half inches. No fever had been present nor were there any rashes at any time.

On physical examination, the pustule had healed with formation of a fine reddened scar 1 mm. in diameter and the rubbery slightly tender mat of nodes previously described was palpable. No skin test was done because of the clear cut history and findings, and no treatment was prescribed.

Case II: S. M. B., five-year-old white female had a history of sudden onset of swelling in right inguinal glands two weeks before and a temperature of 106° F on the first day which had gradually subsided over a week. A white blood count done elsewhere was 15,500 with a normal differential, and a tuberculin patch test was negative. The swelling had increased in size daily since onset despite two injections of penicillin totaling 800,000 units and five days of aureomycin therapy. The child had a kitten which she habitually held in her lap and which had scratched her lightly over the lower abdomen and thighs several times before the onset of her illness.

Physical examination was essentially negative except for the presence of a two-inch by one-inch reddened mat of moderately tender nodes in the right inguinal area. These nodes were fluctuant and 4 cc. of reddish-brown pus were aspirated. This pus was bacteriologically sterile and from it a Frei type antigen was made, by the method of Foshay.[2] This was injected intradermally, and 48 hours later there was erythema one and one half inches in diameter with a central area of vesiculation which over the next few days progressed to umbilication with superficial slough. Injection of the same material into two controls gave no untoward reaction at 48 hours. No treatment was suggested.

Discussion

Since it has been shown[3] that the animals which carry this disease are not themselves ill and do not react to the specific antigen, it must be assumed that they act only to spread the disease by passive mechanical transmission. That this is true is borne out by the fact that a clinical picture similar to this disease has been seen following pricks by thorns, splinters, bones, etc. in patients who had no contact with cats.

The incubation period varies from three to seven days from the original scratch to development of the initial lesion consisting of papule or pustule at the site of scratch. This initial papule or pustule may be very indolent in its healing. In from seven to 42 days thereafter, appearance of swollen nodes begins. Any nodes may be involved depending on the site of inoculation.

The tendency is for gradual decrease in swelling with or without suppuration. Healing leaves no scar. Complications are few, although concurrent encephalitis has been reported.[4] The differential diagnosis is that of any regional adenitis, including tuberculous adenitis, tularemia, lymphogranuloma venereum, infectious mononucleosis, sarcoidosis, Hodgkin's disease, sodoku and pyogenic adenitis.

It has been the impression of some investigators that aureomycin and/or terramycin are effective in shortening the course of the disease and preventing suppuration. However, it is rather doubtful that these drugs are at all effective in the well-established case.

It is felt that if the possibility of this disease is borne in mind that much unnecessary medical treatment or surgical biopsy may be prevented. For a more complete review of the subject, the reader is referred to the recent publications of Daniels and MacMurray.

REFERENCES

1. Mollaret, P., Reilly, T., Bastin, R., and Tournier, P., La d'ecouverte du virus de la lymphoreticulose benigne d'inoculation. Presse. Med. 59:681, 59:701, 1951.
2. Foshay, L., (1951) *What's New*.
3. The'lin, F., Martin-du-pan. R., New observations of disease due to cat scratches. 40:74, 1951. Praxis, Bern.
4. Stevens, H., Cat scratch fever encephalitis. Am. J. Dis. Chil. 84:218, 1952.
5. Daniels, W. B. and MacMurray, F. G., Catscratch disease; non-bacterial, regional lymphadenitis, Arch. Int. Med. 88:736, 1951.
6. Daniels, W. B. and MacMurray, G., Catscratch disease; non-bacterial, regional lymphadenitis: A report of 60 cases. Ann. Int. Med. 37:697, 1952.

ATTEND THE A. M. A.
San Francisco - - June 21-25

ℳedical Grand Rounds

Case Presentation:

CONGENITAL HEMOLYTIC ANEMIA

JAMES M. COLVILLE, M. D., TED CLEMENS, Jr., M.D.
and ROBERT F. MORGAN, M.D.

On August 18, 1953, this 62-year-old white man was admitted to the University Hospital for the second time.

Chief Complaint: 1. An ulcer on the left shin for 50 years.

2. Anemia for six months.

Present Illness: At the age of 12, or 50 years prior to admission to this hospital, the patient was kicked in both shins by a person who was wearing brass-toed boots. Trauma was indicated by bruises approximately 4 centimeters in diameter over the anterior aspects of both tibiae. These lesions sloughed resulting in draining, ulcerating areas on either tibia. A few months later these areas were operated upon by a physician who subsequently told the patient that he had osteomyelitis of both lower tibiae. The areas did not heal and have continued to drain until the present time. In 1949 the patient was hospitalized at another hospital in Oklahoma City for infection which had spread from the original site of osteomyelitis in the right lower tibia to involve the right knee. A mid-thigh amputation of the right leg was performed. The ulcerating area on the left was skin-grafted shortly thereafter, but the graft did not take and the bone was scraped and regrafted. The area again broke down and has continued to drain yellowish material until the present time.

Six months prior to the admission to this hospital, the patient underwent a left lumbar sympathectomy in an attempt to speed the healing of the ulcer on the left tibia. The patient stated that at that time he was found to be anemic and received three blood transfusions before surgery and two blood transfusions after surgery. Following the

THE AUTHORS

Authors of Medical Grand Rounds, University Hospital, are James M. Colville, M.D., Ted Clemens, Jr., M.D., and Robert F. Morgan, M.D. Doctor Colville graduated from Cornell University School of Medicine and served internships and residencies at New York Hospital and also in the U. S. Air Force from 1950-1953. He is now chief resident in the Department of Medicine, University Hospital.

Doctor Clemens was graduated from the University of Oklahoma School of Medicine in 1952. He interned at Wisconsin General Hospital and is now resident in medicine, University Hospital.

Doctor Morgan was graduated from the University of Oklahoma in 1952 and is now interning at University Hospital.

operation, blood studies and gastric analysis were performd. The patient did not know the results of these studies but was told that he had pernicious anemia and was treated with parenteral liver, at first twice a week, and later, once every two weeks. Early in the course of liver therapy his blood picture improved. However, continued treatment did not produce further improvement in his anemia and he was subsequently sent to the University Hospitals with a note that the diagnosis of pernicious anemia was doubtful and that the last blood count approximately two weeks before admission had shown a hemoglobin of 9 grams per 100 cc of blood and a red blood cell count of 2.8 million red cells per cubic millimeter. There had been no signs or symptoms of anemia in this patient and he specifically denied glossitis, paresthesias.

Past History

Forty years prior to admission, at age 22, the patient had had pneumonia which was followed by generalized icterus. Thereafter with nearly every upper respiratory tract infection, he became jaundiced. Approximately three years prior to admission, he had typical symptoms of peptic ulcer. An upper GI series revealed "a touch of ulcer". On medical management, the symptoms improved.

Family History: Ths patient has a sister, age 70, who is living and apparently well. However, it has been noted that every time she suffers an upper respiratory tract infection, she become icteric.

System Review: Essentially non-contributory.

Physical Examination: T. 98.6; P. 18; B.P. 110 mm. of mercury, systolic, 70 mm. of mercury, diastolic. General: the patient was a well developed, well nourished white male who appeared to be chronically ill. There was a right mid-thigh amputation. Skin: the skin was generally sallow with a faint icteric tint. Eyes: the sclerae were slightly icteric. Tongue: was normal in appearance. Examination of the heart and lungs was essentially normal. Abdomen: the spleen was palpable 8 centimeters below the left costal margin with a sharp, smooth edge which was slightly tender; the liver was palpable approximately 5 centimeters below the right costal margin and was non-tender. Examination of the extremities revealed a well-healed mid-thigh amputation on the right. There was ankylosis of the left ankle and a large area of discoloration covering 75 per cent of the anterior, medial and lateral aspects of the left lower leg with three large denuded and ulcerating areas draining a serosanguineous material. Neurological examination was essentially normal.

Laboratory: Laboratory work on admission included the following: Red blood cell count, 3.2 million per cubic millimeter; hemoglobin, 10 grams per 100 cc.; hematocrit, 25 per cent; white blood cell count, 7,150 per cubic millimeter. Admission urinalysis showed 2+ protein and occasional white cells per high power field. Serum bilirubin: total 3.6 mgms. per 100 cc. with 0.175 per cent in the direct fraction and 3.45 mgms. per cent in the indirect fraction. Fasting gastric aspiration: total acid, 35 degrees; free acid, 15 degrees. Congo red test: 14.1 per cent retention in one hour. This was interpreted as a negative test. Gum biopsy

for amyloidosis was negative. Red blood cell fragility test: Patient's hemolysis was 86 per cent complete in concertration of 0.4 per per cent saline. Control: hemolysis was 13.8 per cent complete in concentration of 0.4 per cent saline. Peripheral blood studies repeated ten days after admission revealed: questionable spherocytosis; reticulocyte count of 6.1 per cent; hemoglobin, 12.4 gms. per cent; red blood cell count, 3.26 million per cubic millimeter; white blood cell count 9,700 per cubic millimeter, and hematocrit 31.5 per cent. Twenty-four hour fecal urobilinogen was 72.4 Ehrlich units per 100 gms. of stool. Indirect Coombs test, negative. Bone marrow examination revealed hypercellularity with erythroid elements constituting 78.3 per cent of the nucleated cells; 24-hour incubation of the Red Cell Fragility Test confirmed the previous examination. Further smears of peripheral blood showed 27 per cent reticulocytes and definite spherocytes.

The patient's 70-year-old sister was asked to come in for examination and blood studies. Examination revealed that she was markedly jaundiced and her spleen was palpable 5 centimeters below the left costal margin. She has been getting along quite well through the years and showed no signs or symptoms of the anemia confirmed by examination of peripheral blood. Her red cells had markedly decreased resistance to hypotonic saline.

Course: In view of the above findings of this man, it was felt that the diagnosis of congenital hemolytic anemia had been well established and that splenectomy was indicated. Accordingly, approximately one month following admission to this hospital, (9/10/53), the patient was operated upon and a large, tense spleen was removed without undue difficulty. In addition, the gall bladder was removed because it was chronically inflamed and contained stones. The spleen weighed 970 grams and microscopically showed acute passive hyperemia. Postoperatively, the patient's course was smooth. On the 14th postoperative day the red cell count was 4.6 million per cubic millimeter; hemoglobin, 16 grams per cent; reticulocytes, 0.6 per cent; white cell count 11,600 per cubic millimeter; serum bilirubin, 1.0 mgm. per cent. The ulcer on the surface of the left tibia did not change markedly following surgery, and as of December 18, 1953, there appeared to be minimal healing without evidence of active infection. Skin grafting is planned.

Discussion

This patient represents a typical case of congenital hemolytic anemia or spherocytic jaundice. His family history reveals that one sibling has had similar signs and symptoms for many years. The patient has had intermittent jaundice, chronic leg ulcers, splenomegaly and anemia for approximately 50 years. His present laboratory findings are compatible with a diagnosis of congenital hemolytic anemia. They will be discussed. When the diagnosis of hemolytic anemia is established, it is of utmost importance that all available members of the family be examined for spherocytosis. There may be close relatives who have spherical erythrocytes, but who have not manifested the disease clinically. The episodic nature of the disease itself may confuse the diagnostician. A patient seen in a quiescent period of the disease will frequently not show all of the striking abnormalities in laboratory tests which the present case demonstrates.

Given a patient with chronic anemia in whom the indices are normochromic, the finding of an elevated reticulocyte count suggests the possibility of a hemolytic anemia. The history, physical, and initial laboratory findings in the case at hand suggest such a process. The clinician must then differentiate the congenital from the acquired type. The acquired type may be divided into two categories, primary or idiopathic acquired hemolytic anemia, and hemolytic anemia secondary to any of a variety of malignancies, such as leukemia, lymphosarcoma, Hodgkin's disease and others. It is important, therefore, to exclude these diseases early in the study of any hemolytic anemia. If one be present, the basic problem is that of the primary disease process and treatment is governed accordingly.

The laboratory findings are of prime significance in differentiating the congenital from the acquired hemolytic anemia. These procedures are aimed at determining whether the primary defect is present in the erythrocytes or whether there is another explanation for hemolysis, such as a circulating hemolysin or an aggressive sequestration of red cells by the spleen. In congenital hemolytic anemia, the defect is in the red blood cell itself, which is spherical rather than biconcave.[1] That this abnormally shaped cell is the primary cause of the anemia has been shown experimentally in a variety of ways. When red blood cells from a normal person are transfused into an individual with congenital hemolytic anemia the transfused cells have a normal life span.[2] Conversely, when red blood cells from a patient with congenital hemolytic anemia are transfused into a normal recipient, the transfused erythrocytes survive only approximately 15 days. The spherical erythrocyte of congenital hemolytic anemia is more readily hemolyzed by hypotonic saline than is the normal red cell. Clinically, the two simplest and most informative laboratory tests are examination of peripheral blood for spherocytes and measurement of the osmotic fragility of the patient's red blood cells.

In certain types of acquired hemolytic anemia, the defect is due either to the presence of an auto-antibody adsorbed on the patient's red blood cells or to an auto-antibody in the serum, or to both. This concept is supported by transfusion experiments, which show that the fate of the transfused cells is the reverse of the situation in congenital hemolytic anemia. When cells from a normal person are transfused into a patient with acquired hemolytic anemia, the transfused cells have a shortened life span.[2] Conversely, when red blood cells of a patient with acquired hemolytic anemia are transfused into a normal person, the transfused erythrocytes have a normal life span. Clinically. the presence of an auto-antibody is detected by a positive Coombs test.[3]

The basis of the Coombs test is as follows: red blood cells from a patient are washed in saline and to these washed cells, rabbit anti-human serum is added. If hemolysis ensues, the test is positive. The mechanism for this test is that an antibody which is not washed off by saline is adsorbed on the affected red blood cell. This adsorbed antibody reacts with rabbit anti-human globulin to produce hemolysis. The indirect Coombs test detects an auto-antibody in a recipient's serum. Red blood cells from a normal person are incubated with the patient's serum and following this incubation the direct Coombs' is performed.

Here the auto-antibody in the serum is adsorbed on the normal individual's cells during incubation and subsequently these cells are hemolyzed by the antihuman rabbit serum. The antigenic stimulus for the production of these auto-antibodies is unknown. In acquired hemolytic anemia, the osmotic fragility of the red cells is normal during quiescence, but may be irregularly increased during a crisis. Thus, the test is variable and often not informative. Here, too, the cells are normal in shape.

Various theories have been proposed for the pathogenesis of the hemolytic crisis in congenital hemolytic anemia. The precise mechanism is still unknown. Dameshek believes it due to a humoral substance secreted by the spleen.[4] Owrens of Norway believes it due to an acute and transitory aplasia of the bone marrow with subsequent anemia occurring rapidly because of the shortened life span of the red cell.[5] Although Owrens' clinical observations are interesting, further confirmation of this hypothesis is needed.

The treatment of hemolytic anemias may be considered under two categories: those aimed at supporting the patient through a crisis and those aimed at eradicating the disease. Transfusions given at frequent intervals may be a life-saving matter in a sharp crisis. More frequently there is a slow but relentless progression of the anemia with blood transfusions being necessary but less pressing. If possible, transfusions should be delayed until the basic laboratory tests have been satisfactorily completed. The interpretation of the direct and indirect van den Bergh and of the level of the fecal urobilinogen is very difficult if whole blood has been given. Many physicians and surgeons prefer to delay blood in cases coming to splenectomy until the abdomen has been opened and the splenic pedicle clamped. This attitude has been prompted by the added gravity of a possible transfusion reaction in a patient with hemolytic anemia. Indeed, the opinion has been current that such patients show an increased tendency to have transfusion reactions. With a wider understanding of various blood sub-groups, and hence better typing of blood as to its compantbility, the incidence of reactions in hemolytic anemia, as in other circumstances, should be reduced. Certainly the most meticulous and thorough care in typing and cross matching blood to be given to a person with a hemolytic anemia is in order. In either congenital or acquired hemolytic anemias, spontaneous remissions may follow such conservative management, but the unpredictability of such remissions leaves the physician small comfort.

If the hemolytic process is thought to be the result of an antigen-antibody reaction, the use of ACTH or corisone is logical. Experience with these hormones in selected cases of acquired hemolytic anemia has been gratifying.[6] If a remission can be induced, it is safe to anticipate success by similar management of subsequent crises. All too frequently, however, the remission lasts only so long as the patient is taking the drug.

Definite treatment for congenital hemolytic anemia is splenectomy. If all splenic tissue, including accessory spleens, is removed, almost 100 per cent of the patients can be expected to return to permanent good health.[7] The operation does not alter the basic defect of the erythrocyte, but does remove the organ concerned with its rapid destruction. In the acquired variety, only 50 per cent or less of the patients will be benefitted by splenectomy.[7] In the malignant lymphomata and other malignancies, where the spleen is infiltrated, increased sequestration and phagocytosis by the spleen may result in a severe acquired hemolytic anemia. Here splenectomy may offer dramatic improvement in the patient's general condition.

Finally, one should be aware of the increased incidence of biliary pigment stones in patients suffering from chronic hemolytic anemia.[8] It is not uncommon to find gall bladder disease and not hemolytic anemia directing the patient to the physician. When such is the case, both processes should be treated surgically. Because any stressful situation may precipitate a hemolytic crisis, splenectomy and then cholecystectomy are often recommended.

REFERENCES

1. Haden, R. L.: J. Lab. and Clin. Med., 26:65, 1940.
2. Loutit, J. F., and Mollison, P. L.: J. Path. and Bacteriol., 58:711, 1946.
3. Singer, K. and Motulsky, A. G.: J. Lab. and Clin. Med., 34:768, 1949.
4. Dameshek, W., and Bloom, M. L.: Blood, 3:1381, 1948.
5. Owren, P. A.: Blood, 3:231, 1948.
6. Dameshek, W., Rosenthal, M. C., and Schwartz, L. I.: New England J. Med., 244:117, 1951.
7. Zuelzer, Wolf W.: J. Pediat., 41:4, 1952.
8. Pemberton, J. de J.: Ann. Surg., 94:755, 1931.

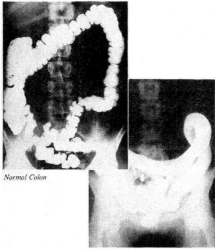

Normal Colon

Atonic Colon

Ulcerative Colitis

Smoothage and Bulk in Correcting Constipation

To initiate the normal defecation reflex,
the "smoothage" and bulk of Metamucil® provide
the needed gentle rectal distention.

Once the habit of constipation has been established, due to any of a large number of causes, it becomes a major problem. Self-medication with irritant or chemical laxatives, or repeated enemas, usually causes a decreased, sluggish defecation reflex and may result in its complete loss.

Rectal distention is a vital factor in initiating the normal defecation reflex, and sufficient bulk is thus of obvious importance in restoring this reflex. Metamucil provides this bulk in the form of a smooth, nonirritating, soft, hydrophilic colloid which gently distends the rectum and initiates the desire to evacuate. Metamucil demands extra fluid, imparting even greater smoothage to the intestinal contents.

It is indicated in chronic constipation of various types—including distal colon stasis of the "irritable colon" syndrome, the atonic colon following abdominal operations, repressions of defecation after anorectal surgery and in special conditions such as the management of a permanent ileostomy. Metamucil is the highly refined mucilloid of Plantago ovata (50%), a seed of the psyllium group, combined with dextrose (50%) as a dispersing agent.

The average adult dose is one rounded teaspoonful of Metamucil powder in a glass of cool water, milk or fruit juice, followed by an additional glass of fluid if indicated.

Metamucil is supplied in containers of 4, 8 and 16 ounces. It is accepted by the Council on Pharmacy and Chemistry of the American Medical Association. G. D. Searle & Co., Research in the Service of Medicine.

Association Activities

PRESIDENT'S LETTER

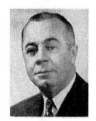

Another year has rolled around, and much too fast to have allowed time for all the work allotted to me. Many of the good resolutions have not been carried out; but perhaps it is better thus. Every President starts out with vigor, and mellows with age. I sincerely hope that it has not all been in vain.

Any failures, or shortcomings, that may have occurred, have not resulted from lack of cooperation of the Executive Office, or from the Membership. Allow me to give credit to our Executive Office, the Executive Secretary, and his worthy assistant for the energetic enthusiasm, and efficient service in the affairs of The Oklahoma State Medical Association.

Permit me, also, to again mention my immediate predecessor, Dr. Alfred Sugg, who did so much to help me during my preceptorship.

To my successor I offer sincere thanks for his valuable assistance during my year as President. I also offer appreciation to my Committees, and their excellent Chairmen, who have performed their arduous tasks of handling the detailed problems of the Association. I must pay especial tribute to the Public Policy Committee, and its Chairman, Dr. R. Q. Goodwin, and his ever ready Legislative Chairman, Dr. Malcolm Phelps.

Last, but not least, and probably the most deserving of all, the enthusiastic Membership that has arisen to every call of duty to maintain a better Association, and for better health of the citizens of Oklahoma. We, the doctors of Oklahoma will now, and in the future, be the watchdogs over the health problems of this great State of ours.

I sincerely offer my loyal support to my successors, for whatever it may be worth.

John E. McDonald M.D.

President

The *known* clinical advantages of rapid absorption,

wide distribution in body tissues and fluids, prompt

response and excellent toleration, *proved* by the

extensive experience of physicians in successfully

treating many common infections due to susceptible

gram-positive and gram-negative bacteria, rickettsiae,

spirochetes, certain large viruses and protozoa, have

Terramycin®

established *proved*

Brand of oxytetracycline

as a broad-spectrum antibiotic of choice

Have You Heard?

HENRY H. TURNER, M.D., Oklahoma City, was guest speaker at the annual meeting of the Missouri State Medical Association April 7. He spoke on "Endocrine Disorders of Childhood."

CLYDE KERNEK, M.D., formerly of Holdenville, writes that he is still serving as resident in surgery at the New England Center Hospital, Boston 11, Mass. His address is 32 Riverdale Road, Wellesley 82, Mass.

FORMATION OF THE OKLAHOMA ALLERGY CLINIC in the Pasteur Medical Building, 711 N.W. 10th St., Oklahoma City, has been announced by George S. Bozalis, M.D., Dick H. Huff, M.D., Vernon D. Cushing, M.D., and George L. Winn, M.D.

ROSCOE WALKER, M.D., Pawhuska, was recently honored with a barbecue and celebration given by his home town in observance of his 41 years of medical practice there. More than 400 friends and neighbors were present.

J. GUILD WOOD, M.D., Weatherford, was recently the subject of a feature story in the Daily Oklahoman about his hobby, raising orchids. Doctor and Mrs. Wood estimate they have given more than 100 orchids away a year since they became interested in the hobby.

ROY L. COCHRAN, M.D., was recently honored with a surprise birthday party at his office in Caddo. He was 64 and has practiced in Caddo for 35 years.

H. E. GROVES, M.D., University of Oklahoma School of Medicine graduate, and recently discharged from the U. S. Navy, has joined the Foster Clinic at 318 W. Commerce, Oklahoma City.

RANCH ACRES MEDICAL CENTER at 31st and Harvard in Tulsa has recently opened. The one story building of Colorado pink stone, resembles a clubhouse. The comfortable reception room features a wood burning fireplace. Physicians and dentists located in the center are Doctors Henry A. Brocksmith, James W. White, Loren V. Miller, J. K. Lee, Robert E. Wright, Gifford H. Henry, William S. Jacobs, Oliver H. Thompson, T. C. Covington, Jr., Jack D. Pigford, H. F. Mount and John F. May.

LEB. E. PEARSON, M.D., was recently featured in an article in his home town recounting his experience during 50 years of medical practice.

GEORGE BAXTER, M.D., Shawnee, was presented a gold 25 year service key by Oklahoma Baptist University, which he has served as physician for a quarter of a century.

JACK P. MYERS, M.D., recently discharged for the military service after serving two years in Italy, has joined the Buell Clinic in Okmulgee.

J. J. BILLINGTON, M.D., has opened a clinic in Stigler.

EDWARD M. SCHNEIDER, M.D., formerly of Tulsa, has been apointed chief of the gastroenterolgy section of the Veterans Administration hospital in Oklahoma City.

JOE L. DUER, M.D., Woodward, represented the O.S.M.A. at a meeting of the American Medical Education Foundation in Chicago recently.

J. HOYLE CARLOCK, M.D., Ardmore, addressed the Ryonis Club in that city recently on the medical angle of poliomyelitis.

W. N. OXLEY, M.D., formerly of Texhoma, has joined the Smith-Buford Clinic in Guymon.

D. C. RYAN, M.D., has recently moved from Antlers to Duncan where he joined the Lindley Hospital staff.

LOYD LONG, M.D., Ardmore, headed the Heart Fund Drive in that city.

N. H. COOPER, M.D., formerly director of the Kay County Health Department in Ponca City, is now director of health activities of the Welfare and Health Council of New York City.

FOUR MCALESTER PHYSICIANS have recently received their Board certification. They are S. L. Norman, M. D., Ben T. Galbraith, M. D. and C. K. Holland, Internal Medicine, and Bruce H. Brown, M. D., Radiology.

HARL N. STOKES has been named the administrator of Capitol Hill General Hospital in Oklahoma City. New owners of the hospital are A. R. Jackson, M.D., John R. Little, M.D., Ralph O. Clark, M.D., Marshall Opper, M.D., Charles F. Engles, M.D., J. M. Cannon, M.D., Paul B. Rice, M.D., (now deceased); J. T. McInnis, M.D., E. E. Shircliff, M.D., C. F. Foster, M.D., Scott Hendren, M.D., and Vance A. Bradford, M.D.

LT. COL. RICHARD J. BRIGHTWELL (MC) has been elected a Fellow of the Royal Society of Medicine, London. His address is: Hdq. Third Hospital Group, APO 240, USAF, c/o Postmaster, New York. Col. Brightwell is due to rotate back to the States in August.

SIR ALEXANDER FLEMING delivered the annual Alpha Omega Alpha address at the University of Oklahoma School of Medicine April 22.

W. C. GILLIAM, M.D., 85 year old Spiro physician, was honored by his fellow townspeople on his birthday.

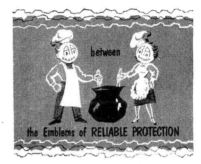
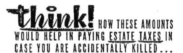
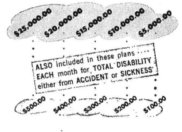

Deaths

H. C. COCKERILL, M.D., 1871-1954

H. C. Cockerill, M. D., Mooreland, died January 25, following a heart attack.

Doctor Cockerill was born at Villeaca, Ia. July 14, 1871. He established his medical practice in Mooreland in 1903. He was a member of the Masonic order having received his 50 year pin in that organization in 1946, also a member of the Mystic Shrine, the Scottish Rite Consistory and Odd Fellows lodge and the Methodist church.

WILLIAM B. HARNED, M.D., 1876-1954

William B. Harned, M. D., Walters, died January 26 of coronary thrombosis.

Doctor Harned, who had practiced medicine for more than 52 years, came to Oklahoma in 1907. He practiced at Chattanooga until 1917 when he went into military service. He was discharged as a lieutenant colonel. From 1932 to 1940 he was on active duty in CCC work. He resumed private practice in Walters and had practiced there since except from 1945 to 1947 when he practiced in Grandfield.

E. E. LAWSON, M.D., 1876-1954

E. E. Lawson, M. D., for 30 years a Medford physician, died January 12 in an Enid hospital.

Doctor Lawson was graduated from the University of Baltimore school of Medicine. In 1902, Doctor Lawson came to Oklahoma and opened his office at Carrier. He later practiced at Gage, Seiling, Oakwood and Helena. He served with the army medical corps in World War I.

EDWARD F. DAVIS, M.D., 1881-1954

Edward F. Davis, M.D., Sulphur, died March 15 after several years illness.

Doctor Davis was born in Dent, Ohio, and graduated from the University of Cincinnati Medical School in 1902. He spent a year in Peoria, Ill., before coming to Oklahoma City in 1903. He later studied at the University of Vienna, Austria. During World War I, he served as a captain in the medical corps. He moved to Ardmore in 1941 and later moved to Sulphur.

PATRICK HENRY MAYGINNIS, M.D., 1871-1954

Patrick Henry Mayginnes, M. D., pioneer Tulsa physician, died January 19 after a long illness. Doctor Mayginnes retired in 1948 after practicing 51 years in Oklahoma. He practiced in Cushing before coming to Tulsa in 1908.

Doctor Mayginnes was graduated from the St. Louis College of Physicians and Surgeons in 1897. He was an Honorary Member of the Oklahoma State Medical Association.

WALTER HARDY, M.D., 1870-1954

Walter Hardy, M. D., Ardmore resident for 72 years, died February 16 in an Ardmore hospital.

He was graduated from Washington University School of Medicine in St. Louis in 1897. Doctor Hardy was born April 11, 1870 in Arkansas.

He was a life member of the Oklahoma State Medical Association, a Mason, a fellow of the American College of Surgeons, and a charter member of the First Methodist Church.

R. D. CODY, M.D., 1873-1954

R. D. Cody, M. D., pioneer Centrahoma physician, died February 1 after a week's illness.

Doctor Cody had practiced in Centrahoma since 1904 until his retirement in 1951. He had been presented an O.S.M.A. Fifty Year Pin last year.

GEORGE W. SCOTT, M.D., 1911-1954

George W. Scott, M.D., former Tishomingo physician, died April 1 at his home in Irving, Texas.

Doctor Scott was born in 1911 and graduated from the University of Arkansas medical school in 1939. He practiced in Tishomingo from that time until 1952 when he moved to Texas except for a period during World War II when he served as a captain in the medical corps in the South Pacific.

(Continued on Page 144)

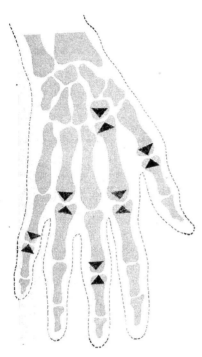

in

arthritis

and allied

disorders

Rapid Relief of Pain
usually within a few days

**Greater Freedom
and Ease of Movement**
functional improvement in a significant
percentage of cases

No Development of Tolerance
even when administered over
a prolonged period

BUTAZOLIDIN

(brand of phenylbutazone)

Its usefulness and efficacy substantiated by numerous published reports,
BUTAZOLIDIN has received the Seal of Acceptance of the Council on
Pharmacy and Chemistry of the American Medical Association for use in:

- Gouty Arthritis   • Rheumatoid Arthritis
- Psoriatic Arthritis   • Rheumatoid Spondylitis
- Painful Shoulder (including peritendinitis, capsulitis, bursitis and acute arthritis)

Since BUTAZOLIDIN is a potent agent, patients for therapy should be selected
with care; dosage should be judiciously controlled; and the patient should be regularly
observed so that treatment may be discontinued at the first sign of toxic reaction.
Descriptive literature available on request.
BUTAZOLIDIN® (brand of phenylbutazone), coated tablets of 100 mg.

GEIGY PHARMACEUTICALS
Division of Geigy Chemical Corporation
220 Church Street, New York 13, N.Y.
In Canada: Geigy Pharmaceuticals, Montreal   357

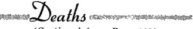

Deaths

(Continued from Page 142)

J. B. LANSDEN, M.D., 1877-1954

J. B. Lansden, M.D., Greer county physician for many years, died March 5 following an illness of six months.

Doctor Lansden was born at Livington, Tenn. and attended the University of Nashville and the University of Tennessee and graduated from the University of the South, Sewanee, Tenn., in 1901. He practiced in Willow Grove, Tenn. until 1913 when he moved to Granite.

He had received a 50 Year Pin and Life Membership.

Survivors include the widow of the home, two sons and a daughter.

P. N. CHARBONNET, M.D., 1890-1954

P. N. Charbonnet, M.D., formerly of Tulsa, and a Life Member of the Oklahoma State Medical Association, died recently at the Boston Club in New Orleans where he had made his home for several years.

Doctor Charbonnet was born in 1890 and was graduated from Tulane University in 1916. His specialty was obstetrics and gynecology.

J. R. BRYCE, M.D., 1873-1954

J. R. Bryce, M.D., Kiowa county's first practicing physician and a pioneer teacher of Jackson county, died March 12 after a long illness.

A native of Georgia, he came to Oklahoma in 1888. He practiced at Mountain Park and Snyder before retiring in 1943.

JULIAN FEILD, M.D., 1884-1954

Julian Feild, M.D., pioneer Enid physician, died March 16 in an Enid hospital. He had been in ill health since last summer.

Doctor Feild was born in Little Elm, Texas and came to Enid shortly after the opening of the Cherokee Strip in 1893. Doctor Feild attended Oklahoma University and graduated from Jefferson Medical College, Philadelphia in 1907. He retired from practice about seven months ago. He was active in medical and civic organizations and was a member of the First Presbyterian church, past president and charter member of the Enid Rotary club and past master of Enid Lodge No. 80 A. F. and A. M.

Surviving are his widow of the home, three daughters, two brothers and two sisters.

PAUL B. RICE, M.D., 1904-1954

Paul B. Rice, M.D., Oklahoma City, died March 22 after suffering a heart attack 10 days previously.

Doctor Rice was born in Lawton. He graduated from Oklahoma City University in 1925 and received his medical degree from the University of Oklahoma in 1938.

Prior to studying medicine, he taught high school and was athletic coach. He practiced for a short time in Antlers before coming to Oklahoma City in 1942.

He was a Mason and a member of the Methodist church.

He is survived by the widow of the home, two daughters, his mother and a sister.

THOMAS FLESHER, M.D., 1876-1954

Thomas Flesher, M. D., Edmond, died December 20, 1953, in an Oklahoma City hospital of acute leukemia.

Doctor Flesher was the subject of "Dr. Flesher Day" held two years ago in Edmond when nearly 400 persons turned out to honor him. He was presented with an O.S. M.A. Fifty Year Pin at that time.

Doctor Flesher was born February 10, 1876 in Reedsville, Ohio. He was graduated from Keokuk Medical College, Iowa (now the University of Iowa Medical School) in 1901. The following August he moved to Edmond and had practiced there since that time.

He was a member of the Masonic Lodge, a member of the board of the First Methodist church. He had served as city physician and was school physician at Central State College.

WILL C. WAIT, M.D., 1881-1954

Will C. Wait, M. D., McAlester, died January 20 following a heart attack suffered at the home of a patient.

Doctor Wait was the first prison physician in Oklahoma. He was superintendent for four years of the state reformatory for Negro boys. In 1935 he was named superintendent of the Oklahoma Tubercular Sanitarium at Clinton. He returned to McAlester in 1938.

Doctor Wait was born at Somerset, Kentucky May 20, 1881 and came to Pittsburg county in 1906 after graduating from the medical department of Central University in Kentucky.

(Continued on Page 146)

Meats-in-a-Can
and Kitchen-Cooked Meats...
Comparative Nutritive Values

From a practical dietary standpoint, meats-in-a-can—preserved by commercial canning—are nutritionally interchangeable with meats of like variety prepared in the home.[1] For taste appeal, for economy and "keeping" quality, and for household convenience, meats-in-a-can are advantageous in many respects.

As the comparative data here shown indicate, kitchen-prepared meats and similar meats-in-a-can are closely alike in the amounts of various nutrients they provide

COMPARATIVE COMPOSITION OF KITCHEN-COOKED AND COMMERCIAL-CANNED MEATS
(Nutrient Amounts per 100 Grams)

	*Kitchen-Cooked Ham[2]	**Canned Ham[3] (Chopped, Cured)	Kitchen-Cooked Beef Round[2]	Canned Roast Beef[2]
Water	50%	50%	59%	60%
Protein	21 Gm.	20 Gm.	27 Gm.	25 Gm.
Fat (ether extract)	28 Gm.	20 Gm.	13 Gm.	13 Gm.
Niacin	4.0 mg.	4.3 mg.	5.5 mg.	4.2 mg.
Riboflavin	0.21 mg.	0.19 mg.	0.22 mg.	0.23 mg.
Thiamine	0.46 mg.	0.40 mg.	0.08 mg.	0.02 mg.

*Values after conversion from 42% to 50% water basis.
**Values after conversion from 58.69% to 50% water basis.

Experimental studies have shown that the processing which meats-in-a-can undergo leads to little if any greater vitamin losses than does home-cooking of similar cuts of meat. In general, meats-in-a-can retain of their original vitamin content approximately:

60 to 80 per cent of thiamine
90 to 100 per cent of riboflavin
90 to 100 per cent of niacin
80 per cent of biotin
70 to 80 per cent of pantothenic acid.[4,5]

During storage for customary periods, at usual warehouse temperatures, meats-in-a-can show little, if any, further vitamin loss except in thiamine. Even thiamine, a highly thermolabile vitamin, was 52 per cent retained in pork-in-a-can after ten months' storage at 80° F. Retention of the vitamin was notably greater when the canned pork was stored at 38° F.

Since meats-in-a-can are thoroughly cooked in processing, they may be consumed as purchased, merely warmed or mildly cooked. When the meat is moderately cooked in preparation for consumption, little or no further loss in vitamins need to occur.

Recent studies show that meats-in-a-can are excellent sources of needed amino acids.[6] The 18 amino acids determined in these studies appeared in similar ratio and amounts in canned beef, pork, and lamb as in the respective fresh or home-cooked meats.

1. Howe, P. E.: Foods of Animal Origin, Handbook of Nutrition, American Medical Association, ed. 2, Philadelphia, The Blakiston Company, 1951, p. 637.
2. Watt, B. K., and Merrill, A. L.: Agricultural Handbook No. 8, United States Department of Agriculture, 1950.
3. Schweigert, B. S.; Bennett, B. A.; Marquette, M.; Scheid, H. E., and McBride, B. H.: Food Res. 17:56 (Jan.) 1952.
4. Rice, E. E., and Robinson, H. E.: Am. J. Pub. Health 34:587 (June) 1944.
5. Schweigert, B. S.: Am. Meat Inst. Foundation, Circular No. 8, Nov. 1953.
6. Schweigert, B. S.; Bennett, B. A.; McBride, B. H., and Guthneck, B. T.: J. Am. Dietet. A. 28:23 (Jan.) 1952.

American Meat Institute
Main Office, Chicago ... Members Throughout the United States

Medical Societies Around the State

Okmulgee-Okfuskee

R. M. Bird, M. D., Oklahoma City, associate professor of medicine at the University of Oklahoma School of Medicine, was a recent speaker at the Okmulgee-Okfuskee Medical Society when it met in Henryetta. Doctor Bird spoke on "Treatment of Leukemia."

Present at the meeting were the following physicians: Bob Alexander, Carlton E. Smith, Sam Leslie, John W. Deaton, I. W. Bollinger, M. L. Whitney, M. L. Peter, S. B. Leslie, A. S. Melton, G. Y. McKinney, W. C. Jenkins, C. M. Ming, Ted Clements, A. L. Buell (President), Jack P. Myers and R. D. Mercer.

Craig-Ottawa

Officers were elected at a meeting of the Craig-Ottawa Society held in Miami. Officers are J. M. McMillan, M. D., Vinita, President; Eugene Highland, M. D., Miami, Secretary; and Kenneth Lane, M. D., Vinita, Vice-President.

Caddo

New officers of the Caddo County Society elected at a meeting held at the Anadarko Hospital are: E. T. Cook, Jr., M. D., President; Burl Stone, M. D., Secretary; both of Anadarko; and W. L. Dickson, M. D., Cement, Vice-President.

Eleventh District

The annual dinner meeting of the 11th Councilor District was held recently in Durant. John McDonald, M. D., O.S.M.A. President, discussed medical problems at the state and national level. The scientific program was presented by William E. Barnett, M. C., Dallas, who spoke on "Cardiac Arrhythmias". Alfred Baker, M. D., Durant, Councilor, presided at the meeting.

Deaths

(Continued from Page 144)

WILLIAM ALLISON MORELAND, M.D., 1877-1954

William A. Moreland, M.D., pioneer Idabel physician, died February 26 after a four weeks illness.

Doctor Moreland was born May 23, 1877, at Elligay, Ga., and had resided in Idabel since 1903. He was a graduate of the University of Chattanooga, Tenn. Doctor Moreland was a veteran of World War I. He was a charter member of the Idabel Legion post, a member of the Baptist church, a Mason and a Shriner.

He is survived by the widow, two brothers and a sister.

E. L. COLLINS, M.D., 1873-1954

E. L. Collins, M. D., for 55 years a practicing physician in Panama, Okla. died March 1 at the age of 81.

Doctor Collins was born in Gasper, Ala. November 7, 1873, and settled in LeFlore county soon after his graduation from the University of Alabama School of Medicine.

Doctor Collins was active in medical organizations, was treasurer of the school board for 46 years, and a member of the Lions Club.

VIRGIL BERRY, M. D., 1866-1954

Virgil Berry, M.D., Okmulgee, died March 10 after a two year illness.

Doctor Berry was born March 14, 1866, at Salem, Ind. Following his medical education, he practiced in Salem for a time, later moving to Springfield, Ill. He moved to Wagoner and later to Wewoka. He moved to Okmulgee in 1909. He served in the army Medical Corps in World War II.

Four children, one brother and three sisters survive.

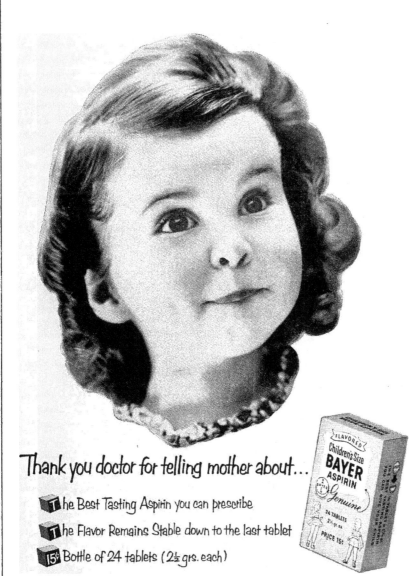

Thank you doctor for telling mother about...

■ The Best Tasting Aspirin you can prescribe

■ The Flavor Remains Stable down to the last tablet

15¢ Bottle of 24 tablets (2½ grs. each)

We will be pleased to send samples on request

THE BAYER COMPANY DIVISION of Sterling Drug Inc., 1450 Broadway, New York 18, N. Y.

Book Review

THE TURNING OF THE TIDES. Paul W. Shafer and John Howland Snow. The Long House Publishers, Inc., P. O. Box 1103, Grand Central Annex, New York 17, N. Y. 1953.

This little volume of 187 pages and a workable index dealing with the philosophy of education, is most significant. It has to do with our individual liberty and the freedom of our country. To physicians, whether or not they have children, its significance is obvious.

Without freedom of thought and action, medicine cannot function efficiently.

It is a documented statement of the socialistic, collectivist movement in our schools which amounts to a subtle blow to the future integrity of our government and our American way of life. The book should be read by every literate citizen of the United States and explained to every illiterate individual who can appreciate the security provided by our Constitution and the Bill of Rights.

For a period of approximately 50 years, organized advocates of the Bismarckian socialistic code developed in Germany and the similar Fabian philosophy in Great Britain have insidiously and artfully invaded our schools with their dangerous doctrines and destructive motives.

The opening paragraphs give an account of a meeting in New York City in a loft above Pecks Restaurant, on September 12, 1905, for the organization of the Intercollegiate Socialist Society. Two pages over we find that John Dewey, progenitor of progressive education, had organized the Progressive Education Association and the American Association of University Professors.

With these and other organizations in operation, the story runs through three parts with crescendo trends toward socialism with the hopeful turning of the tides as portrayed in the fourth part.

Is it not time for the American people to rise up and protect themselves and their

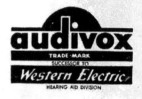
children by swelling the "turning tide" and engulfing the ominous movement in a powerful undertow.

Our sovereign freedom is our children's birthright. Indifference and procrastination at this time may rob them of the priceless gift of personal liberty.

This is not the first time we have faced danger. Our chief danger is procrastination. The words of John Adams, *Boston Gazette*, 1763, seem appropriate:

"The true source of all our suffering has been our timidity. Let us dare to read, think, speak and write. Let every order and degree among the people arouse. Let the pulpit resound. Let the bar proclaim. Let every sluice of knowledge be opened and set a-flowing."

Let every good American read the book, check conditions in his own community and act accordingly. — *Lewis J. Moorman, M.D.*

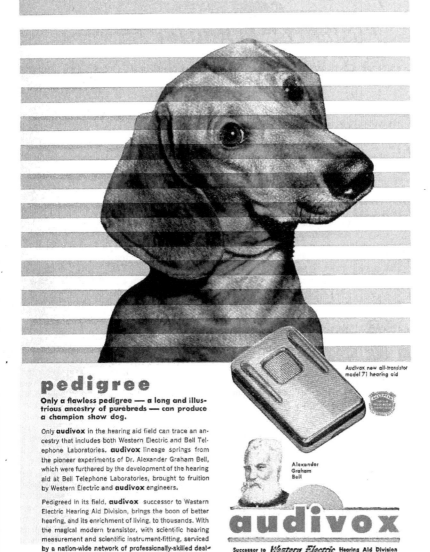

pedigree

Only a flawless pedigree — a long and illustrious ancestry of purebreds — can produce a champion show dog.

Only **audivox** in the hearing aid field can trace an ancestry that includes both Western Electric and Bell Telephone Laboratories. **audivox** lineage springs from the pioneer experiments of Dr. Alexander Graham Bell, which were furthered by the development of the hearing aid at Bell Telephone Laboratories, brought to fruition by Western Electric and **audivox** engineers.

Pedigreed in its field, **audivox** successor to Western Electric Hearing Aid Division, brings the boon of better hearing, and its enrichment of living, to thousands. With the magical modern transistor, with scientific hearing measurement and scientific instrument-fitting, serviced by a nation-wide network of professionally-skilled dealers, **audivox** moves forward today in a proud tradition.

TO THE DOCTOR: Send your patient with a hearing problem to a career Audivox and Micronic dealer, chosen for his interest, integrity and ability. There is such an Audivox dealer in every major city from coast to coast.

Audivox new all-transistor model 71 hearing aid

Alexander Graham Bell

audivox

Successor to *Western Electric* Hearing Aid Division

INDIAN OBJECTS *in a* CLEVELAND MUSEUM

HOWARD DITTRICK, M.D.

The Oklahoma State Medical Association has undertaken a most praiseworthy project of gathering together archives and materials that make up the story of medicine in Oklahoma. This problem comprises not only the experiences of pioneer physicians, an endeavor common to the history of all states, but also an unusual tale, that of primitive medicine among some of the western Indian tribes. I am unable to supply the secretary with any information or material relating to the Indians of Oklahoma. Perhaps a description of some Indian customs and possessions connected with our museum may suggest methods of further exploration.

A worthwhile magazine, published in Santa Fe and called El Palacio, frequently contained references to Indian Medicine. For example, mention was made of bandages for the head and splints for fractures, the latter made of reeds woven together. A method of reducing a dislocated hip was rather amusing. A lean and lanky horse was deprived of water for several days. The patient with the dislocation was then placed on its back and his feet were tied together under the horse's belly. The horse was then urged to drink water freely. Pressure outward and downward had a corrective effect on the dislocation. Flint knives were used to open an abscess of the breast and dried grasses were inserted for drainage. In many natural history museums collections of bags used by the Medicine Man reveal strange superstitions.

Among our possessions is a figurine coming from Arctic Siberia, made of walrus ivory. It can be disjointed beneath the arms and bits of hair or clothing belonging to the sick patient, introduced. The shaman in an effort to transfer the disease from the patient, leads in a ritualistic dance about the doll.

One of the Haida Indians in British Columbia carved a figure in black slate. The posterior surface represents a patient presumably consulting one of his deceased ancestors. On the anterior surface he appears to have recovered from his illness, although his leg has been amputated and he is wearing a crutch.

The Ojibways of Ontario are represented by a wood rack in which the papoose was securely bound, the rack then being attached to the mother's back. Another method of transporting the baby was in a basket made of birch bark, the baby being held in the basket by means of buckskin laced together with leather tongs.

Ohio had its own tribe, the Mound Builders. We have a skull from a member of this tribe, with a magnificent set of teeth. A display of flint knives and other instruments that came from Ohio's Flint Ridge was presented to the Museum by the Ohio State Museum in Columbus.

In Oklahoma you are probably familiar with many Navajo examples of Indian Medicine. The doll that is secured in the Ojibway rack has the features and dress of a Navajo baby. Another fetish, made of a specially shaped stone was handed down from father to son. It is dressed as a child with decoration of mother of pearl, turquoise, beads and bird feathers. It was given a place of honor in the home, and in return good health was ensured to all the family.

The San Blas Indians of Panama hung fetishes over the head of the patient's bed to keep away evil spirits. Two such figures are of carved wood. In driving away these evil influences the Medicine Man employed music from drums and flutes. A drum that was used for this purpose is one of our treasures. It appears that the Scotch attempted to establish a colony among the San Blas, and when this was disbanded, before 1800, the Scotch physician remained behind

(Continued on Page 152)

for greater safety in streptomycin therapy...

DISTRYCIN

Squibb Streptoduocin
Streptomycin and dihydrostreptomycin in equal parts

Distrycin has an important advantage over streptomycin. It has the same therapeutic effect but ototoxicity is greatly delayed. Since the patient is given only half as much of each form of streptomycin as he would have on a comparable regimen of either one prescribed separately, the danger of vestibular damage (from streptomycin) or cochlear damage (from dihydrostreptomycin) is significantly lessened.

Signs of vestibular damage appear in cats treated with Distrycin as much as 100 per cent later than in animals given the same amount of streptomycin.

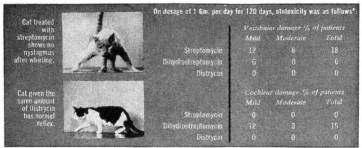

On dosage of 1 Gm. per day for 120 days, ototoxicity was as follows*:

Cat treated with streptomycin shows no nystagmus after whirling.

Cat given the same amount of Distrycin has normal reflex.

	Vestibular damage % of patients		
---	Mild	Moderate	Total
Streptomycin	12	6	18
Dihydrostreptomycin	6	0	6
Distrycin	0	0	0
	Cochlear damage % of patients		
	Mild	Moderate	Total
Streptomycin	0	0	0
Dihydrostreptomycin	12	3	15
Distrycin	0	0	0

*Heck, W.E.; Lynch, W.J., and Graves, H.L.: Acta oto-laryng. 43:416, 1953.

Distrycin dosage is the same as for streptomycin. In tuberculosis the routine dose is 1 Gm. twice weekly, in conjunction with daily para-aminosalicylic acid or Nydrazid (isoniazid). In the more serious forms of tuberculosis, Distrycin may be given daily, at least until the infection has been brought under control.

SQUIBB

a leader in streptomycin research and manufacture

'Distrycin'® and 'Nydrazid'® are Squibb trademarks

Distrycin is supplied in 1 and 5 Gm. vials, expressed as base

'Medicine And You' Is Panel Topic

Panel discussions on "Medicine and You" are being sponsored by the Oklahoma County Medical Society and the Oklahoma City Libraries. Offered free as a public service, the discussions are held each Tuesday in the Oklahoma City Main Library. Oklahoma County Medical Society members participate in the discussions.

Topics which have been or will be discussed are "You and Blood Pressure," "You and Nerves," "You and Anesthetics," "You and Drugs," "You and Headaches," and "You and Allergies."

The seven member medical committee who helped outline the experimental series is: Tullos O. Coston, M. D., Chairman, C. M. O'Leary, M. D., R. Q. Goodwin, M. D., Richard E. Carptenter, M. D., R. Gibson Parrish, M. D., George S. Bozalis, M. D., H. V. L. Sapper, M. D., and Henry G. Bennett, Jr., Society President.

Newcomers To Tulsa Get Medical Care Facts

The Tulsa County Medical Society has prepared a "welcome to new-comers" pamphlet. A copy is mailed direct from the Society to each new resident of the city.

The top of the first page is ornamented by a caduceus, followed by a simple welcome message which includes the following: "We hope that we can, with the information contained in this folder, help to dispel some of the confusion which you may encounter as a new resident of Tulsa—particularly in regard to medical and hospital care."

The second page, under the head of "Medical Services," gives the number of physicians, with an approximate number of general practitioners and specialists; laboratories, both pathologic and x-ray, etc. Also the number of hospitals, general and otherwise, listing their facilities, etc.

On the third page, advice on how to select a doctor is offered. Early selection is advised, whether or not one is immediately needed, and the advantages of early contact —and offering the help of the society in selecting a doctor, if desired.   -   *

There is also a paragraph on voluntary hospital and medical care plans, including Blue Cross and Blue Shield. Information is presented about how to transfer membership and how to enroll.

On the back page is "A Word About Fees," the advisability of discussing them in advance with the physician and procedure if it is felt the fee is our of line—and at the bottom of the page is a statement as to the make-up of the Society.

History of Medicine

(Continued from Page 150)

to care for the sick. The Indians became attached to him and after his death made a wood effigy of him, with the features and kilts of a Scot. This fetish attained a high polish from often being applied to affected areas of sick members of the tribe.

Two reproductions from the Museum of Middle American Research have medical significance. One shows a Mayan woman who is a decided hunchback. The other is a stamped figure, used in some ceremony in connection with childbirth. A Cleveland dentist made some dental inlays for the Museum similar to those of jade, obsidian and gold displayed in the National Museum in Mexico City.

Our largest display of Indian material dates from the pre-Columbian period and represents the art of pottery among the Colombian, Peruvian and Mexican tribes. Some of the pieces were buried with the dead, others were evidently used as votive offerings. Nearly all of these terra cottas represent pathologic conditions. Many of the figures are characteristic of the hunchback, due to tuberculosis of the spine. Diseases of the skin are represented as yaws, syphilis, and mycosis fungoides. Other figures show idiocy, cirrhosis of the liver, goiter, epilepsy, rickets, and pain in various parts of the body.

The list of many of the Indian objects in the Cleveland Museum has been enumerated in the hope that it may prove helpful by pointing out types of material that may be discovered and that may throw some light on the Indian influence on the History of Medicine in Oklahoma.

DO YOU AGREE?

Do you like "Your Doctor?" We'd like to have your opinion. In fact we'd like your personal vote of confidence. Won't you drop us a note soon or, better still, help us "spread the word" by using the coupon below to give someone a gift subscription?

A handsome letter personally signed by the editor naming you as the donor will be sent with each gift subscritpion.

"Your Doctor" is written and edited in cooperation with the Oklahoma State Medical Association.

JOSEPH H. LINDSAY, M. D.
CORNER DRUG BUILDING
DEWEY, OKLAHOMA

April 6, 1954

TELEPHONES:
OFFICE 235
RESIDENCE 266

Mr. Paul A. Andres
Paul Andres Publications, Inc.
1334 First National Building
Oklahoma City 2, Oklahoma

Dear Mr. Andres:

It has been my privilege to receive the recent copies of your publication "Your Doctor" for my reception room.

There has long been a need for such a magazine in this area. Any attempt to establish a better relationship between the patient and the doctor should certainly be commended.

Your choice of material for this publication has been excellent, and I wish to extend my thanks to you for your efforts. Keep up the good work!

Sincerely yours,

Joseph H. Lindsay, M. D.

Circulation to 222 Oklahoma Communities

Your **Doctor** *a magazine for patients*

A Public Relations Magazine
Exclusively for
Oklahoma Medicine

"Your Doctor" is sent complimentary to your reception room every six weeks. You have a "captive audience" waiting there daily. "Your Doctor" is designed to turn the time of this captive audience YOUR personal public relations advantage. Here's your chance to spread the word even further.

GIVE A GIFT SUBSCRIPTION NOW TO:
Schools and libraries
• Favorite Patients
• Newspaper editors and reporters
• Hospitals and sanatoriums
• Medical students, internes, nurses
• Friends and physicians in other states
• Public opinion leaders in commerce and industry

Clip here

The PAUL ANDRES PUBLICATIONS, Inc.
1334 First National Building
Oklahoma City 2, Oklahoma

Yes, I agree, "Your Doctor" is filling a definite medical public relations need in Oklahoma. Please bill me $3.50 for a year gift subscription to be sent in my name to:

Send magazine to.........................

Address ....

City and State.........................

Send Bill to:

Name.........................

Address ....

City and State.........................
Please list additional subscriptions on separate sheet

1954 County Medical Society Officers

Society	President	Secretary-Treasurer
Alfalfa	Nova L. Morgan, M.D., Cherokee	George A. Hart. M D., Cherokee
Atoka-Bryan-Coal	A. C. Fina, M.D., Atoka	Seals L. Whitely, M.D., Durant
Beckham	Phil J. Devanney, M.D., Sayre	Donald Lehman, M.D., Elk City
Blaine	Kenneth Godfrey, M.D., Okeene	Virginia O. Curtin, M.D., Watonga
Caddo	E. T. Cook, Jr., M.D., Anadarko	B. E. Stone, M D., Anadarko
Canadian	C. Riley Strong, M.D., El Reno	James P. Jobe, M.D., El Reno
Carter-Love-Marshall	John Pollock, M.D., Ardmore	Clyde Tomlin, M.D., Ardmore
Cherokee-Adair	P. H. Medearis, M.D., Tahlequah	G. W. Buffington, M.D., Tahlequah
Cleveland-McClain	George A. Wiley, M.D., Norman	F. C. Buffington, M.D., Norman
Comanche-Cotton	W. F. Lewis, M.D., Lawton	G. G. Downing, M.D., Lawton
Creek	Louis A. Martin, M.D., Sapulpa	Thomas D. Burnett, M.D., Sapulpa
Custer	C. J. Alexander, M.D., Clinton	Glenn P. Dewberry, M.D., Clinton
East Central	D. Evelyn Miller, M.D., Muskogee	Maurice C. Gephardt, M.D., Muskogee
(Muskogee, Sequoyah, Wagoner, McIntosh)		
Garfield-Kingfisher	John R. Taylor, M.D., Kingfisher	Roscoe C. Baker, M.D., Enid
Garvin	W. H. Smith, M.D., Lindsay	Hugh H. Monroe, M.D., Pauls Valley
Grady	B. B. McDougal, M.D., Chickasha	Arnold G. Nelson, M.D., Chickasha
Grant	R. W. Choice, M.D., Wakita	F. P. Robinson, M.D., Pond Creek
Greer	Dwight D. Pierson, M.D., Mangum	J. B. Hollis, M.D., Mangum
Hughes-Seminole	W. E. Jones, Jr., M.D., Seminole	Andy N. Deaton, M.D., Wewoka
Jackson	E. A. Abernethy, M.D., Altus	E. W. Mabry, M.D., Altus
Jefferson	Jose Abelarde, M.D., Waurika	Lee Pullen, M.D., Waurika
Kay-Noble	E. H. Arrendell, M.D., Ponca City	John Gilbert, M.D., Ponca City
		C. D. Northcutt, Exec. Secty., Ponca City
Kiowa-Washita	J. B. Tolbert, M.D., Mountain View	M. Wilson Mahone, M.D., Hobart
LeFlore-Haskell	C. S. Cunningham, M.D., Poteau	G. J. Womack, M.D., Wister
Lincoln	Harold T. Baugh, M.D., Meeker	Ned Burleson, M.D., Prague
Logan	Webber Merrell, M.D., Guthrie	J. E. Souter, M.D., Guthrie
Northwestern	M. K. Braly, M.D., Woodward	M. C. England, M.D., Woodward
(Beaver, Dewey, Ellis, Harper, Woodward)		
Okfuskee	N. E. Gissler, M.D., Okemah	M. L. Whitney, M.D., Okemah
Oklahoma	Henry G. Bennett, Jr., M.D., Oklahoma City	Elmer Ridgeway, Jr., M.D., Oklahoma City
		Alma O'Donnell, Exec. Secty., Medical Arts Bldg., Oklahoma City
Okmulgee	A. L. Buell, M.D., Okmulgee	S. B. Leslie, Jr., M D , Okmulgee
Osage	P. H. Haralson, M.D., Fairfax	W. A. Geiger, Jr , M.D., Fairfax
Ottawa-Craig	J. M. McMillan, M.D., Vinita	John E. Highland, M.D., Miami
Payne-Pawnee	Harold Sanders, M.D., Stillwater	C. W. Moore, M.D., Stillwater
Pittsburg	Ben T. Galbraith, M.D., McAlester	Sam Dakil, M. D.,McAlester
Pontotoc	Orange Miller Welborn, M.D., Ada	David Cozzens Ramsay, M.D., Ada
Pottawatomie	John R. Hayes, M.D., Shawnee	Clinton Gallaher, M.D., Shawnee
Rogers-Mayes	Bert Morrow, M.D., Salina	William Bynum, M.D., Pryor
Stephens	Jack Gregston, M.D., Marlow	W. R. Cheatwood, M.D., Duncan
Texas-Cimarron	*Not Reported*	James E. Morgan, M.D., Guymon
Tillman	R. L. Fisher, M.D., Frederick	O. G. Bacon, M.D., Frederick
Tri-County	A. E. Hale, M.D., Idabel	Thomas E. Rhea, M.D., Idabel
(Choctaw, McCurtain, Pushmataha)		
Tulsa	Wilkie D. Hoover, M.D., Tulsa	Charles G. Stuard, M.D., Tulsa
		Jack Spears, Exec. Secty., Medical Arts Bldg., Tulsa
Washington-Nowata	H. E. Denyer, M.D., Bartlesville	J. H. Lindsay, M.D., Dewey
Woods	*Not Reported*	T. D. Benjegerdes, M.D., Alva

Editorials

'Caritas Medici'

The Special Article in this issue of the Journal under the above title by William Bennett Bean is worthy of a careful reading. It sounds a warning and calls for a return to the time tried principles of medical care.

The author, William Bennett Bean, M. D.[1] edited the *Aphorisms of Osler* collected by his distinguished father, Robert Bennett Bean (1874-1944), who, as a student and graduate, worked in close association with William Osler. Obviously, "Caritas Medici" comes down through father and son from the abiding spirit of the world's greatest exponent of bedside medical care.

William Bennett Bean is now Professor of Medicine and Head of the Department of Internal Medicine at the State University of Iowa College of Medicine and holds many other important positions.

Those who fail to read this arresting address will miss a santifying experience.

A New Department in the Journal

To extend the service the *Journal* can give its readers, a department of case reports was started in the May issue. The purpose has to do with both the writer and the reader.

The writer will report on his observations of a particular case or cases. They need not be original or unusual, but should not only be of interest to the readers of the *Journal*, but should be helpful in his practice. The cases reported in this issue illustrate the point. Cat Scratch disease reported in last month's Journal is not uncommon, but it goes unrecognized because little has been written about it in publications that are readily available to the average practitioner. An unexplained lymphadenopathy suggests extensive diagnostic procedures. If Cat Scratch disease is kept in mind and the small indolent lesion in the area is searched for, much uneasiness and unnecessary studies can be avoided.

1. Sir William Osler, Aphorisms from his Bedside Teachings and Writings. Collected by Robert Bennett Bean, M.D. and edited by William Bennett Bean, M.D. Henry Schuman, Inc., New York. 1950. Price $2.50.

The writer or reporter may be a keen student, may love to teach and may be an extraordinarily good observer. His work, however, may be so general in nature that he does not have the opportunity for a wide searching experience in any one field. It is difficult for him to write convincingly of subjects. His observations on individual cases however, may be most impressive. This department should be used by him to satisfy his urge to teach. The thought of possible reporting should make his studies of patients more complete, his recording a matter of pen and ink instead of capricious memory and should discourage loose thinking.

The reader not only learns the lesson intended by the case report, but he compares the method of study and approach to the problem with that of his own. He may gain a certain new respect for the reporter and he should say to himself that there are studies that he himself should report. The *Journal* is particularly anxious to have material that has a special bearing on practice in this area.

The Editorial Board asks only that the material be in good form, of fairly general reader interest and medically sound. This department should bring reports from many places over the state.

Social Security

The April issue of the *Nebraska State Medical Journal* pungently poses a question which has been editorial vogue in our own *Journal* since the days of Bob Wagner. Bodily, we lift the editorial for the benefit of our readers:

"Doctors, like all other citizens, should be aware of the following facts:

"—Over $7 billion was spent by the Federal Government for Social Security, health, and welfare, in 1953.

"—A recipient of the meager old age benefits must sacrifice his benefits if he earns more than $75 per month in his effort to supplement them.

"—An alien working in the United States may become eligible to receive maximum benefits of $85 per month by paying as little as $81. He may then return to his home land, marry, raise a family, and receive these benefits for himself and family for life. He may do this with no restriction on his earnings.

"Between 1940 and 1953, the number of recipients of OASI benefits living abroad increased from 100 to 30,145.

"—Over six million persons paid Social Security taxes without receiving any benefits.

"—Over half a milion aged persons receive the minimum, $25 monthly, and only 53,000 receive $85.

"Do you want Social Security?'

Bob Wagner, who helped Franklin D. Roosevelt and Harry Hopkins load us with this system so destructive of initiative, self competency, honor and integrity, was born in Nastatten, Germany, where no doubt he inherited the Bismarckian philosophy of Social Security which, after helping to wreck the leading nations of Europe, is now gnawing out our own vitals, spiritual and economic. If we don't want more Social Security, why don't we do something about it. One of the most significant admonitions found in the Bible appears in just two words —say so"!

Currently the International Labor Organization under the guise of increased Social Security through the treaty gap has been trying to bring about complete government control of medicine.

Do you want this to come about? If not, "say so"!

Blue Cross and Blue Shield

The 1953 Annual Reports of Oklahoma Blue Cross and Blue Shield present a heart warming picture. Numerically and graphically, they depict the phenomenal progress of a voluntary service designed to help in time of need. Truly it may be sad that these agencies are friends indeed.

This great service has been made possible through the combined voluntary efforts of forward looking laymen and members of the medical profession. Particularly are the participating laymen to be commended. The medical profession is organized and maintained with service in mind, even though its members must make a living as they serve but they too must have credit for making these services possible.

These interesting and clearly delineated reports, between blue and silver covers, should have a wide reading. It requires little imagination to see the silver lining, and to envision the sense of security inherent in the mere fact of membership with its liberal and comprehensive coverage. Add to this the sustained sense of security, the sum total of actual service, both medical and surgical within the sheltering walls of the hospital, take into account the saving of mental and nervous strain, otherwise inevitable, and you have a fair appreciation of the abiding satisfactions vouchsafed through the good offices of the Cross and the Shield.

he Torch that has been lighted must be kept burning for the benefit of all who need its light and its guidance.

Brick Without Straw

Treating disease without understanding the patient as a whole and his immediate environment in relation to the world in which he lives is like making brick without straw. Accepting the new term for an old practice, medicine must be not only psychosomatic but mundane as well.

Not only must physicians consider stomach and guts, the heart and its conduits, the lights and liver, the genitorinary system, the pancreas, the spleen and the adrenal cortex, but that more abundant cortex wherein dwells the mysterious psyche which with a strange potency orders our existence, conditions our response to environment and obviates the danger of utter chaos.

Socrates set the example and Hippocrates became the first exemplar and teacher of what we call psychosomatic medicine. If psychiatrists had been medical historians we might have escaped the new term and the public spared a shattered faith with the puzzling query, why did it take physicians so long to find out what everybody with a modicum of gray matter knows by both intuition and experience. Always the mind has influenced the body and bodily defects and dysfunctions have conditioned the mind.

In a broad sense, all this means that the successful physician must know "the old humanities as well as the new science." His medicine must be steeped in culture. The bricks must have straw, not chaff.

Scientific Articles

Incidence and Treatment

GASTRIC DIVERTICULA *of the* STOMACH

VIRGIL RAY FORESTER, M.D., Oklahoma City

The rarity of gastric diverticula is still obvious. Brown, Bissonnette, and Alvea[1] reported a series of 30 cases collected from an estimated 60,000 roentgen ray examinations of the stomach. Cheney and Newell[2] reported three cases in 3,445 roentgengrams. Rivers et al.[3] reported 25 cases out of 91,532 roentgen examinations.

Most cases are found in the adult though apparently diverticula can occur at any age. Sinclair[4] reported a diverticulum in a four months old baby.

Reports in the literature are not in agreement as to who first described gastric diverticula. According to Martin[5] Baillie made the first authenic report in 1793. Voigtel is quoted as crediting Helmot[5] with the first description in 1804.

Gastric diverticula are classified as true or false. True diverticula are considered to be congenital. To be so classified they must contain all the coats of the stomach. A roentgengram showing the rugal folds to radiate into the diverticulum will aid in making the differentiation (Fig. 1).

False or acquired diverticula are further classified as traction or pulsion. The traction type may result from some extragastric disease. The pulsion type can occur from intragastric pressure.

Two sites in the stomach have a predilection for the occurrence of diverticula — the pyloric area and, more frequently the cardiac area. At the cardia, the diverticulum will usually be just below the entrance of the esophagus into the stomach, on the posterior surface and near the lesser curvature. Diverticula less frequently occupy other sites of the stomach.

THE AUTHOR

Virgil Ray Forester, M.D., the author of "Gastric Diverticula of the Stomach: Their Incidence and Treatment," was graduated from the University of Oklahoma in 1945. He served his internship and residency at Kings County Hospital, New York. During World War II, he was in the service and was a captain.

Keith[7] has proposed an explanation for the frequency of involvement of the cardiac area by suggesting a weakening of the musculature and therefore unusual straining probably encourages development of an outpouching. Bockus[8] does not agree with this explanation, for if it were so, he believes that gastric diverticula would occur much more frequently.

A pre-operative or pre-roentgenologic diagnosis is seldom made, although Lahey and George[9] have reported making one. Diverticula are frequently overlooked during an roentgen examination, especially when the stomach is completely filled with barium at the onset. Results are best if the patient is in an upright position and takes a small amount of barium at the start (Fig. 2).

If one has overlooked the diverticulum early in the examination, he may first suspect its presence on noting a rather large fleck of barium remaining in the stomach in the three hour film (Fig. 3).

To differentiate between a true diverticulum and a peptic ulcer or an ulcerating malignancy is not always easy. Buckstein[10] lists the following features for the roentgen diagnosis of gastric diverticula:

1. In the vast majority of cases, the diverticulum originates on the posterior wall near the lesser curvature, high up in the cardiac region of the stomach.

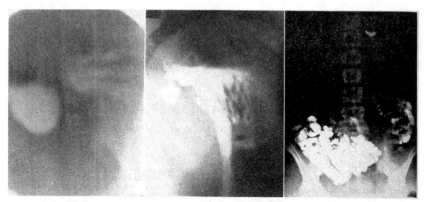

| Fig. 1 | Fig. 2 | Fig. 3 |

2. The diverticulum is perfectly smooth in outline.

3. Particularly significant is the demonstration of a narrow smooth neck communicating with the stomach. In rare instances the neck may be wide.

4. When the patient is erect, the diverticulum will often look like a miniature gastric air bubble.

5. Strands of normal mucosa may be seen entering the diverticulum from the stomach.

6. In cases of gastric diverticulum in which the neck is markedly narrowed, barium may be retained in the pouch at 24 hours, long after the rest of the stomach has emptied in a normal manner.

7. Gastroscopic examination is a valuable adjunct to diagnosis, especially in differentiating between a diverticulum and an ulcerating neoplasm.

Most diverticula of the stomach are asymptomatic. Complications may be encountered in the form of massive hemorrhage, epigastric pain, perforation, and inflammatory changes in the form of peri-diverticulitis.

Since most diverticula are asymptomatic,

treatment for the usual case is not indicated. If the symptoms are mild, a bland diet and anti-acid powders will usually afford some relief. Postural drainage should be tried along with the other palliative methods. If symptoms are severe, surgical excision should be recommended. Although the diverticulum is usually high in the cardia, its removal is not usually difficult as it is for diverticula of the duodenum where the presence of the pancreatic and common bile ducts make the removal hazardous.

REFERENCES

1. Brown, Charles H., et al.: Diverticulum of the stomach, Gastroenterology 12: 10, (Jan.) 1949.

2. Cheney, G. and Newell, R. R.: Large diverticulum of the gastric cardia, Am. J. Dig. Dis. and Nutrition, 3:920 (Feb.) 1937.

3. Rivers, A. B., Stephens, G. A., and Kirklin, B. R.: Diverticula of stomach, Surg. Gynec., and Obs., 60:106 (Jan.) 1935.

4. Sinclair, N.: Congenital diverticulum of the stomach in infants, Brit. J. Surg., 17:182 (July) 1929.

5. Martin, L.: Diverticula ef the stomach, Ann. Int. Med. 10:447, (Oct.) 1936.

6. Helmot, J. B. Van, quoted by Voital, F. G.: Handbuch der path, Anatomie. Halle, 1804-1805, p. 512.

7. Keith, A.: Diverticulum of the alimentary tract of congenital obscure origin, Brit. M. J., 1:375 (Feb. 12) 1910.

8. Bockus, H. L., Gastroenterology, W. B. Saunders Company, 1947, vol. 1, p. 770.

9. Lahey, F. H., and George, S. M.: Diverticulum of the alimentary tract, S. Clinic North America, 6:747-765 (June) 1926.

10. Buckstein, Jacob: Digestive Tract in Roentgenology, Philadelphia, J. B. Lippincott Co., 1953, vol. 1, p. 299.

Associate Professors

Several Faculty Members of the School of Medicine have been promoted from assistant professor to associate professor. They are: Dr. Robert Schneider, Department of Medicine; Dr. Phillip C. Smith, Department of Preventive Medicine and Public Health, and Dr. Sam C. Smith, Department of Biochemistry. Their appointments are effective July 1, 1954.

PAROVARIAN CYSTS

DIXON N. BURNS, M.D., Tulsa

THE AUTHOR

Dixon N. Burns, M.D., wrote "Parovarian Cysts." Doctor Burns, who has practiced in Tulsa since 1952, was graduated from Vanderbilt University Medical School in 1945. He received his B.A. in 1942. Before beginning his practice in Tulsa, he served in the army as a captain. His specialty is obstetrics and gynecology.

Development: Formation of the human urogenital system begins with the pronephros, which consists of about seven pairs of rudimentary pronephric tubules, formed as dorsolateral sprouts from the nephrotomes of the seventh to the fourteenth mesodermal segments. The solid nodules begin to hollow out and open into the coelom cranially and caudally into the lateral wall of the cloaca; they become paired and form the pronephric ducts. Degeneration of the tubules begins early and is soon complete, but the pronephric ducts persist and serve as the main excretory ducts of the second set of kidneys, the mesonephros.

The mesonephros retains the ducts of the pronephros and develops many tubules, the ducts being called mesonephric ducts or Wolffian ducts. As the tubules enlarge they bulge ventrally into the coelom and produce a urogenital ridge on each side of the dorsal mesentery. This ridge is then divided into a lateral mesonephric ridge and a medial genital ridge. The majority of the tubules degenerate, only a few remaining. In the male these are used as exretory ducts of the spermatic system, but in the female they serve no useful function.

The median or genital ridge develops an area of thickened epithelium with the cranial end remaining open; the caudal end progresses to the cloaca-development of Mullerian or paramesonephric ducts completes the development of the fallopian tubes cephalad, the distal portions uniting to form the uterus and cervix.

The ovary, which develops from the urogenital ridge, migrates caudally and acquires the mesovarium, which is separated from the mesonephros only by a longitudinal furrow. The mesonephric tubules are closely grouped in the most lateral third of the mesovarium and extend up through the lateral mesosalpinx. The mesonephric duct is found close to the musculature of the ovi-

Presented before the General Session at the Annual Meeting of the Oklahoma State Medical Asso-. ciation April 15, 1953.

duct; it is convoluted, has its own discrete muscular investment that is usually heavier than the mesonephric tubules.

During the progress of the paramesonephric ducts.cephalad the cranial end shows multiple invaginations, some of these tubules remaining in the adult, having no direct continuity with the remainder of the duct. These are believed to develop into accessory oviducts; when both ends are closed and degeneration of the tubules occurs, they form the. hydatid of Morgagni.

Thus in the embryo the mesonephric duct and about 80 mesonephric tubules are a part of the urinary apparatus called the mesonephros. As the definitive kidney is formed the lower one-third of the duct and 10 or 15 tubules are all that remain. In the male these are used in the spermatic system, but the female makes no further use of these structures. It is from the parovarium (the vestigial remnant of the sexual portion of the wolffian body) with its main duct, and the 10 to 20 tubules extending toward the hilum of the ovary and the mesosalpingeal border of the tube, that the parovarian cysts develop.

Gross Appearance: Cysts developing from small tubules are small with thin translucent walls, often being multiple and perhaps papillomatous. Those arising from large ducts may reach a size of 20 centimeters in diameter. The cyst can always be recognized by its position between the tube and the ovary, the ovary being intact, and the tube stretched over the upper border of the tumor. They are often ovoid with a thin wall, enclosed between the layers of the mesosalpinx. The cavity is usually unilocular and contains a clear fluid of low specific gravity.

Microscopic Characteristics: The lining epithelium is a single layer of cuboidal or low columnar cells with a layer of smooth muscle and connective tissue beneath. Those cysts of paramesonephric origin are a miniature replica of the epithelium lining Fallopian tubes.

Symptoms: No example of malignant change is known, and the only symptoms are the result of growth of the tumor with resulting pressure effects or of twisting and degeneration. There are two reported cases of labor obstructed to the extent that operative delivery was necessitated.

Clinical Characteristics: A clinical study of 20 cases shows the oldest patient to be 52, the youngest 19. There was no evidence that these cysts were a cause of menstrual irregularities. Three married women gave a history of infertility; two had severe rheumatic heart disease, the third patient had a congenitally absent right ovary, occluded right tube, and a 10 centimeter left parovarian cyst. Two patients had experienced abortions; one had two living children and two abortions; the other had one living child and one criminal abortion.

Pre-operative diagnosis was; ovarian cyst, 14; fibroid, three; appendicitis, one; tubal pregnancy, one; parovarian cyst one. In two instances the cysts were bilateral. Size varied from three to 20 centimeters in diameter.

A 52-year-old patient had been subjected to supra-vaginal hysterectomy eight years previously for fibroid tumor.

The only post operative complication encountered was a uretero-vaginal fistula which healed spontaneously, aided by ureteral dilation.

Surgical Principles: These patients are very often young women of reproductive age requiring conservation of ovarian function.

Injection of normal saline into the broad ligament about the cyst frequently allows blunt removal of the tumor without jeopardizing ovarian blood supply. The ureter is in close proximity and should be palpated before removal of the cyst to insure the integrity of the urinary system.

Conclusions

Parovarian cysts are infrequently seen and diagnosed.

Symptoms result only from pressure or torsion.

No adverse effects upon reproduction or menstruation were noted.

There was one post-operative complication among 20 patients — a uretero-vaginal fistula, which healed spontaneously.

REFERENCES

1. Greene, R. R., Gardner, G. H., and Peckham, B. M.: American Journal of Obstetrics and Gynecology. 55:930, 1948.
2. Novak, Emil: Gynecological and Obstetrical Pathology. W. B. Saunders Company, Philadelphia, 1940.

Exhibit Available

Persons in your home town suffering from clogged heads or draining noses will be especially interested in the new exhibit—"Sinus Trouble" — which the AMA Bureau of Exhibits now is offering to state and county medical societies for local showings at fairs and similar public gatherings. Depicting the location of the sinuses, diagnostic procedures and latest treatments now followed by physicians, this exhibit is available for immediate bookings through the Bureau, 535 N. Dearborn, Chicago 10, Ill.

Report of Three Cases

HUMAN HYPODERMAL MYIASIS

BEN H. NICHOLSON, M.D., PHIL E. SMITH, Sc. D.
and WALTER H. DERSCH, JR., M.D.

That human hypodermal myiasis is a clinical problem in Oklahoma is apparent from the following case studies:

Case 1: D. C., the three-year-old son of a western Oklahoma farmer was admitted to Wesley Hospital on November 5, 1951, because of enlarged glands in his neck and groin and swelling of the left leg.

He had been well until about three months before when he developed large nodes in the neck which in a few days subsided only to reappear three weeks before admission. At the same time the glands in his groin were enlarged and the left leg was swollen from the upper thigh to below the knee. He used the leg, however, as if nothing were wrong. The swelling subsided in two and one-half weeks. The referring physician could not explain the disability but did find a 45 per cent eosinophilia.

There was nothing pertinent in the past or family history that was obtained at this time.

Physical examination showed some enlargement of the cervical, axillary and epitrochlear nodes and a somewhat greater enlargement of the inguinals. The left thigh measured 1 to 2 cm. larger than the right.

The only significant roentgen ray or laboratory finding was a moderate leukocytosis (10-15,000) with an eosinophilia that ranged from 10 to 52 per cent. All efforts to explain the eosinophilia on the basis of any of the usual causes or any of the collagen diseases were of no avail. Because the father had to go home to harvest a maize crop, he was discharged to return for further study with the thought that some type of allergic phenomena was in operation.

He was re-admitted to the hospital on December 11, 1951. At this time there was a broad band of swelling, redness and induration across the lower abdomen extending to the inside of the thigh on both legs and with slight swelling of the penis and

THE AUTHORS

Three authors, Ben H. Nicholson, M.D., Oklahoma City; Phil E. Smith, Sc.D., Oklahoma City; and Walter H. Dersch, Jr., M.D., Shattuck, collaborated in the case report on "Human Hypodermal Myiasis." Doctor Nicholson, whose specialty is pediatrics, was graduated from Vanderbilt in 1928. He is with the Pediatric Department, Oklahoma City Clinic. Doctor Smith is a member of the Department of Preventive Medicine at the University of Oklahoma School of Medicine. Doctor Dersch practices at the Newman Clinic in Shattuck and his specialty is internal medicine. He was graduated from the University of Oklahoma in 1945 and served as a captain in the army from 1946-1948.

scrotum. Further studies were unrewarding except for the finding of strongyloides in the stools. Since strongyloides may cause such an eosinophilia, he was discharged with this as the doubtful impression.

Four months later the father wrote that the boy had developed two "risins" on his head and that when these were opened a worm was expressed from each.

Case 2: H. L., the two-year-old son of a western Oklahoma farmer was admitted to Wesley Hospital on August 8, 1953, because of swelling of the right eye.

He had been well until four months before when recovering from measles he developed a swelling of his right cheek and several 2 cm. erythematous wheals on his shoulders. At the same time there was puffiness of his forearms but all the swelling was gone in four or five days. Five weeks later he developed several swollen areas on his face, head and neck. Again they disappeared in a few days. Three times during several weeks prior to admission, the patient's eye had been swollen shut. Improvement had been apparent each time in about three days. At no time did he seem to be sick or to feel bad.

Physical examination revealed a well developed normal boy except for marked periorbital edema of the right eye with protrusion of the eyeball. The pupils reacted equally to light and accommodation and subsequent examination of the fundi showed no abnormality. The white blood count varied between 12 and 22,000 and the eosinophils from 27 to 42 percent. No explanation for the periorbital edema or eosinophilia was found in x-ray studies of the skull, sinuses or chest. Other laboratory studies were unproductive. The swelling about the right eye disappeared and the left became similarly affected during his hospital stay. Because of the possibility of migrating cutaneous larvae and an allergic reaction to them, the patient was treated for a time with Cortisone and Hetrazan. For a time there seemed to be some improvement, but on August 30, the mother wrote that his eye had swelled again and on that day his throat and neck were very sore and "his tongue was swelled until it stuck out of his mouth. It was thick enough that his teeth rested on it." For this he had been treated with Cortisone at home, she wrote. Nothing else was heard from him until December 28, 1953, when the mother wrote that he had developed a bump on the right side of his head above the ear which the father thought looked like a cow's warble. When the doctor opened this he expressed a larva the size of a match stick about three-fourths inch long.

Case 3: J. C., a seven-year-old white male was first seen at the Newman Clinic on December 11, 1953. The patient had experienced a painful swelling of the posterior aspect of the left thigh three weeks prior to the initial examination. This subsided within a few days but a similar lesion appeared on the left buttock about two weeks later. This too subsided within a few days. The day before coming in for examination, the scrotum had become swollen and painful. At the time of examination the scrotum was red, quite tender and edematous, the edema extending into the left inguinal region. There was a serosanguineous discharge coming from the scrotal area. With gentle pressure a larva 13 mm. long and 2 mm. wide at the middle was expressed from the draining area in the scrotum. This larva form has not yet been identified.

Discussion

Flies of the genus *Hypodermis*, the heel flies or ox warble flies, have larval stages called cattle grubs. Two species are found in the United States, *Hypoderma lineata* and *Hypoderma bovis*. The former species is more widely distributed and has been recorded from Oklahoma; the latter is more northerly in its distribution. Although cattle are the normal hosts, humans are occasionally parasitized.

In the normal life cycle the adult flies, which are somewhat robust and bee-like in appearance and more or less covered with bushy hair, lay eggs on the hairs of cattle, usually on the legs. This is normally in the summer or fall. Within a week the eggs hatch and the small larvae move to the skin and enter hair follicles or they may bore directly into the skin. The larvae migrate to various parts of the body but finally appear on the backs of cattle in early January to late April. When mature, the grubs make their way out of the swollen area, drop to the ground and pupate. Adult flies emerge later in the summer.

Most case histories of human infestation reveal some association with cattle during the summer or fall preceding the attack. Parasitism is accompanied by severe discomfort, and the results may be serious or even fatal. Adults are often attacked, but the number of cases among children is proportionately very high.

The first symptoms usually occur during the winter months. The wanderings of the larvae are usually upward and the path of the larvae may be followed by the localized or swollen area. When the individual larva is ready to molt it produces indurated swellings, and since man is an abnormal host it may move to the surface several times before it perforates the skin. Sometimes the small larvae enter the eye and such parasitism may result in the loss of the eye.

Other reviews of case histories and details of the life cycle are summarized by James, 1947 and Matheson, 1950.

BIBLIOGRAPHY

1. James, M. T., The Flies that cause Myiasis in Man; U. S. Dept. of Agriculture, Misc. Publications No. 631, 1947.
2. Matheson, Robert, Medical Entomology, Ithaca, N. Y., 1950.

Clinical Pathologic Conference

HOWARD C. HOPPS, M.D., and ROBERT H. FURMAN, M.D.

DOCTOR HOPPS: We are very happy to have Dr. Robert Furman of the Oklahoma Medical Research Foundation to discuss the clinical aspects of our case for today. Doctor Furman has at his disposal only that information about the case which has been provided to each of you in mimeographed form.

Protocol

Patient: E. A., 64 year white widow.

Chief Complaints: Weight loss, nervousness, swelling of feet, pounding of heart, intermittent abdominal pain and chest pain.

Present Illness: Except for the gradual loss of 45 pounds during the past two years, the patient was in fairly good health until two months prior to hospital admission. At this time she had "flu". She described this very vaguely and was not sure she had fever. The acute illness lasted about 10 days but was followed by a non-productive cough, malaise, weakness, tachycardia and palpitation, orthopnea and paroxysmal nocturnal dyspnea. The occasional slight swelling of her ankles, which she had had off and on during the year previously, became more marked and persistent. She became much more nervous than she had been previously and this was one factor in her frequent episodes of tachycardia and palpitation. However, these were also brought about by exertion, overeating, or lying flat on her back. Two or three times a week these episodes were accompanied by left chest pain described by the intern as "angina-like". Sometimes the pain would involve her back also. During the two months prior to admission the patient mentioned occasional dull epigastric pains which usually occurred after "eating too much." Sometimes this pain would "throb with the heart beat." In spite of the statement of weight loss the

patient stated that her appetite was very good.

Past History: The patient had the usual childhood diseases, also malaria in 1907. She denied any operations or other illnesses. She was married 25 years, but had no pregnancies. She lived in town, drank well water and raw milk. She suffered from insomnia for seven or eight years. One year prior to admission she had intermittent dysuria and incontinence for one month. She had been constipated for years and used laxatives every two weeks regularly.

Family History: The patient's mother died of tuberculosis at age 65. The patient was living with her at the time. The patient's father died of "old age" at 80. One brother died of "gland trouble". One sister died of unknown cause and another sister was living and in good health.

Physical Examination: Pulse was 120; R. 18; T. 99°; BP 180/96 - 200/90. The patient was described as a well developed, well nourished white female who appeared chronically ill with evidence of marked recent weight loss. She weighed 97.5 lbs. (she was 5' 2".) She was depressed and anxious although fairly alert and cooperative. Neck veins were distended and tortuous, with visible pulsations. The thyroid was enlarged approximately three times, very firm, smooth, and symmetrical. Funduscopic examination revealed no abnormality save arterio-venous nicking. The tongue was covered with a heavy dark brown furry coat. Breasts were atrophied and contained no masses. There was moderate dorsal kyphosis. Many small moist rales were heard in both lung bases. The heart was enlarged and its border was 2 cm. outside the left MCL. The PMI was very diffuse in the sixth interspace and the entire precordium moved with each beat. The rhythm was irregularly irregular. Grade II systolic murmurs were heard at the aortic area and

The University of Oklahoma School of Medicine. Presented by the Department of Pathology and Medicine.

transmitted into the neck and left arm. A_2 was less than P_2. A grade II or III blowing presystolic murmur was heard at the apex and transmitted into the axilla. The liver was palpable two fingerbreadths below the costal margin. There was a palpable mass in the epigastrium (questionably liver). Pelvic and rectal examinations revealed no abnormalities. There were no palpable lymph nodes. Extremities were not remarkable except for 1+ pitting edema of the ankles and feet and a coarse tremor at all times. A tremor was also noted on protrusion of the tongue. Deep tendon reflexes were slightly hyperactive; there were no pathologic reflexes. Sensory and motor functions were not especially remarkable except for generalized weakness.

Laboratory Data: Voided urine had a sp. gr. of 1.019, pH 6.5, and contained 1-3 WBC/h.p.f.; it was negative for protein and sugar. The Mazzini was negative. Hemoglobin was 11.5 gm. per cent. WBC's were 7,000 with a normal differential. Total protein was 6.5 gm. per cent ($A/G = 4/2.5$). A stool examination was positive for occult blood, negative for ova and parasites. A serum bromide was negative. A fasting serum cholesterol was 83 mg. per cent. Chest x-ray showed only moderate enlargement of the heart in its transverse diameter with straightening of the left border and calcification of the aortic knob. Fluoroscopy revealed slight enlargement of the left ventricle and moderate enlargement of the left auricle and right ventricle. A 2 cm. calcification was noted in the left side of the pelvis. An arm to tongue circulation time was 18 seconds. Venous pressure was 230 mm. saline. An electrocardiogram taken two days after admission showed incomplete right bundle branch block and auricular fibrillation with a rapid ventricular rate (120/min.) Another ECG taken four days later was similar.

Clinical Course: The patient was started on a regimen of bed rest, parenteral vitamins, an 800 mg. Na diet, ammonium chloride, and mercuhydrin. She was given enemas as needed for constipation, seconal as needed for sleep, and aspirin as required for headache. Digitalization apparently had no effect and she continued to have a radial

pulse deficit of 10-20/minute. During the first six hospital days the patient lost 10 and a half pounds (presumably fluid).

On the sixth hospital day she became quite restless and had left chest pain. This was not relieved by sublingual tablets or nitroglycerine, and 15 mg. of morphine sulfate was administered hypodermically. This allayed restlessness and the patient went to sleep. The following morning she was restless, moaning (chest pain?) and semi-comatose. Intravenous fluids were given with caution. Temperatures previously ranged below 100° until the eighth hospital day when rectal temperatures were recorded above 103°. Aside from admission blood pressures the only ones recorded are in the nurses notes and these ranged from 190/0 to 140/0 during the last several days of life. The patient developed increasing rhonchi and dyspnea, unrelieved by oxygen and stimulants. She died on her eighth hospital day.

DOCTOR FURMAN: It seems almost certain from the protocol that the patient suffered from hyperthyroidism and presumably thyrocardiac disease. The findings of weight loss, nervousness, tremor, weakness, tachycardia, auricular fibrillation, increased blood pressure, and palpitation all point to thyroid over-activity. Particularly significant is the statement that the appetite was good in spite of the weight loss. This does much to strengthen our attitude regarding hyperthyroidism and is against the possibility of malignancy, particularly carcinoma of the stomach, since in the latter situation weight loss is associated with anorexia. The physical examination further corroborates our suspicion by demonstrating an enlarged thyroid. We note also the low serum cholesterol level of 83 mg. per cent. The electrocardiogram shows auricular fibrillation and incomplete right bundle branch block. The latter is compatible with right ventricular hypertrophy.

The description of the blowing presystolic murmur at the apex makes mandatory the diagnosis of mitral stenosis, although the typical presystolic murmur is described usually as "rumbling" in character. The systolic murmur heard at the aortic area is of uncertain significance. It is difficult to believe that it represents aortic stenosis in view of the blood pressure and the absence of a thrill in this area. It is possible that these murmurs represent functionally unimportant calcific aortic stenosis and therefore this possibility cannot be excluded. It is of interest that when we examine the chest films there is no evidence of calcification either in the mitral or aortic valve area.

It would seem established then that we are dealing with a patient who has both hyperthyroidism as well as rheumatic heart disease with mitral stenosis. We are not disturbed by the absence of a history of previous rheumatic fever since one-fourth to one-half of the patients discovered to have rheumatic heart disease fail to give such a history. It is of interest to observe that hyperthyroidism, which can occur at any age, and mitral stenosis, are both disorders which have a definite predilection for the female.

In this patient, who now can be said to have suffered from both rheumatic mitral stenosis and hyperthyroidism, we find clear cut evidence of cardiac failure, and evidence suggestive of coronary insufficiency. It is of interest to note that the pain which the intern described as "angina-like" presumably was not typical and we also note with interest that the pain would "involve her back." This pain was of recent origin, having been described as occurring only two or three weeks prior to the hospital admission. Two months prior to admission the patient complained of epigastric pain which "would throb with the heart beat." The significance of this pain will be discussed later. One is presented with the problem now, in connection with the congestive failure, of deciding whether the failure was on the basis of "thyrocardiac disease," rheumatic heart disease, or possibly a combination of both. It would seem most likely that the congestive failure developed as the result of the combination of both disorders, since when congestive failure develops in hyperthyroid individuals we find it most often associated with coronary artery disease, hypertension or rheumatic heart disease. This of course is especially true of the patient under 40 years of age. While rheumatic heart disease alone would be sufficient explanation for the presence of auricular fibrillation, one must bear in mind, of course, that hyperthyroidism *per se*

can be a cause for auricular fibrillation and congestive failure.

We seem to have established, so far, the diagnosis of thyrocardiac disease, rheumatic heart disease and congestive heart failure.

Turning now to the consideration of the pain, one is tempted to diagnose coronary atherosclerosis in view of pain suggestive of angina pectoris, but we certainly have enough evidence to justify the assumption that the coronary insufficiency (assuming that the "angina-like" pain was true angina) resulted from a combination of the factors already described rather than atherosclerosis primarily. Furthermore, we tend to consider hyperthyroidism and the low cholesterol levels, characteristic of this disorder, as being anti-atherogenetic, and it is quite possible that we will find that this patient had relatively little coronary artery disease. After all, signs and symptoms of coronary insufficiency arise whenever the myocardial blood flow is sufficient, regardless of the mechanism responsible for the insufficiency of blood flow.

Turning now to a consideration of some of the factors which are a little bit more difficult to evaluate, we find first of all that this patient had hypertension, primarily systolic, which persisted even "during the last several days of life." We are forced to rely on the nurses notes in this regard however, and the blood pressures recorded range from 190/0 to 140/0 and are rather perplexing in regard to the diastolic level. This drop in diastolic pressure suggests aortic insufficiency or a "wide-open peripheral vascular bed," evidence for either of which is lacking. One wonders if there is some relation between this rather unusual blood pressure, the atypical chest and abdominal pain and the aortic murmur. The radiation of the chest pain to the back and the throbbing quality of the epigastric pain in the presence of hypertension suggests the possibility of aortic dissecting aneurysm. The physical signs of dissecting aneurysm are certainly not distinctive but such signs as gallop, friction rub, etc., are usually absent (in the absence of myocardial infarction) and the cardiac sounds are usually normal. The chest x-ray may show some mediastinal widening but inspection of the film in this case fails to reveal such widening. The elevated blood pressure commonly found in individuals with dissecting aneurysm often is maintained until very shortly before death. If the nurses notes are to be relied upon in this connection, it would seem that this patient more or less exhibited this phenomenon, and one wonders if the zero diastolic could have resulted from the dissection preceding in a retrograde fashion and destroying function of one or more aortic valve cusps. The evidence for this is rather tenuous. We would like to be able to support this thinking with observations on the quality and level of pulse and pressure in the extremities, and in the absence of this information can only suggest this as a possibility. Against it of course, is the lack of any description of a diastolic murmur in the aortic region. The abdominal mass in the epigastrium might have resulted from leakage of blood from the aorta during dissection resulting in hematoma formation. However, in view of the scant support for dissecting aneurysm I think it more prudent to assume that this mass was liver.

The presence of hypertension, of course brings to mind the possibility that this could be of the so-called "essential" variety. In addition, coarctation of the aorta must be considered, especially since we have raised the question of dissecting aneurysm, since aortic dissection is not uncommon in coarctation. A glance at the chest film fails to reveal any evidence of rib notching, and although this diagnostic roentgenographic finding may be absent, it is almost always present, and in this instance I think we are safe in ruling out this possibility. It is not unlikely that the hyperthyroidism *per se* was responsible for the primarily systolic hypertension noted in this patient.

The terminal episode suffers for want of a more adequate description and documentation, but it seems that the preterminal period was characterized by a continuation of pain, a persistence of relatively high blood pressure levels and an absence of fever until the last day. The increasing rhonchi and dyspnea described in the protocol suggest progressive cardiac failure. The chest pain, of course, could represent further dissection. If death was associated with dissecting aneurysm then bleeding into the pericardium and/or mediastinum might represent the

cause of death. Again we have insufficient evidence to be at all dogmatic in this regard. Death may well have occurred as the result of cardiac failure.

My final clinical diagnosis: (1) Thyrocardiac disease, (2) Rheumatic heart disease and mitral stenosis. I am not able to exclude the possibility of: Dissecting aneurysm of the aorta.

Pathologic Findings

DOCTOR HOPPS: This moderately emaciated, pale, elderly female had dry skin and poor turgor. The peritoneal cavity was opened to reveal a somewhat smaller than normal liver which, on the left, was depressed a bit because of a low diaphragm. The liver did occupy the epigastrium and it appeared that this was the basis for the palpable epigastric mass described. The pleural cavities were not remarkable nor was the pericardial cavity; (there was no hemopericardium). The heart weighed 315 gm. You will recall that this was a rather small woman so that this weight may represent slight hypertrophy. The left ventricle was moderately thickened, averaging 1.8 cm, additional evidence of hypertrophy. Valvular orifices were within normal so far as their measurements were concerned. The pulmonic valve cusps and tricuspid valve cusps were within normal limits, but the mitral valves presented beadlike fibrous thickening, especially at the line of closure, as is seen often in rheumatic fever, and there was moderate thickening and increased opacity of the chordae tendineae. There was slight fusion of the commissures of the aortic valve and slight calcification of the bases. These changes were not marked and it is doubtful that they would have produced more than slight mitral insufficiency. There were no abnormalities here that might explain a diastolic pressure of 0, and I think that the most reasonable explanation for the diastolic pressure was that it was taken by a nurse who probably missed the slight change in tone which indicated the true diastolic pressure. The myocardium was somewhat flabby and, particularly in the septum and the left ventricle, cut surfaces revealed minute foci (1-2 mm.) of whitish discoloration suggesting interstitial fibrosis. There was no evidence of old or recent infarction and no patchy fibrosis to suggest arteriosclerotic heart disease. The aorta was not remarkable except for a rather slight atherosclerosis. The lungs exhibited slight nodularity, suggesting slight bronchopneumonia, and also changes compatible with slight chronic passive congestion. The liver weighed only 915 gm. (approximately two-thirds normal). There was increased fibrosis here suggesting very early Laennec's cirrhosis, and that is what we found miscroscopically. The spleen was moderately enlarged, weighing 200 gm. There was hardly enough chronic passive congestion (microscopically) to explain this almost two-fold increase in size, and I think we should attribute it to thyrotoxicosis. We did find evidence in the thyroid to support the diagnosis of thyrotoxicosis. This woman's thyroid weighed 42 gm., as compared with an average normal of 22 gm. for this age. It was multi-nodular and microscopic sections revealed hyperplasia of the thyroid tissue and of lymphoid tissue too, which is morphologic evidence of thyrotoxicosis. The other organs were not particularly noteworthy.

From the findings which I have presented so far, we don't have adequate explanation for many of the patient's manifestations and for her terminal course. However, explanation was provided when we examined the heart microscopically. To our surprise we found that the heart of this 64 year old woman exhibited *active rheumatic myocarditis* with multiple small inflammatory foci and marked degenerative change of muscle, approaching necrosis in occasional minute foci. These were the minute foci of whitish coloration that grossly suggested fibrosis.

Our final pathologic diagnosis was:

Rheumatic fever, active, with marked degenerative changes of myocardium and multiple foci of necrosis (apparently secondary to arteritis)

Hyperplasia of thyroid, nodular with lymphoid hyperplasia (thyrotoxicosis)

Congestion, passive — acute and chronic, of viscera

Parenchymatous degeneration of liver, marked, with interstitial fibrosis — early Laennec's cirrhosis

Osteoporosis, marked.

Discussion

DOCTOR FURMAN: This is certainly an unusual and a very interesting case. I'm wondering whether or not at least part of the degenerative changes in myocardium might be the result of thyrotoxicosis. Some years ago Doctor Goodpasture described changes rather similar to these as an effect of thyrotoxic heart disease.

DOCTOR HOPPS: This possibility was given careful consideration, Doctor Furman. The demonstration of focal granulomatous lesions in the heart representing a typical Aschoff bodies seemed conclusive evidence of a rheumatic process. It is certainly possible that the heart presents a mixture of effects and that at least a portion of the degenerative change resulted from thyrotoxicosis.

Book Review

CHILDREN OF DIVORCE. J. Louise Despert, M. D. Doubleday and Company, Inc., Garden City, New York, 1953

Doctor Despert has written a very provocative book primarily designed for the layman and specifically for those who are contemplating or going through divorce and is concerned with the impact of divorce upon the children involved. Her straightforward and common sense approach is replete with illustrative examples, including the eventual outcome in each case. Physicians would do well to acquaint themselves with this book in which there is much material that can be used in advising parents how to handle their divorce in order to produce the least amount of trauma on the children. It also sets forth some excellent examples of how enlightened communities can provide counseling service through the courts for couples contemplating divorce.

—*John P. Colmore, M. D.*

CARITAS MEDICI

WILLIAM BENNETT BEAN, M.D., Iowa City, Iowa

The occasion of the installation of an Alpha Omega Alpha chapter is a fitting time to take a broad view of some of the central problems of morals, ethics, and humanities in medicine. This honor society, emphasizing scholarship, has grown in stature because it recognized students with especially high qualities. It is an honor to present this address and I begin it by congratulating your Alma Mater on this symbol of excellence and you who have been chosen to uphold what should be every physician's ideal "to be worthy to care for and heal the sick."

II. A dozen themes crossed my mind as possible topics for my talk, and I have chosen one made up of Latin words because it not only defines the mores of the physician of good will but embodies a rich expression with the savor of the early morning dew still upon it. The expression bedside manner, more sinned against than sinning, captures some of the meaning. *Caritas* through vagrant changes gives us charity and care and carries implications of love and tenderness and dearness. But *caritas medici*, a physician's *caritas*, means more. It is that vigilant and humane insight and care, compact of wisdom, and spirit, which the doctor owes his patient, be it for discipline or sympathy. This concept Francis Peabody epitomized beautifully for us in this statement that "The secret of the care of the patient is in caring for the patient."

III. One of the rare major intellects modern medicine has produced, Wilfred Trotter, has given me a theme. He says:

> The passage of time has tended more and more to clear up these lingering confusions of an anthropocentic biology, and thought is gradually gaining courage to explore, not merely the body of man but his mind and his moral capacities, in

Delivered in Oklahoma City, May 1, 1953, at the installation of a chapter of Alpha Omega Alpha of the Medical School of the University of Oklahoma.

the knowledge that there are not meaningless intrusions into an otherwise orderly world, but are partakers in him and his history just as are his vermiform appendix and his stomach, and are elements in the complex structure of the universe as respectably established there, and as racy of that soil as the oldest saurian or the newest gas.

IV. The capacity to offer criticism and the willingness, one might say the temerity, has become increasingly rare in our age of conformity. I say as did Lord Bacon in his preface to "The Elements of the Common Laws in England" that

> I hold every man a debtor to his profession, from the which as men of course do seek to receive countenance and profit, so ought they of duty to endeavor themselves, by way of amends, to be a help and ornament thereunto. This is performed, in some degree by the honest and liberal practice of a profession; when men shall carry a respect not to descend into any course that is corrupt and unworthy thereof; and preserve themselves free from the abuses wherewith the same profession is noted to be infected. But much more is this performed, if a man be able visit the strengthen the roots and foundation of the science itself, thereby not only gracing it in reputation and dignity but also amplifying it in profession and substance.

V. For those whose cortex is not congealed (and in these humoral days I must specify cerebral, not adrenal cortex), there is fascination in speculating about what future medical historians, say 50 or even 500 years from now, will think of us. Each age mercifully thinks of itself as being the best and by definition is the most modern and contemporary. Without being morbid or melodramatic I will point to certain features of modern medicine which should be of special concern to you who by natural endowment or hard work have demonstrated qualities of scholarship and leadership. Physicians as a group are no longer distinguished for their contributions to or knowledge of humane letters. The curious concentration upon accumulating data, the mesmerization in developing techniques, the hypnosis of applying tests, have all inevitably tended to separate the individual physician further and further from contact with the patient. In any art or craft the nearness of the artisan and material is measure of its validity, and in the art of medicine this nearness of patient and physician must be maintained in spirit as well as in substance. Moral values, historically the binding link between the good physician and his patient, have been relegated to a corner or thrown bodily out the door at no little hurt to the proper aim of medicine.

VI. If sudden catastrophe comes and puts an end to our modern society without quite extinguishing it, who will be the Hippocrates or the Galen of the ensuing dreary ages of darkness? What handful of current medical books would you select to dominate by dogma a future when advance is frozen? Or perhaps will the future hold that these, our times, are themselves veritable dark ages, that the concentration on fact and method of the modern conveyor-belt practice of medicine has so depersonalized us that we are not even as humane physicians as were the barber-surgeons of bygone days?

VII. I hold as first premise that physicians and most members of our contemporary professions, by forsaking humanism and the feeling for continuity with history have debased themselves to the role of technicians in a trade school age. Even without religion and the spirit of wonder which we too often dismiss with childhood, human nature escapes the raw crassness of a molecular vision of man and life if it is imbued with historic sense and humanistic spirit. Secondly, if we have not some creed and acceptance without proof every man is slave to his own intellect. He cannot honestly venture beyond the near reefs of what he himself has proved. Whatever the individual brilliance and talents, the life of man is bounded by pressures and time which do not much exceed the Psalmist's three score years and ten. If modern man must build his own tower, unaided by the past, small wonder that it is often a tower of Babel. We must all take what good and what solace we can from the vast concourse of history to avoid incessant repetition of error long exposed and participation in futile races already lost. Thirdly, I submit that morals and manners

are different expressions of the same principle, a principle which though it may not thrive on a base of history and humanism cannot come into being without them. The present-day physician by his training in the laboratory and his devotion to the totems of a "scientific" age risks losing contact with the historic role of the physician. In the rush of everyday work his manners have vanished and he is made uneasy by a dim but haunting consciousness of a want of moral force or moral standards.

VIII. Let us without fear or favor look back at the training of the medical student of today. His preliminary learning at home, whatever it may have been, certainly did not include cultivation of a knowledge of the classics. Very probably there was no deep spiritual force. The standard education of the grammar school and the high school or prep school stressed in the great current American tradition sports, teamwork, cooperation. He did not get rigorous discipline in any field. Compare the education of the founding fathers of the republic whose training was designed to fit them for active participation in the society of the day, training in the art and science of thinking rather than the squirrel-like activity of accumulating vast quantities of facts. Graduation implied mastering the three elements of the trivium, grammar, logic, and rhetoric, and the four elements of the quadrivium, the four liberal arts, music, astronomy, arithmetic, and geometry. Their mastery was tested by the defense of a proposition or thesis against any and all comers. Think how far we have fallen from the aims expressed some 20 years ago about just one of the aspects, namely, competence in rhetoric, which included

teaching us how to elevate our wisdom in the most amiable and inviting garb and to give life and spirit to our ideas and to make our knowledge of the greatest benefit to ourselves and others, and lastly, how to enjoy those pure intellectual pleasures resulting from a just taste for polite letters, a true relish for the sprightly wit, the rich fancy, the noble pathos and the marvelous sublime shining forth in the works of the most celebrated poets, philosophers, historians and orators with beauties ever pleasing, ever new.

And what does the college training, the preprofessional experience of the physician of today include? A vast concentration of the sciences, chemical, physical, mathematical, biological, with a minimum of anything that could be included under the ancient trivium and quadrivium. In fact, where these arts stand today is exquisitely illustrated by the scorn we have cast on the word trivium by our own trivial. Then the training in medical school with its initial emphasis on the basic sciences delays cultural growth by not approaching any preclinical field as a science in its own right but merely as applied to the future training in the medical school. Finally, by the time the undergraduate medical student arrives at the bedside it is no wonder that he experiences great difficulty in thinking of the sick patient as a person at all instead of the cumbersome vehicle of marvelous lesions and curious processes or as a psychosomatic complex Medical school training could scarcely be less conducive to the one possible salvation at this stage; namely, a true interest in medical history.

IX. And now you are come to the time of graduate training, the internship, the residency, and, for some, fellowships, research, teaching, and for all the final incarceration in the minutiae of practice of administration. What chance is there for you today in our system of collectivist training when we are enthralled by one of the unhappy aspects of our aging and security-minded society, namely the influence of the specialty boards on graduate medical training. My views are sufficiently well known to this audience not to need further elaboration. Therefore I merely comment that it is sad enough to be confined in the miserable cage of conformity but doubly sad that so many are in love with the cage. I for one have not been unmindful of Horace's query, *Quis custodes ipsos custodiet*, or, to paraphrase in the words of a popular song of yesteryear, "Who'll take care of the caretaker's daughter when the caretaker's busy taking care?"

X. With this background little wonder that there is so much emphasis on money, on expensive cars, on a life measured by bank account, television, and a conservative view which is retrograde in outlook and stifles with precocious senility. The vapidity of medical writing which reflects very little logical or rigorous thought indicates that the cultural potential of physicians, instead of leading, has fallen below the average. Anyone forced by editorial obligations to read

critically many medical papers is struck by the singular and consistent absence of form, a vast desert of data with the rare oases of prose all too often the dried up water holes of the alkali plains.

XI. And what thesis do I propound from a view of the history of humane letters as it bears upon the profession of medicine today? It is simple. It has no sanctions beyond some familiarity with the accumulated experience of the past. From the Renaissance onward developments in medicine illustrate the extreme difficulty that man has always had when accumulations of facts, the raw data of science, so overload the intellect that logic goes flabby from overwork in systematizing knowledge. Imagination is shackled, perhaps by fatigure or by not having the time needed for meditative gestation. In any event, we have seen the stringency of the austere rationalism of the Middle Ages and the old urbanity of Greek rationalism fade out before the immense and monolithic aggregations of contemporary fact. How truthful were the words of Artemus Ward — "The researches of so many eminent scientific men have thrown so much darkness upon the subject that if they continue their researches we shall soon know nothing."

XII. Henry Adams is a good example of the disorder of thought that is inevitable with the deep pessimism of a purely material concept of life. To him life was the vaguely disturbing hum of a top running down. Compare William James's meditative view of the significance of the second law of thermodynamics. He was concerned not so much with the total volume and duration of energy as with its distribution and the work it produced. He readily granted that the destination of mundane travel might be zero but nonetheless the scenery was magnificent and if the ultimate end was extinction the penultimate might be the millennium.

XIII. Another example of the dilemma of contemporary man in his efforts to deal with masses of accumulated data is Selye's Procrustean endeavor to equate disease with stress, for here surely neorationalism has gone soft with a surfeit of miscellaneous facts which cannot all be acted upon by intellectual digestive juices and reduced to a final simple concept. Not the least distressing aspect is the pessimistic implication of the stress thesis; namely, that life is disease, since existence without stress is inconceivable. This implication is none the less gloomy because it is so subtle. Is this an unduly somber reading of the contemporary scene? The world is about us for those to read who will.

XIV. The fruitful and great tradition of Western society has been the worth of the individual and the freedom of the soul, and our society has drawn strength and sustenance from the inner revelations of saint and artist. It will continue at its own hazard if it abandons this source of inspiration for external manipulation and purely mundane solution of its problems. The great leader whose creative personality transforms and elevates mankind will be increasingly rare in the ordered society we are entering with its drastic suppression of everything which tends to escape from the dominant norm of its stereotype. Indeed, in such a situation, salvation of the individual is replaced by the security and welfare of the collective or common man. As physicians we risk becoming repair men and mechanics for that bleak abstraction 'The Common Man," whom the small-volt engineers serve up to us as an engine slightly more complex than their electrical turtle. No hot-brained physicist with his transistors and cybernetics is going to hoodoo *me* out of *my* mind, such as it is, or, in the words of Walshe,

interpret for me in terms of microvolts and feedback mechanisms in the brain, the sonnets of Shakespeare, the Primavera of Botticelli, or the going out to death of Captain Oates in the dark wastes of the Antartic. There are more things in heaven and earth than are revealed by an amplifying valve.

XV. Primitive man, loaded with taboos, blocked in on all sides by fear and superstition, was finally freed by the emergence of intellect and the advance of knowledge. Indeed, science itself, by enlarging the scope of human choice, actually contributes to human freedom, for no one can choose what he is ignorant of. As an example from everyday life, the necessity for obeying traffic regulations is not looked upon as a serious loss of freedom because of the great potential which is opened up by employing the paraphernalia of an automotive age. I think the prophets of doom have looked too dimly

upon the possibilities of human intellect and instincts combining for a practical solution of our problems. But it should be remembered that intelligence leaves its owner no less impelled by instinct than his simpler evolutionary ancestors. It merely enlarges the capacity for varied response.

XVI. Somewhere between intelligence and instinct we find habit, which is most useful because it releases the energy for intellectual exercise from ordinary matters, allowing it to concentrate on the exceptional, the novel, and the changed. Instinct is the imbedding of such responses within the genetic mechanism that controls natural development, but it too, can play a part in liberating the intelligence from routine. Therefore, properly adjusted instinct and intelligence may be, and indeed must be, harmoniously combined.

XVII. My plea is that somewhere into a habit pattern we put good manners and morals, that we recognize not only intelligence and emotions, but, I add and I urge, spirit.

XVIII. Let me wander off into another bypass for a moment. It is not surprising that devotees of the psychosomatic have not seized upon the innumerable references by perceptive writers of the past to illustrate better than most of them do today in what is too often arid and graceless prose the concepts they aim to codify into a new branch of medicine? Smollett in his remarkable book, "Humphrey Clinker," has this passage in which Squire Bramble writes to Dr. Lewis,

I find my spirits and my health affect each other reciprocally—that is to say, everything that decomposes my mind, produces a correspondent disorder in my body; and my bodily complaints are remarkably mitigated by those considerations that dissipate the clouds of mental chagrin—The imprisonment of Clinker brought on those symptoms mentioned in my last, and now they are vanished at his discharge.—It must be owned, indeed, I took some of the tincture of ginsing, and found it exceedingly grateful to the stomach; but the pain and sickness continued to return, often at short intervals till the anxiety of my mind was entirely removed, and then I found myself perfectly at ease.

XIX. It is curious and disheartening how we have neglected spirit as well as literature all these years. The melancholy absence of spirit from much psychosomatic emphasis today merely exemplifies a geneal trend. It is tragic that in some places the psychosomatic school, with such potential for good, should have been developed and popularized so much by the nonhumanistic scientist rather than have arisen from a view of the patient which included spirit with mind and body. When medicine was split off from the church, duplicating the old cleavage of physician from priest, the apothecary surgeon had in his care the mind and body. The parson or priest was left with care of the soul, and his employment was contingent on failure of the physician. The strange controversy of science versus religion added injury — as though music was to be judged by the tone deaf or painting by the color blind. The low place accorded to the spirit today is measure of our perverse inability to deal with nonmaterial, nonobjective phases of existence, perhaps a reversion to the conceptual level of matter rather than energy.

XX. As a foremost attribute of spirit I reckon morals and the practical everyday correlate manners. In its simplest aspect physicians encounter it in relations and interrelations with patients. The teacher-student association should sustain the same pattern and ideally so should the investigator-subject relation. With so much science we have tended to relegate the practical arts of medicine to the lowest place on the totem pole. These arts represent a traditional and special body of common sense knowledge in action. As Knowledge expands, the general principles governing these arts may emerge and slowly the arts become transformed into applied science. Until this happens their employment is critically necessary. This involves certain intellectual arts. They demand special mental aptitudes, the fruit of training and experience, which show up in the fine clinician as in a connoisseur and in the poor one as in a dilettante.

XXI. I will quote now some paragraphs from a convocation talk I gave several years ago to medical students.

Let your concern be for excellence in manners in dealing with colleagues, teachers, friends, and patients. Undergraduate students have not escaped the corroding blight of modern times and modern education, that of unkindliness and selfishness. In the protracted adolescence of modern society our hunger for pleasure and happiness finds expression in boorishness, vulgarity, and petty meanness which is especially distressing and hazardous in professions concerned with health. It is disheartening to note man's inhumanity to man in any place but it is particularly so where it affects the sick and the miserable. All too often a doctor, a nurse, an orderly or others caring for the sick exhibit meanness, short temper, or maybe just some trifling lack of consideration which may nullify the efforts of brilliant science and technical virtuosity. In manners the simple rule of putting yourself in another's place will indicate what should be done. Thought and consideration for others will alleviate some of the pains of neurotic preoccupation with self which prevails so widely. With the emphasis on considerateness it is even possible that politeness may grow into courtesy and courtesy into the dignity and refinement which constitute excellence in behavior.

In the selection and cultivation of your friendships remember that subtle qualities rather than superficial ones are of importance. To a surprising degree your friends influence you and mold your habits and character. In your associates be content with nothing less than the best. Avoid the flashy, the vicious, and the shallow. Good company elevates whether it be in the people you associate with or in the books you read. Indifferent company is retarding and dulling. Bad company weakens and ultimately cripples.

Another admonition concerns integrity and intellectual honesty. In professions which depend on personal relationships and of course in all others there is no substitute for absolute integrity. A baneful tendency of some of your education up to now has been that as students you have lined up in a hostile and separate camp on the one side, with your teachers and instructors in another, and made sport of getting away with what you could in petty deceits. Dishonesty corrodes. You cannot compartmentalize its sphere and be honest in all save one or a few sections. In learning a profession the substitution of another's knowledge in default of your own is a malignant deceit which may destroy your usefulness because it later endangers those coming to you for help and comfort. In the various branches of the medical and health profession those infected with dishonesty may survive for a time, but sooner or later the blight will damage others and so destroy them.

Among the many problems which concern us, your fellow students, who by accident of chronology happen to be teaching, is the age old problem of the proper balance between education in facts and education in methods, between technics and knowledge, between ways and wisdom. Contrary to what you may suppose, scientific facts are not final and eternal but change with our growing understanding. They are knotty difficult things, and all of us at certain stages must learn a great many of them by sheer force of memory before we can integrate them into the broad pattern of what we are learning. You must never be satisfied with the mere accumulation of facts but rather try to get an understanding of their relations one to another. Be concerned not only in the acquisition of a storehouse of facts, a knowledge of technics, drugs, and doses, but in an appreciation of their true significance as they relate to the various branches of professional activity in which you will be engaged. Unless you achieve excellence not only in knowledge but in the art and craft of a profession, an integration and synthesizing of your facts, it becomes a mere business. The art of what you practice has to do with personal relations, and success in such matters depends on high standards of excellence being kept in view at all times.

How are such standards to be sustained? To recall the aphorism ascribed to Hippocrates, "Life is short and art is long, opportunity is brief, experience dubious and judgment difficult." The time is past when spoon feeding can nourish your minds and give the needed sturdiness to the fabric of intellect and character. There is no magic vitamin, no capsule of intellectual chemotherapy, which will serve in the place of the one medicine which gives excellence—hard work, Dr. William Osler's master word. Work, he says, is "a little word but fraught with momentous sequences if you can but write it on the tablets of your heart and bind it upon your foreheads." And how can work enable you to reach your goals? Most readily by cultivating a system, by concentrating and attending. If ever there was a time of scattered attention this is it. Suspended by vague ambitions, prodded by anxiety and baffled by frustration, we seem to have lost the capacity for sharp and exclusive focus of the attention. Without attention there can be no system and system withers without work. Remember this, to reach the narrow end of the distribution curve which marks excellence, you must have an abiding conviction of the need for hard work and the value of system in your work.

XXII. There can be no real need to lay qualities one against another, a comparison of those we should have and those we should suppress. In all our dealings we should be calm, not rough. The patient is by definition sick or thinks he is which is the same thing for our purposes. A calm demeanor may help soothe him. Quietness and poise instead of confusion and noise, kindness instead of thoughtlessness, patience instead of hurry, thoroughness instead of superficial approach. These I think all have their counterpart in morals so that honesty, candor, strength, and integrity dominate the scene.

XXIII. Somewhere during my brief Army experience in the Pacific, I came across a mimeographed sheet of paper with a moving message. The paper, briefly read, has disappeared. Neither the source nor the author is known to me, but I should like to conclude with the words modified as I remember them.

Go calmly amid the daily hurly burly. Remember the peace there is in silence. Be on good terms with people. Speak your truth quietly and convincingly but listen to others; they have their side to tell. Avoid loudness and aggression. Comparisons are to no purpose for there are always greater and smaller persons than yourself. Enjoy your plans as well as your achievements. Keep a vital interest in your own professional life and progress, a real possession in the changing fortunes of time. Do not let dishonesty blind you to the fact that virtue exists. Be true, be yourself, and be true to yourself. Do not feign love, nor simulate affection. Neither be ironic about love. In the face of all disillusionment and disenchantment, it is as perennial as the grass. Grow old gracefully surrendering at appropriate times the things of youth. Do not borrow trouble with dark imaginings. Be gentle. You are a child of the universe no less than the stars and the trees and whether you see it or not no doubt the universe is unfolding as it should. Be at peace with God whatever you conceive him to be. In the noisy confusion of life be at peace with your soul.

XXIV. And finally I end with a quotation from Tennyson's "Idylls of the King," which I think might be as profitable reading for many of us as the latest installment in the mystery of the isotope. I quote:

For manners are not idle, but the fruit
Of loyal nature and of noble mind.

ACKNOWLEDGMENTS
In Lieu of Bibliography

As the perceptive will see, this paper is derived, and, much more than the quotations indicate, it represents the selective quarrying of other men's minds. That some may be moved to explore the easily found sources I am putting down for reference in a sort of skeletal "Road to Xanadu" some of the paths which have been followed. To my parents, among innumerable debts, I owe the love of reading, a care for fine books, and a fascination with the potential beauties of language as a medium for ideas; to my teachers at Episcopal High School, Williams, Reade, Hoxton, and others, the first love of excellence, avidity for knowledge, and the illumination of the classics, and to Barr, Lewis, Metcalf, Luck, Webb, and others at the University of Virginia the disciplines of scholarship in a university setting where honor was the theme of our common dealings and where Jefferson's influence was pervasive in much more than just the grace and dignity of the beautiful buildings. My medical wayfarings, Virginia, Johns Hopkins, Harvard, Cincinnati, and Iowa, of supreme importance, really comprise another story.

I have numbered the paragraphs in order to avoid chopping up the text with distracting reference marks.

II. This theme was taken from F. M. R. Walshe (Arts of Medicine and Their Future [Lloyd-Roberts Lecture], Lancet 2:895, 1951), and some of the words too. His several lucid critiques of the contemporary scene, notably his Harveian Oration (1948) and Linacre Lecture (1950) have been borrowed from freely. Peabody's thin volume, "The Care of the Patient," I find essential reading at least every year.

III. Trotter, in his luminous and sparkling "Collected Papers" and erudite "Instincts of the Herd in Peace and War" has combined deep thought with criticism in a wonderfully elegant and sharp style.

IV. Bacon is just as stimulating and pertinent today as when he wrote, and has much good advice.

VIII. The quotation is from J. J. Walsh's "Education of the Founding Fathers of the Republic."

X, XI. Walshe and Charles Singer have contributed thoughts and some of the words.

XII. Recently published letters exchanged by Adams and James develop this theme.

XIV. The first sentences are almost a quotation from some lost source, and more than the quotation marks indicate came from Walshe.

XV, XVI. Part of this is from the same lost source as XIV.

XIX. This paragraph owes much to George Day's 1952 Hunterian Society Oration "P.P.S." but does not exactly fall within quotation marks.

XX. Osler, Singer, Trotter, and, not least, Walshe had a hand in this.

XXI. In my original convocation talk I acknowledged a debt to Arling and quoted him, but when I later reread one of his papers, which I had heard delivered, I realized how much more was inspired by his ideas and words, which in turn had a debt to Daniel Drake. I have a treacherous memory which may let go dates and doses but fix leech-like on a paragraph or verse. In the process of recall the verse gets identified but sentences or paragraphs lose their provenance and appear unobtrusively in my writing. Such accretions I have tried to recognize, and to this end I have made a card file of underlined passages from a wide and various reading which now, alas, has grown past my capacity to index it.

XXIV. Guinevere, from "Idylls of the King."

There are influences of Alan Gregg, Mayo Soley, Stanley Dorst, Detlev Bronk, and many others which involve attitudes more than words. Perhaps critical readers will notify me of hidden sources and lost references.

Association Activities

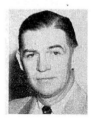

PRESIDENT'S LETTER

The Oklahoma State Medical Association can be justifiably proud of its convention just past. It was very successful on several counts.

The meeting of the House of Delegates was superbly led by its Vice-speaker, Dr. Weldon K. Haynie. Probably the most significant action taken by the House was the revision of the by-laws concerning the Grievance committee. This committee is one of our most worthwhile committees in operation, and has done more to improve public relations than any other single body within the organization. The changing of the by-laws puts the committee on firmer ground by giving its members a better definition of their procedures and powers.

In spite of the rainy weather, the convention was very well attended. The total physician registration was approximately 775, which shows a gratifying interest in the type of program provided. The program committee should be commended for obtaining such interesting and able speakers.

Mr. Graham and Mr. Hart of the Executive office did their usual fine job of seeing that all details were properly handled.

The Oklahoma City papers, the wire services, and television stations gave us excellent and very favorable coverage for the entire convention.

Now, however, is no time for complacency in any part of our program, especially in regard to national legislation, as evidenced by the fact that many professional groups are apparently in serious danger of being compelled to be a part of the Social Security program. If we are to be placed in this position it should be on a voluntary basis.

The coming convention of the A.M.A. in San Francisco, June 21 to 25, should bring forth many interesting reports, and will possibly settle many controversial issues.

President

Amebiasis[1] a "Poorly Reported" Disease

Until serious complications arise,
amebiasis may pass unrecognized and
patients receive only symptomatic treatment.

Although amebiasis is a disease with serious morbidity and mortality, statistics on its incidence[1] are incomplete because its manifestations are not commonly recognized and consequently not reported.

"Vague symptoms[2] referable to the gastrointestinal tract, such as indigestion or indefinite abdominal pains, with or without abnormally formed stools, may result from intestinal amebiasis. Not infrequently in cases in which such symptoms are ascribed to psychoneurosis after extensive x-ray studies have been carried out, complete relief is obtained with antiamebic therapy."

To prevent possible development of an incapacitating or even fatal illness and to eliminate a reservoir of infection in the community, diagnosing and treating[3] even seemingly healthy "carriers" and those having mild symptoms of amebiasis is advised.

Early diagnosis[1] is important because infection can be rapidly and completely cleared, with the proper choice of drugs and due consideration for the principles of therapy. For treatment of the bowel phase these authors find Diodoquin "most satisfactory."

For chronic amebic infections, Goodwin[4] finds Diodoquin to be one of the best drugs at present available.

Diodoquin, which does not inconvenience the patient or interfere with his normal activities, may be used in the treatment of acute or latent forms of amebiasis. If extraintestinal lesions require the use of emetine, Diodoquin may be administered concurrently. It is a well tolerated and relatively nontoxic orally administered amebacide, containing 63.9 per cent of iodine.

Diodoquin (diiodohydroxyquinoline), available in 10-grain (650 mg.) tablets, reduces the course of treatment to twenty days (three tablets daily). Treatment may be repeated or prolonged without

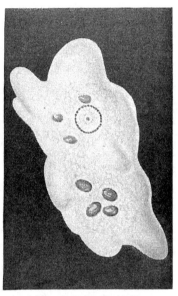

Endamoeba histolytica (trophozoite).

serious toxic effect. It is accepted by the Council on Pharmacy and Chemistry of the American Medical Association. G. D. Searle & Co., 'Research in the Service of Medicine.

1. Hamilton, H. E., and Zavala, D. C.: Amebiasis in Iowa: Diagnosis and Treatment, J. Iowa M. Soc. 42:1 (Jan.) 1952.

2. Goldman, M. J.: Less Commonly Recognized Clinical Features of Amebiasis, California Med. 76:266 (April) 1952.

3. Weingarten, M., and Herzig, W. F.: The Clinical Manifestations of Chronic Amebiasis, Rev. Gastroenterol. 20:667 (Sept.) 1953.

4. Goodwin, L. G.: Review Article: The Chemotherapy of Tropical Disease: Part I. Protozoal Infections, J. Pharm. & Pharmacol. 4:153 (March) 1952.

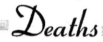

Deaths

E. F. HURLBUT, M.D.
1880-1954

E. F. Hurlbut, M.D., pioneer Meeker physician, died April 3 in Oklahoma City where he had lived for several years.

Born March 13, 1880 in Illinois, he was graduated from the medical school of the University of Illinois. He practiced in Meeker from 1917 until his retirement two years ago because of illness. He was active in civic affairs in Meeker and was a member of the Presbyterian church.

NESBITT L. MILLER, M.D.
1901-1954

Nesbitt L. Miller, M.D., Oklahoma City physician, died May 4, in a New York hospital of cancer.

He was graduated from the University of Oklahoma School of Medicine in 1925. At the time of his death he was president of the Doctors' Dinner Club.

As a highschool graduate at the age of 15, he volunteered for service in World War I and served in France. Later when the 45th division was activated in the '20's, he became a battalion surgeon and later division surgeon as a lieutenant colonel. He was medical director of the Oklahoma City Red Cross. He was a member of the Presbyterian Church.

His widow and two daughters survive.

GLENN FRANCISCO, M.D.
1890-1954

Glenn Francisco, M.D., physician at Enid for many years, died May 13. Doctor Francisco, whose specialty was urology, was graduated from the University of Oklahoma School of Medicine in 1916.

PAUL R. BROWN, M.D.
1876-1954

Paul R. Brown, M.D., pioneer Tulsa proctologist, died March 22 after a week's illness.

Doctor Brown received his medical degree from the University of Maryland in 1901. He began his practice at Danby, New York, coming to Oklahoma in 1902.

He was a veteran of the Spanish-American War where he served as medical sergeant on a hospital ship before going to medical school and was in World War I where he served as a captain. He was born at Fort Shaw, Montana, in 1876.

LEILA EDNA ANDREWS, M.D.
1876-1954

Leila Edna Andrews, M.D., Oklahoma City, first woman physician in the United States to be made a fellow of the American College of Physicians, died April 28.

Doctor Andrews was born in North Manchester, Ind. on August 14, 1876. She received her medical degree from Northwestern University in 1900 and practiced eight years in North Manchester before coming to Oklahoma City.

Her general practice won her wide recognition for her treatment of blood diseases. Doctor Andrews was a member of Alpha chapter at Northwestern University of Alpha Epsilon Iota, national women's medical sorority. She founded a chapter of that sorority in Oklahoma City and from 1923 to 1925 served as national president.

BENJAMIN WINFIELD RALSTON, M.D.
1878-1954

Benjamin W. Ralston, M.D., died March 26 at his home in Commerce. He had been in ill health for four years and had not practiced since 1952.

Doctor Ralston moved to Indian Territory in 1901 and lived in Lindsay before moving to the Tri-State district. He was educated in Nebraska and Kansas and received his medical degree from the University of Kansas School of Medicine. He received an O.S.M.A. 50-Year Pin several years ago.

Survivors include the widow of the home, one son and a grandson.

FRED SHEETS, M.D.
1885-1954

Fred Sheets, M.D., retired Oklahoma City physician, died April 21 of cancer. Graduating from the Chicago College of Medicine and Surgery, he practiced in Bartlesville before coming to Oklahoma City.

MARY RYNDAK, M.D.
1860-1954

Mary Ryndak, M.D., Hobart, early day Oklahoma City physician, died April 20. She had retired from medical practice in 1901.

A native of Hungary, she came to the United States at the age of 18 and received her medical training in St. Louis.

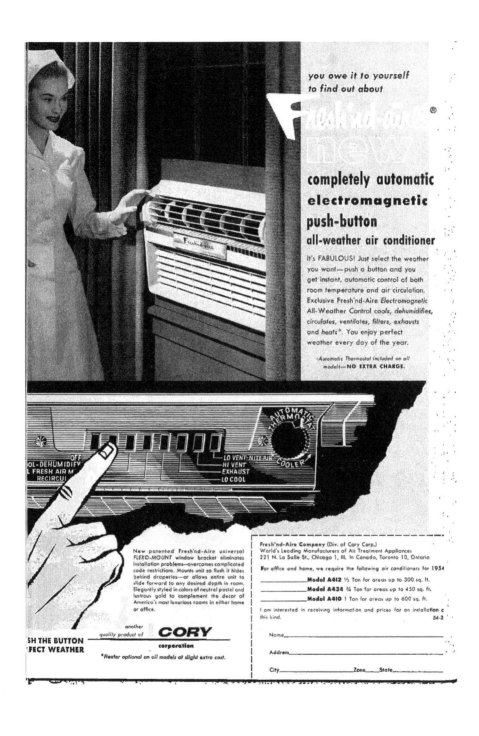

Varied Scientific, Business, Social Program Marks 61st Annual Meeting

Bruce Hinson, M. D., Enid, was installed as President of the Oklahoma State Medical Association at the Annual Meeting held in Oklahoma City May 9-10-11-12. He succeeds John E. McDonald, M. D., Tulsa.

At the House of Delegates session held Sunday, May 9, R. Q. Goodwin, M. D., Oklahoma City, was named President-Elect. Other officers elected were: James Stevenson, M. D., Tulsa, A.M.A. Delegate (reelected); E. H. Shuller, M. D., McAlester, Alternate Delegate to the A.M.A.; C. M. Bassett, M. D., Cushing, Vice-President; and Lewis J. Moorman, M. D., Oklahoma City, reelected Secretary-Treasurer-Editor. Clinton Gallaher, M. D., Shawnee, was reelected Speaker of the House of Delegates; and Keiller Haynie, M. D., Durant, was again named Vice-Speaker.

Councilors Elected

Councilors and Vice-Councilors elected were: District 2, E. C. Mohler, M. D., Ponca City, Councilor; Glen McDonald, M. D., Pawhuska, Vice-Councilor; District 5, A. L. Johnson, M. D., El Reno, Councilor; Ross Deputy, M. D., Clinton, Vice-Councilor; District 8, Wilkie Hoover, M. D., Tulsa, Councilor; Wendell L. Smith, M. D., Tulsa, Vice-Councilor; District 10, Paul Kernek, M. D., Holdenville, Councilor; C. D. Lively, M. D., McAlester, Vice-Councilor; District 11, A. T. Baker, Durant, Councilor; Thomas E. Rhea, M. D., Idabel, Vice-Councilor; District 6, Elmer Ridgeway, Jr., M. D., Oklahoma City, Councilor; P. E. Russo, M. D., Oklahoma City, Vice-Councilor; District 14, J. B. Hollis, Mangum, Councilor; and R. R. Hannas, M. D., Sentinel, Vice-Councilor.

Many Get X-Rays

One of the most successful scientific exhibits was the Chest X-Ray equipment set up by the Oklahoma State Health Department. Approximately 250 miniature chest x-ray films were made of physicians and guests attending.

More than 300 physicians and their wives and guests attended the President's Annual Inaugural Dinner Dance held in the Persian Room of the Skirvin Hotel. Following the dinner and inaugural program, Dick Jurgens orchestra played for the dance. The popular orchestra appeared for the second time this year at an Association annual dance.

The 1955 Annual Meeting will be held in Tulsa.

Minutes of the House of Delegates will appear in the July and August issues of the Journal.

Record Registration

More than 750 physicians attended the three day scientific session May 10-11-12. Additional registration of Auxiliary members, interns, residents, exhibitors and other guests brought the total registration to over 1,000.

Held in the Zebra Room of the Municipal Auditorium, a varied program was presented for the physicians attending. Besides the scientific papers, television programs were presented on surgery, orthopedics, gynecology, medicine, pediatrics and radiology. A clinical pathologic conference was held on Wednesday.

Fifty-six commercial exhibits presenting the newest developments in equipment, supplies and drugs were on display and 21 scientific exhibits were set up for the physicians to visit.

Message Center

As a courtesy to the visiting physicians by the Medical Society of America, a complete message center was set up with lines available for both incoming and outgoing calls for physicians. An innovation at this year's annual meeting, the service proved so successful that the organization plans to make it available at future meetings.

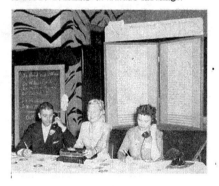

Delegates Instructed

Highlight of the action in the House of Delegates was the discussion of the Cline report regarding osteopathy wherein the House of Delegates instructed the Oklahoma delegates to the A. M. A. to oppose the Cline Report if no amendments could be made to the report. The House of Delegates also authorized the appointment of a Building Committee to explore the possibility of either buying or building a permanent headquarters. The House of Delegates also reaffirmed by resolution its previous stand that the specialties of radiology, pathology and anesthesiology are the practice of medicine and that these specialties should not be practiced by hospitals.

Auxiliary Elects

A complete business and social program was also held for the Auxiliary members attending including a tea, breakfast, and luncheon and style show. During the business session, Mrs. W. R. Cheatwood, Duncan, was installed as President. Mrs. M. L. Henry, McAlester, is the outgoing president and Mrs. E. C. Mohler, Ponca City, was named President-Elect.

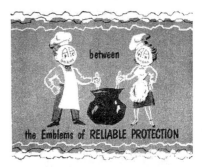
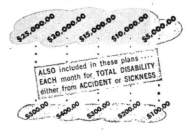

Service Disabilities
Treated At VA Expense

Doctor Charles W. Robinson, Chief Medical Officer, VARO, Oklahoma City, stated that an increasing number of veterans are unnecessarily required to pay for private hospitalization and treatment relative to their service-connected disability. If proper notification is received by the Veterans Administration, such services may be authorized at government expense.

Physicians treating veterans for their service-connected conditions could greatly assist these veterans, according to Doctor Robinson, by contacting the Veterans Administration prior to placing the veteran in a private hospital or rendering out-patient treatment. If it is medically feasible and facilities are available, veterans must be hospitalized in a VA hospital. Emergent cases may receive private hospitalization at government expense provided the Veterans Administration is notified prior to entry in a hospital, and in no event later than 72 hours after admission.

Doctor Robinson pointed out that although Spanish-American War Veterans are entitled to out-patient treatment, they are not entitled to private hospitalization at government expense, and every effort should be made to secure a bed in a VA facility when hospitalization is required.

If the Veterans Administration is not properly notified, a claim for unauthorized medical expense is the only means whereby a veteran may be reimbursed. Eligibility criteria for such claims are hard to meet, and many claims are disallowed. This causes undue hardship in many cases, Doctor Robinson added.

Society Announces Memorial Award

Oklahoma Arthritis-Rheumatism Society anounces the annual Ian McKenzie Award to be given to the medical student, intern, or resident submitting the best presentation for the treatment of arthritis.

This award in the sum of $50.00, has been instituted as a memorial to the late Ian McKenzie, M.D., of Tulsa. Case presentations of less than 5,000 words should be submitted

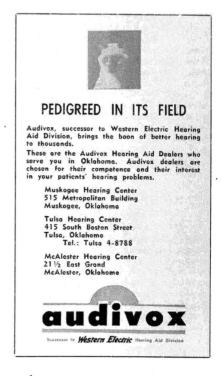
in legible form, preferably typewritten, to Richard W. Payne, M.D., Secretary of the Society, at 625 N. W. 10th St., Oklahoma City, by July 15, 1954.

Dermatologists Elect

New officers have been announced by the Oklahoma State Dermatological Association. Hervey A. Foerster, M. D., Oklahoma City, is President; William Doyle, M. D., Muskogee, Vice-President; and William McCreight, M. D., Oklahoma City, Secretary-Treasurer.

Officers were elected at the annual meeting of the group held Sunday, May 9. Guest speaker was Earl D. Osborne, M. D., Buffalo, N. Y. Sixteen rare skin diseases were presented at the University Hospital followed by discussion. A luncheon was also held for the group.

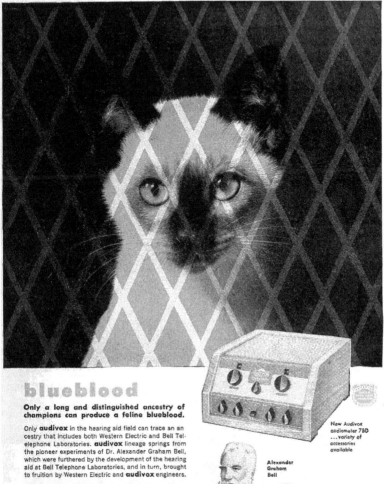

blueblood

Only a long and distinguished ancestry of champions can produce a feline blueblood.

Only **audivox** in the hearing aid field can trace an ancestry that includes both Western Electric and Bell Telephone Laboratories. **audivox** lineage springs from the pioneer experiments of Dr. Alexander Graham Bell, which were furthered by the development of the hearing aid at Bell Telephone Laboratories, and in turn, brought to fruition by Western Electric and **audivox** engineers.

Distinctly a blueblood in its field, **audivox**, successor to Western Electric Hearing Aid Division, brings the boon of better hearing, and its enrichment of living, to thousands. With the magical modern transistor, with scientific hearing measurement and scientific instrument-fitting, serviced by a nationwide network of professionally-skilled dealers, **audivox** moves forward today in a proud tradition.

TO THE DOCTOR: *If you use or need an audiometer* there is in every major city from coast to coast a career Audivox dealer, chosen for his integrity and ability, who will be glad to show you why an Audivox audiometer will serve you best.

New Audivox audiometer 7BD ...variety of accessories available

Alexander Graham Bell

audivox

Successor to *Western Electric* Hearing Aid Division

123 Worcester, St., Boston, Mass.

Have You Heard?

KIEFFER DAVIS, M.D., Bartlesville, was recently elected president-elect of the Industrial Medical Association. TOM HALL MITCHELL, M.D., Tulsa, was appointed to serve as councilor for the Arkansas-Oklahoma district of the association.

E. S. CROW, M.D., Olustee, recently received a 50 year Masonic pin.

R. L. BAKKEN, M.D., has recently completed a 14 month tour of duty in Korea and rejoined the Sisler Clinic in Bristow.

CHARLES ED WHITE, M.D., Muskogee, has been invited to deliver a paper at the International Congress of Gynecology and Obstetrics in Geneva, Switzerland, in July.

I. N. KOLB, M.D., Blanchard, was recently honored by 1,200 townspeople on the anniversary of his 48th year in the practice of medicine.

L. J. STARRY, M.D., Oklahoma City, has been reappointed chief of staff of St. Anthony Hospital. GRIDER PENICK, M.D., was reappointed vice-president and C. R. ROUNTREE, M.D., is secretary.

L. P. HETHERINGTON, M.D., Miami, returned May 5 from an extensive European tour. He was one of 40 doctors making the airborne trip sponsored by the California State Medical Association.

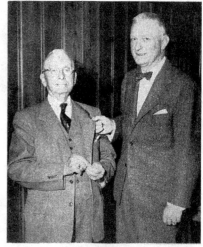

J. F. Renegar, M.D., Tuttle, receives his 50 Year Pin from H. M. McClure, M.D., Chickasha, Councilor for District 13. Doctor Renegar's pin was presented at a meeting of the Grady County Medical Society.

GRANVILLE J. WOMACK, M.D., formerly of Wister, has moved to Heavener.

J. E. MCDONALD, M.D., F. A. STUART, M.D. and JOHN C. DAGUE, M.D., associated in the Orthopedic Clinic in Tulsa, have moved from the Tri-State Insurance Building to the new Utica Square Medical Center.

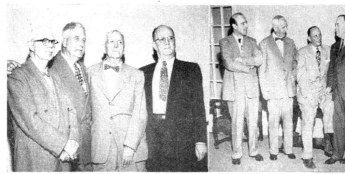

Old time members of the Okmulgee County Medical Society get together at the 50th anniversary of the founding of the society held in April. Pictured left to right are J. C. Matheney, M.D., Okmulgee; M. B. Glismann, M.D., now of Oklahoma City; S. B. Leslie, Sr., Okmulgee; and W. W. Stark.

Pictured in the group at right are left to right: S. B.

Leslie, Jr., M.D., Secretary of the Society; S. B. Leslie, Sr., M.D., oldest practicing physician who is a member of the Society; Dick Graham, Executive Secretary of the Oklahoma State Medical Association; John E. McDonald, M.D., Tulsa, President of the O.S.M.A. at the time the picture was made; and Jack P. Myers, M.D., Okmulgee, youngest member of the Society.

To ease the blow when you say..."No Salt!"....

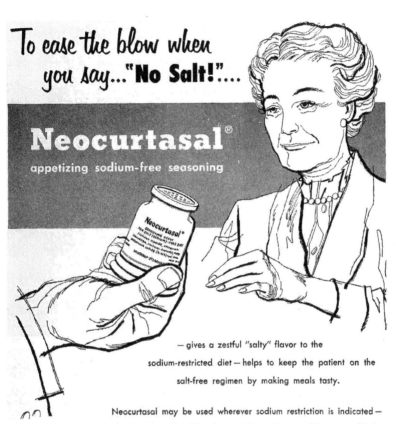

Neocurtasal®
appetizing sodium-free seasoning

— gives a zestful "salty" flavor to the sodium-restricted diet — helps to keep the patient on the salt-free regimen by making meals tasty.

Neocurtasal may be used wherever sodium restriction is indicated — it is completely sodium-free. May be used like ordinary table salt — added to foods during or before cooking or used to season foods at the table.

WINTHROP

supplied in 2 oz. shakers and 8 oz. bottles.

Neocurtasal

"...trustworthy non-sodium containing salt substitute"[1]

Write for pad of diet sheets.

1. Heller, E. M.: The Treatment of Essential Hypertension. Canad. Med. Assn. Jour., 61:293, Sept., 1949.

Neocurtasal, trademark reg. U.S. & Canada

WINTHROP-STEARNS INC.

NEW YORK 18, N. Y. • WINDSOR, ONT.

Hospital Opened

The new Physicians and Surgeons Hospital has been opened in Holdenville. The new privately owned hospital was build adjacent to the Pryor, Johnston and Schaff Clinic.

The hospital is equipped throughout with acoustical tile, air conditioning, and is made of fireproof brick and concrete. It will accommodate 34 adult patients and has six bassinets and four children's cribs.

Pastel shades are used throughout and all furnishing are new and of the latest design. An IBM call system has been installed. There are 26 employes including nurses, technicians, business staff members, cook and

maintenance men. The staff includes the following physicians: V. W. Pryor, L. A. S. Johnston, H. V. Schaff, T. A. Trow and D. H. Cramblett.

With G-E diagnostic x-ray units, you can

start small...

build big!

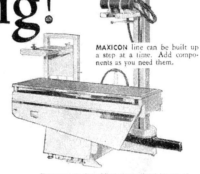

MAXICON line can be built up a step at a time. Add components as you need them.

ONE of the three General Electric diagnostic units shown here will give you the results you have a right to expect within the range of service you need. All provide modern radiographic and fluoroscopic facilities . . . each is built to the exacting standards naturally associated with General Electric.

And remember — you can get any of these units — *with no initial investment* — under the G-E Maxiservice® *rental* plan. What's more, if you want to upgrade or "trade-in" your rented unit, there's no obsolescence loss.

Get all the facts from your G-E x-ray representative.

OKLAHOMA CITY—627 N.W. Tenth Street
TULSA—1101 South Main Street

Progress Is Our Most Important Product

GENERAL 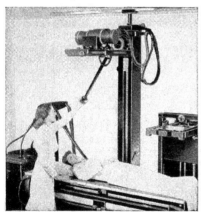 ELECTRIC

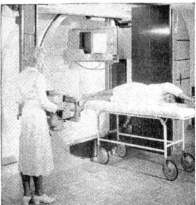

MAXISCOPE® gives you every feature you've sought in conventional x-ray apparatus — fast, consistent results for both radiography and fluoroscopy.

IMPERIAL begins where conventional x-ray units leave off — gives all technics new ease and facility with exclusive features previously unobtainable.

Direct Factory Branches:
OKLAHOMA CITY — 627 N.W. Tenth Street   **TULSA — 1101 South Main Street**

GLYNAZAN

(Brand of Theophylline-Sodium Glycinate)

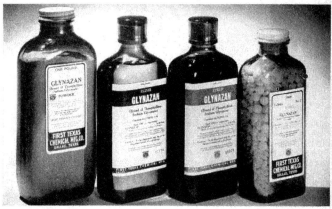

POWDER	ELIXIR	SYRUP	TABLETS
(Equivalent to Theophylline, U.S.P. 50%)	(Glynazan 1 grain per c.c.)	(Glynazan ½ grain per c.c.)	(2½ and 5 grains)

COUNCIL ACCEPTED GLYNAZAN PRODUCTS AVAILABLE FOR PRESCRIPTION USE.

ADVANCING

THEOPHYLLINE THERAPY

A Theophylline Compound exhibiting maximal solubility with minimal gastric iritation. Permits intensive Theophylline therapy in bronchial and circulatory disturbances.

FIRST TEXAS
CHEMICAL MANUFACTURING CO.

1903 - 1954: Celebrating 51 Years of Making FINE PHARMACEUTICALS

1810 N. Lamar   Dallas

Editorials

The University of Oklahoma
On the Student Matching Board

Junior Student William J. Dickerson, University of Oklahoma School of Medicine, has been selected for service on the Board of Directors of the National Intern Matching Program, Inc. The two undergraduates sitting on this national board are selected in the following way. One is elected by the Student American M e d i c a l Association House of Delegates and one at large, chosen from those placed in nomination by the Junior c l a s s of their respective schools. These nominations are supplemented by letters from the members of the school and University Hospital staffs.

Since only two students are appointed and this is the second year of operation, the University of Oklahoma School of Medicine and the fortunate nominee are to be congratulated.

Also worthy of note is the fact that Dickerson is now serving as President of the local chapter of Phi Beta Pi. Oklahoma anticipates the exercise of sound judgment and administrative ability with commendable modesty in each of these responsible positions.

Roentgen Ray Screening
A Striking Demonstration

In this issue of the *Journal* there is a news story concerning a fine bit of cooperation between the State Health Department and the State Medical Association, for the purpose of demonstrating the importance of Roentgen ray screening surveys and the routine screening of all hospital admissions.

The story presents a statistical study of the 220 films taken during the State Meeting and it is accompanied by a picture showing the type of equipment recommended for routine service in general hospitals. Two of our members appear in the picture. You may guess who they are.

Small Print

When yielding to the glowing appeals of protagonists of life, health and accident insurance companies, beware of the small print in the proposed contracts. Often the company's safeguard is in the small print. Even so, it's well for the policy holder to know just where the small print cuts him off.

It is said that government contracts offering subsidies, even for the construction of hospitals, carry surprises in small print. Only those having a sharp eye and a keen mind can afford to sign.

International Health
And World Peace

Worthy of note is the mounting interest in international health and the general participation in international and World Medical organizations and allied agencies.

The May 19 and 29 issues of the *British Medical Journal* report the section meeting of the American College of Surgeons in London and the latter comments editorially on the splendid spirit of cooperation in behalf of world wide human weal. Emphasizing the latter, the editorial calls attention to the fact that many of the avid participants had already attended medical meetings in Glasgow, Edinburgh and Leeds and, as if these were not enough, some of them had hurried on to meetings in France, Belgium and Italy. This represents only a part of the spring crop. International medical meetings and symposia are being held in various sections of the world throughout the year. Unfortunately, some have conflicting dates but never a serious conflict in purposes.

Does this insatiable urge for increased knowledge and skills stem from selfishness? In a sense, yes, it means increased knowledge and individual efficiency, but in the last analysis, it is for better care of the afflicted throughout the world. No secrets are harbored, no harmful, selfish motives are entertained. Physicians know that what is good for one is good for all and that the peoples of the world have a right to demand the best that can be provided by the best minds and the highest skills of the medical profession.

Compare this frank spirit of cooperation and all the revealing exhibition of existing knowledge freed from the last vestage of selfish motives with the Geneva Peace Conference. Obviously, what government needs today is an Hippocrates to put the welfare of the people first; a self-effacing Oath committing all to the preservation of law and the pursuit of peace.

Lest We Forget

In connection with the American Medical Education Foundation's plea for funds to obviate the danger of government subsidies for medical schools, there seems to be a melancholy lack of gratitude and loyalty that so few physicians respond.

In the past, as at present, medical education was given largely at public expense. Physicians have paid liberally in time and effort for their medical education but tuition and fees fell far short of actual costs. Largely they owe their income and their position in society to the University that made possible their medical education.

Does the slender response represent a low percentage of gratitude? May it justly be attributed to a lack of understanding?

The address is: American Medical Education Foundation, c/o American Medical Association, 535 North Dearborn, Chicago 10, Ill.

Why not send a check and help keep the medical schools free from government control. Your gift may augment the general fund or it may be designated for the school of your choice.

Non-Service Connected V. A. Hospitalization

Early in November, the Veterans Administration announced a new policy with reference to the hospitalization of veterans suffering from non-service connected conditions.

After so much agitation, it is good to have the following definite declaration.

Formerly the applicant with non-service connected complaints only had to declare that he was not financially able to pay hospital costs and he was admitted. Now ac-

ccrding to a recent A.M.A. Washington report, the veteran who makes such a declaration must answer the following definite questions:

"What is the total current value of your property, both real and personal?"

"What is the current amount of your ready assets in the form of cash, bank deposits, and savings bonds?"

"If you own real property, what is the approximate amount of the unpaid mortgage or other indebtedness owed thereon?"

"What are your average monthly expenditures including your mortgage payments and all other personal expenses including expenses for your dependents?"

"What was your average monthly net income for the last six months from all sources?"

No doubt every good American citizen, veteran or civilian, will agree that this new policy is reasonable and fair for all.

Unfortunately, some citizens of the United States are not too conscientious in response to such questions. Those able to pay and yet willing to say no under the original plan may be equally ready to give a false answer to the searching questions provided under the new policy.

Apparently the veteran is not placed under oath and the V.A. hospital administration provides no social service investigation designed to discover the facts.

It is unfortunate that the few who thoughtlessly or willfully fail to tell the truth make discussions such as this necessary. What we need today is old-fashioned honesty in all places — high and low.

The Matter of Lay Medical Publicity

Today the non-medical public is vitally interested in everything that relates to health, public health or individual health. The people have a right to know and the medical profession stands ready to supply the established facts. But the medical profession has not given enough thought as to when medical knowledge is ready for public consumption; how it should be dispensed and in what dosage. Some medical discoveries are so breathtaking they should be given to the public in graduated doses increasing as tolerance is developed.

Education of the public in things medical is the proper function of the physician in his individual capacity and through organized medicine. By education, training and experience he knows better than anyone else the answer to the above problems and questions. Better than anyone else he knows the mind of the public, therefore, the probable response to medical truths. He knows that these truths must be accepted and digested by a heterogenous public made up of at least three generations, mentally ranging from morons to the highly intellectual, physically from the fatally ill to the medically sound, economically from the indigent to the fabulously rich. The physician knows it is not easy to prepare medical information in digestible form for such a multifaceted populace.

Should the American Medical Association in cooperation with state and county organizations work out a plan for legitimate effective lay medical publicity on the high level now in effect between physician and patient of carefully considered authencity and of measured quality and quantity with national and local committees for implementation, or should the present haphazard methods continue to stand in the way of the public's legitimate right to the truth and the physician's obligations to the people and to his own self respect.

Today much of the lay medical publicity is produced by lay science writers naturally under the urge for news. As a result there is much premature lay medical print. As a result, possibly, through no fault of the lay writer, after the truth is distorted, unwarranted claims are presented, false hopes are aroused or unnecessary fear results according to the nature of the alleged possibilities, good or bad. Since from the news viewpoint, euphoria rather than anxiety makes the story, there is a tendency to play up rather than to play down. Thus readers may be lifted into a seventh heaven or occasionally by a misplaced or misunderstood word or by accurate reporting of unfavorable truths they may be plunged into the purgatory of despair. Many examples could be cited. Let the unwarranted euphorial of frenzied tuberculous patients dancing in the wards of tuberculosis hospitals over the prematurely exaggerated claims for a now well known antibiotic in the treatment of tuberculosis. Passing from unjustifiable Eureka to nerve-racking fear, it is said that at one time the pressing publicity about cancer of the breast augmented the popular cancer-complex to such a degree that many worthy young women created much curiosity by constantly feeling for lumps in their breasts.

Is it not time for the medical profession to counteract untimely, unwarranted and often untrue lay publicity by wisely prescribing medical knowledge in proper form for profitable public consumption?

The Responsibility of Medicine

What is medicine's roll in this heterogeneous, unthinking, inconsiderate, inconstant, irreconcilable, inscrutable, world? With many of the old, unsolved problems and all the new truths and fallacies confronting us with innumerable hazards and certain catastrophic possibilities, why are we running away from unresolved reality to wonder about life on Mars. Would it not be wise to muster every atom of thought and reason and every unit of physical energy for the solution of insecure life on our own confused sphere. Our world is tottering and without the steadying influence of calm and concerted effort, Atlas may lose his balance. In the prolongation of individual life, is medicine hazarding the tangential existence of the race?

Contrary to the law of "survival of the fittest," medicine has been remarkably successful in saving the unfit. This thought poses dangerous speculations but it is in the over all picture and deserves consideration. Through preventive measures, including induced immunity, personal and general hygiene and better living conditions, our chances for survival have been greatly increased. By saving life in infancy, fostering health in adolescence, we have produced a hardy but confused youth group. By prolonging the adult's tenure on earth we are pyramiding the old age group. In a society already socio-economically transformed, this prolongation of life with no longer an abiding anchor in the home presents a serious problem which may ultimately become insurmountable. Paradoxically enough, modern magical therapy brings not only added comfort, and often prompt recovery with a great saving of life but obvious unpleasant and occasionally unobserved and unappraised side effects yet to be weighed, classified, and recorded for the benefit of both patient and physician. Returning to the plight of the aged, we may say that because of miracle drugs, the once dependable, respectable disease, lobar pneumonia, has lost cast and can no longer be counted on as the old man's friend. When it was running true to form, often with its desensitizing toxemia, it offered the spent, elderly victim an easy way "across the bar."

The premature, frenzied mirth with wild ward dances in certain tuberculosis hospitals upon the unfortunate announcement of a new anti-tuberculosis drug further emphasizes the physicians responsibility. That promising drug and others in the same category have compromised with the wary tubercle bacillus, often conferring resistance that counteracts their inhibiting effects. This leaves us wondering what may happen to the next generation infected with these same drug-resistant tubercle bacilli. Is it possible that some day the same wards in sorrow and tears may witness the funeral march?

Should these disturbing situations find a sensitive spot in the doctor's consciousness? Whether justifiable or not, there is some comfort in Mark Twain's philosophical suggestion that we may spank a troublesome conscience into passive submission.

Space will not permit more. But these examples should help us to realize, in part, the possible paradoxical meaning of scientific advances, and the inherent good and evil always facing the physician regardless of his knowledge and skill.

Today all physicians, whether they realize it or not, are faced with the appalling responsibility of atomic energy. Just what is the physician's roll? Without his consent or volition, this problem has become world wide. Literally, the torch of scientific reasoning was lighted by the "sleepless, critical spirit" of Greek physicians in the Fifth Century B. C. Through succeeding centuries, it has gone ahead of advancing civilization spurring the rise ana decline of governments, nations and races, to blaze the trail for new and greater achievements. Is it not possible that

medical science may yet find a way through the threatening advances of scientific knowledge in this highly mechanized age. Though confused and troubled, it's a great good world quite worth saving. This is reveille for physicians, the bugle sounds the challenge. Medical science must continue to meet the issues as they arise in the course of civilization.

Mind and Body

Unfortunately, specialization in medicine tends to separate the inseparable and set apart organs and functions which cannot normally operate alone.

Now comes the American Psychiatric Association advocating the amendment of State Medical Practice Acts to definitely include in the definition of the practice of medicine "the diagnosis and treatment of mental and nervous diseases and disorders." This to safeguard those so afflicted from diagnosis and treatment by whose who are not M.D.'s.

Since the days of Hippocrates, physicians have understood that they should deal with the human organism, as a composite whole considering and satisfying the mind while diagnosing and treating the body. Until psychiatry became such a highly differentiated specialty and psychosomatic medicine, merely a new term for an old concept, came to our attention, nobody ever thought of separating mind from body for purposes of therapy.

Certainly the mind belongs to medicine and just as the body must have medical care when it departs from the normal, likewise the abnormalities of the mind demand diagnosis and treatment at the hands of the physician. If he chooses to delegate certain phases of management and medication to trained non medical workers, that is his responsibility.

Only the physician should be legally qualified and legally responsible for the treatment.

The wonder is that there should be any question about such an obvious matter of responsibility. But if existing medical practice acts fail to make clear this responsibility, they should be changed.

Scientific Articles

Diagnosis and Treatment of
BACKACHE -- *from the Standpoint*
of the General Practitioner

CARLO SCUDERI, M.D., Chicago

Introduction

The scope of this paper is a discussion of the etiology, the pathology, and the diagnosis and treatment of backache that is not produced by fractures. Since fractures constitute an entirely different phase of the problem and are easily diagnosed in most instances; they are not included in this discussion of the backache that forms a real problem as far as diagnosis and subsequent treatment and rehabilitation of the patient is concerned.

It would be a fair assumption to state that among the general practitioners in the State of Oklahoma, probably thousands of individuals are examined for back complaints every month. Many of them are successfully treated and return to their former type of work without disability. Every day a few of these cases find themselves in civil suits throughout the country. The cost of the medical care of cases that get well and the cost of the final settlement of cases that come to court, runs into hundreds of thousands of dollars in the State of Oklahoma alone.

General Overall Plan for Arriving at an Accurate Diagnosis

No one has any monopoly on how to make an accurate diagnosis of back complaints, however, there are certain routine procedures that serve everyone well. If they are followed systematically one is apt to arrive at a better diagnostic acuity, than if the patient is gone over haphazardly without any

Read before the Oklahoma Academy of General Practice in Tulsa, Oklahoma, February 16, 1954.

THE AUTHOR

Carlo Scuderi, M.D., Chicago, wrote the article on "Backache." Doctor Scuderi is associate professor of surgery at the University of Illinois and surgery at Cook County Graduate School. He is also senior attending surgeon at Cook County Hospital and chairman of the department of orthopedic surgery at St. Elizabeth's Hospital and Columbus Hospital in Chicago.

systematic arrangement of the examination. Perhaps it is advisable to classify the most outstanding groups of etiology of back complaints so that one has an idea beforehand what the most probable diagnoses are apt to be. We must also take for granted that there is a very minute and insignificant group which could be classified under miscellaneous. These have such an insignificant association to the problem of backache that one can pass them off with a minimal amount of discussion. Such things as enlargement of the prostate, constipation, rectal fissures, retroversion of the uterus, renal colic, etc. do give symptoms of backache, but their diagnostic problem is not too difficult. If a patient is given a thorough examination beforehand these additions can be eliminated very quickly. Then one terminates with the following classification of backache:

1. Sprain.
2. Episacral lipomae.
3. Congenital malformations.
4. Osteoarthritis.
5. Aggravation of a pre-existing condition.
6. Ruptured intervertebral disc.
7. Psychosomatic backache.

History

It is very important that a careful detailed history be taken at the first examination. This frequently clinches the diagnosis and puts one on the right track, as well as saving time for the patient and money for the employer. If the history is taken by an assistant or the nurse, it should be carefully checked item by item by the surgeon to be sure all the pertinent facts are included.

Sprains

A sprain gives a very definite history of specific accident followed by the onset of pain and discomfort to the lower back with or without radiation into the legs. The peculiar thing about most back sprains is that the greatest intensity is immediately at the time of the accident or within an hour or two thereafter. Then the intensity of the discomfort gradually decreases as time goes on.

Epi-Sacral Lipomae

The episacral lipoma is the herniation of a small mass of fat through the deep fascia in the back, in the vicinity of the sacro-iliac joint. As a rule it has a pedicle that runs down to the sacro-iliac joint capsule and articulation. The story of most epi-sacral lipomae is that the onset was insidious and the pain becomes progressively worse, and especially on lying on the back. On palpation of the area there is a definite trigger point of pain and discomfort and it is very well localized to one area. Activity in itself, in most instances does not seem to aggravate the condition.

Congenital Malformations

There are many congenital malformations of the lower back, the most common are as follows: Spina bifida, spondylolisthesis, pre-spondylolisthesis, sacralization of the transverse process of the fifth lumbar vertebra, hemi-vertebrae or abnormal articular facettes at the lumbo-sacral junction. The history in most of these cases is that the patient has gone along quite well until he reached the 20th or 25th year. Then he begins to undertake heavier activities or athletic endeavors as football, baseball and hockey; and he notices that as time goes on the discomfort of the back becomes worse and the duration of the discomfort prolonged. It definitely has a relationship with muscular activity and exertion. Most of these people with congenital malformations of the back do not recognize this fact until they are in college or shortly thereafter. A young healthy individual who slowly begins to have back discomfort with increased activity somewhere in the vicinity of the 20th year is apt to give the above type of history and information. These cases do best under rest.

Osteoarthritis

The history in osteoarthritic cases is uniformly the same. The patient is somewhere in the fourth, fifth or sixth decade of life and usually is somewhat obese. He finds that the first thing in the morning he has difficulty in getting up, stooping over to tie his shoes and in getting to the washroom. However, as the day goes on and he increased his activities his back motions improve and the back discomfort decreases.

Aggravation of a Pre-Existing Condition

All too frequently following an accident with low back strain and discomfort, the point is brought out of aggravation of a pre-existing condition. These may be any one of the malformations of a congenital type or osteoarthritic changes of the back that have existed for a considerable period of time prior to the date of the alleged injury. If it can be definitely shown that the patient apparently was carrying on his normal activities and following this additional strain to the back, he develops pain, discomfort and physical findings that incapacitate him; it is fair to assume that there is an aggravation of a pre-existing condition. If one should actually find an increased forward slippage of the vertebra in a spondylolisthesis, comparing pre- and post trauma X-rays, this also is fair assumption of aggravation of a pre-existing condition. Sometimes in elderly people who have marked osteoarthritic backs who sustain an injury and actually show a fracture of an osteophyte; or very rapid growth of an osteophyte within a few months following low back injury, it is fair to assume from a medical standpoint that this patient has justifications for a diagnosis of an aggravation of a pre-existing condition. This point is a source of a great deal of litigation and confusion especially in the civil courts.

Ruptures of the Intervertebral Discs

These cases give a more or less uniform history but not always the same. They occur in young healthy individuals with good back musculature who do heavy physical work. At a very specific time they sustain a back strain followed by an acute discomfort in the back with or without some immediate radiation into the buttocks and leg on one side. The case may also have a back strain with acute back discomfort in the lumbosacral region, and then in the subsequent few days slowly develop pain and discomfort and radiation down the leg with associated numbness. This condition as a rule becomes aggravated by coughing and sneezing. The history of the case is that the disease is progressive. As time goes on the patient gets worse instead of better, as is the usual case in back sprains.

Psychosomatic Backache

This type of backache presents a real problem. In most instances it is very difficult to come to an accurate diagnosis of psychosomatic backache. As a rule the history is that of an individual who has been off work frequently for rather trivial, insignificant causes and his family life is none too happy. He is emotionally unstable and does not seem to carry his load through life. One finds very frequently that the other members of the family takes care of the finances, the organization of the home and the care of the children. This individual as a rule has a work record that is not too satisfactory. Suddenly one day he gives a history which may or may not be questionable of a back injury and finally begins to get medical care and a lot of extra attention which he never had before. In many instances the patient begins to like this type of life and finally decides consciously or subconsciously that his back discomfort is not going to get well. He enjoys being at the status at which he finds himself when he first sees the doctor. This is an escape mechanism and in the minds of some people, solves their worldly problems. In many such instances there is actually a down and out psychiatric element, and in other instances there is a tremendous element of malingering.

Physical Examination

Every patient who comes to a doctor with a complaint of backache is entitled to a very careful examination. In order to do this successfully all of the clothes must be removed to permit a thorough examination, yet keeping enough to cover the patient and prevent unnecessary personal exposure. The male patients can conveniently strip and put on a loin cloth. The female patients should remove any corsets or girdles they may be wearing, but can leave their slip, bra and panties on.

The entire back and lower extremities must be visible to the examining physician. One should carefully note the position of the back, the muscle tone and any atrophy. In addition such things as the tilt of the pelvis, the appearance of the gluteal structures and circulation of the legs should be observed. The patient should be asked to go through the normal ranges of the back motions to decide whether there is any restriction, pathological spasm or atrophy. These motions are: forward flexion, hyperextension, lateral flexion and lateral rotation to both sides. Careful notes must be made of all these factors for subsequent checkup at a later date. The patient should be instructed to walk and while he does, one takes note of the gait, whether or not there is a shifting of the pelvis, and does he have full motions of the hips, knees and ankles at their articulations. Also the general appearance of the muscles of the thighs and calves should be noted, and checked for muscle tone and atrophy. The patient should be carefully watched when he gets on and off the examining table, and whether he has difficulty in getting into the various positions during the examination.

Various forms of low back tests are employed to determine any pathological findings. Everyone in this group is well acquainted with many of the orthopedic low back tests. The author uses the following seven: Lasegue, Kernig, Fabere, anterior and posterior torsions, lumbo-iliacs and the lumbosacral. The positivity of these tests are graded from one to four, the least positive being one plus and most positive being four plus, and if painless it is considered negative. This is recorded on the chart.

At this stage it might be mentioned that it would be beneficial to those who are interested to read a very small booklet by Mennell entitled *Backache*. It is most beneficial as far as the examination of the patient is concerned and manipulation of the back in some instances for the relief of chronic low back discomfort.

The circumferences of both legs should be carefully checked in the mid thigh and mid calf area to determine any disproportion between the two sides. One should test sensation both by pin prick and stroking with cotton of both legs to determine any hypesthesia or anesthesia of either leg that follows nerve root dermatone distribution.

The Achilles and patellar reflexes must be carefully checked as a decreased Achilles or patellar reflex has a definite clinical significance, especially if there is a question of a ruptured intervertebral disc.

X-Rays

Good detailed X-rays of the lumbar spine and lumbosacral region are most important in coming to an accurate diagnosis. Every case that presents itself with a backache should have careful films taken of the spine. Anteroposterior and lateral views of the lumbar spine and a coned film of the lumbosacral region are imperative. In certain cases if there is some question after seeing the anteroposterior and lateral views, an oblique view should be taken to bring out the articular facettes and the pedicle especially of the fourth and fifth lumbar vertebrae. One should not be satisfied with cloudy, indistinct X-ray films. One must be able to see the finer bone trabeculations and all of the details that are necessary to come to an accurate diagnosis. Nothing is more expensive and more misinformative than poor X-ray films.

Treatment

Sprains: One must have a common understanding of what pathology constitutes a sprain. It is actually a tearing and disruption of the continuity of the fascia, ligaments and sometimes the muscle fibers in the area that is injured. Subsequent to this tearing a resulting hemorrhage occurs with localized edema and soft tissue infiltration which produces swelling. After a few days a reaction of the tissue occurs so that it is more friable, appears somewhat waterlogged and microscopically the cells show actual edema. If one believes that this pathology is true then manipulation, massage and heat only aggravate the condition; producing more edema and more local hyperemia with more bleeding and more edema. Therefore if a diagnosis is made of a sprain the author does not feel that the injection of Novocain and manipulation is justified, as it aggravates the existing condition. Therefore immobilization is most important. Of all the methods that we have at our disposal the use of a small plaster jacket is probably the best, as it gives the firmest immobilization and cannot be removed by the patient.

The use of adhesive is only of a temporary nature, as it loosens after a few hours and in most instances produces blebs or a dermatitis to the skin of the patient's back. The wearing of a back brace or corset is not too satisfactory because it permits removal too frequently. In many instances especially in warm weather the patient prefers to discard it until he returns to see the doctor, therefore delaying his healing process. Once a cast is applied it is felt it should remain on about four to six weeks at which time the pathology of the soft tissue should adequately heal. Then the individual can be given heat, massage and graduated exercises to increase the amplitude of motion of the back and restore the muscle tone. The patient should not be confined to bed with the torso cast but should be permitted to be up and around doing whatever he desires, providing of course it does not include stooping and heavy lifting. Under this regimen practially all sprained backs can be effecaciously cured the first time within a period of about four to six weeks.

194

Epi-Sacral Lipomae

The epi-sacral lipoma can be readily felt over the sacro-iliac joint. Pressure produces pain similar to the one the patient has been complaining of and sometimes there is radiation down the leg along the distribution of the sciatic nerve. The injection of about 5 c.c. of Novacain in most instances will produce complete relief if this is the pathological cause of the backache. This relief may run from four to thirty-six hours. In some cases after injection with Novocain on two to three occasions, for some unknown reason, the p a i n and discomfort in this area completely and permanently disappears. Whether or not it is a rupture of the capsule of the lipoma by the injections, is not known but actual relief does occur. If, however, there is only temporary relief after the injection of Novocain and then recurrence of discomfort when the effects wear off; the removal of this lipoma is indicated and can be done very well. Those who have had experience with removal of episacral lipomae know that the lipoma is usually larger than it feels on the surface and always runs down to the sacro-iliac joint capsule, having a pedicle which must be carefully dissected if one expects to obtain a cure. The fatty tissue has a tendency to bleed and unless good hemastasis is obtained a secondary hematoma forms which is bothersome to the patient, but not necessarily harmful. The period of hospitalization as a rule is not more than 12 to 24 hours. In cases with accurate, correct diagnosis the cure is permanent and simple.

Congenital Malformations

Here we have a problem of a condition that has existed prior to the man's employment and subsequently after an injury is brought to the surface so that it is diagnosed, recognized and becomes a source of question of treatment and litigation. If careful pre-employment X-rays are taken this will eliminate a large percentage of these cases because they are not employed or they are put into a type of employment where back stresses and strains are not apt to occur. Once, however, a man becomes an employee and sustains an injury with symptoms to the back, the company is respon-sible for the return of his condition to one of well-being. If the congenital malformations are of mild type and if the individual's work is of a non-strenuous nature, very frequently these conditions can be treated successfully; by the use of canvas lumbosacral supports with rigid metal stays or by the use of low back braces, with limitation of the amount of activity which the patient should undertake. If, however, under conservative management and guarded activity of a person's employment the condition does not improve, the question arises as to permanent fixation of the area. A fusion eliminates the weakness and motion of the area thereby giving them a solid bony mass in the area, and in most instances if this is carried out successfully it results in a permanent cure. It is not within the scope of this paper to discuss the various forms of spinal fusions, but they are all known to orthopedic surgeons in the field and the results in competent hands are very gratifying. The incidence of pseudoarthrosis in some instances is higher than in others but one can safely feel that better than 75 to 80 per cent of spinal fusions are successful and do not develop pseudoarthrosis.

Osteoarthritis

The treatment of osteoarthritis is a difficult one, because it occurs in people of advanced age and who are overweight. We know that people do better if they can be made to lose weight and limit their activities so that stresses and strains of the lower back are eliminated, than if they continue doing heavy work. It is also known that these cases do better if they live in a uniformly mild climate that is dry, rather than one where the temperature and humidity ranges are great in a relatively short period of time. With the advent of Cortisone and ACTH, many of these cases can be helped tremendously. Other cases do not respond well to this treatment and one has to rely on the old standbys of salicylates, ascorbic acid, saturated solution of potassium iodide and the removal of foci of infection. An individual who once begins to have trouble with an osteoarthritic spine had best change his type of work so that the least amount of trauma is produced to aggravate this condition, as recurrences are very freqeuent. An actual complete cure of an osteoarthritic back can never be attained.

In certain rare instances it does become necessary if the osteoarthritis is limited to only a small segment of the spine, to do a fusion to eliminate the pain and discomfort of the arthritic area.

Aggravation of a Pre-Existing Condition

Here as in congenital malformations, one is presented with the problem of responsibility of the employee who has a pre-existing condition that becomes aggravated by trauma. This can be divided into two groups, a reversible and an irreversible group. In the reversible group an individual sustains an aggravation, but under adequate medical care he returns to the same status of physical well-being as he was in prior to the back strain or injury. Therefore he may be considered of the same physical status as before the injury was manifested. However, certain types of aggravation of a pre-existing condition are irreversible. In other words, the man's condition regardless of the treatment never returns to its former status, and there is definite progressive increased disability with clinical and X-ray manifestations of changes which can never be brought back to their former status. Probably the best example of all is a spondylolisthesis with definite increased slipping of the vertebral body. If pre-employment or former X-ray films of the lumbar spine are checked against the recent ones, one can find there actually has been a movement forward of the vertebra one-fourth or one-eighth of an inch and that the clinical manifestations become very pronounced and remain persistent. This condition therefore, is one that must be treated at the expense of the employer. Conservative management in these cases is usually of little or no avail and ultimately this type of case requires a spinal fusion in order to stabilize the back.

Ruptures of the Intervertebral Discs

Strange as it may seem, prior to the time that Mixter and Barr brought the ruptured intervertebral disc to the attention of the medical profession, many people formerly had backache with sciatic radiation and got well. Since 1932 the medical profession has become acutely conscious of the fact that the cartilaginous material between the vertebral bodies may herniate and produce back pain with sciatic radiation; and for this reason the diagnosis of ruptured intervertebral disc has been made too promiscuously. One must realize that the cause of backache as a result of intervertebral disc rupture probably constitutes less than five to eight per cent of all acute back injuries with disability. The diagnosis can be made safely if one finds the classical triad of: absent or decreased Achilles reflex, hypesthesia that follows a definite dermatone distribution to the extremity and atrophy of the affected leg. These are three objective findings that can be definitely found by careful examination. Although all ruptured intervertebral discs do not present uniformly similar findings, they are always associated with positive Lesague and Kernig findings on the affected side and myelogram studies will reveal the defect in approximately 90 per cent of the cases. One does not wish to go into the technique of myelography but it is a very safe and reputable test, and should be used in all cases prior to surgery. This point, however, is a means of disagreement with the opinion of other men, but in the author's personal experience it has been a very safe and satisfying method of localization of the lesion and also to confirm that a lesion actually exists.

In the last year the author operated four cases that had negative myelograms but at surgery large herniated discs were found laterally. This, however, constitutes a very small percentage of the over all group study.

When a disc herniation does exist with nerve root pressure there is no conservative management. Surgical intervention is indicated and this should be done at the convenience of the patient. If prolonged procrastination takes place, sometimes irreparable changes occur in the nerve and this could be avoided by operation at an earlier date. In some instances the hypesthesia never disappears and sometimes the Achilles reflex never returns, but these in themselves are not great disabling factors. The patient with a definite ruptured disc with nerve root pressure obtains immediate permanent relief once the pressure is removed from the nerve root. Whether or not an associated spinal fusion should be done with removal of the disc is also a source of tremendous argumentation. Neurosurgeons never fuse a spine and some orthopedic surgeons fuse all spines that have disc removed. Certainly there must be a happy medium between the two extremes. The author personally fuses only about 25 percent of the cases operated for ruptured disc and those have definite evidence of mechanical low back instability. One does not wish to enter into this argumentative subject as it would consume a lot of time, discussion and is not the purpose of this paper.

Psychosomatic Backache

Last but not least, we have the group of cases classified under psychosomatic backache. This is a very difficult group to diagnose and certainly a most difficult group to treat. In order to make a diagnosis of a psychosomatic backache, the objective findings must be negative. The X-ray findings and clinical studies must show nothing that could pathologically give this patient disability. The history must be one that would lead the examiner to believe that there is an emotional or mental side to this problem. However, the patient must be given the benefit of every doubt. A thorough examination and conservative treatment should be rendered and after a period of time if there are no satisfactory results, it is important that a neuropsychiatrist be brought into the picture.

The patient must never be told that one suspects that it is a psychosomatic backache as by doing so, it alienates the cooperation of the patient, the patient's relatives and friends. It has been my experience to always tell the patients that I am sending him to a neurologist and fortunately there are many neuropsychiatrists in large centers. A small note is sent along with the patient presenting the problem, and usually a telephone call directly to the doctor explaining the situation eliminates any mentioning of the psychiatric aspects of the case. If after careful psychiatric study the attending physician

and the consultant feel that this is a psychosomatic back, then one is almost at a checkmate. In these cases it is not good to do too many things of a radical nature as they only seem to aggravate the patient and it is best to diplomatically see that the patient goes elsewhere for medical care. In many instances termination of litigation or a settlement of the case helps tremendously to improve these people from both a physical and emotional standpoint.

A word of warning must be given to everyone. Sometimes the examining physician is prone to make a diagnosis of psychosomatic backache because he is unable to find any pathological cause for the backache; and subsequently some colleagues finds a metastatic carcinoma from the prostate or the patient is found to have an abscess or beginning tuberculosis of the spine. It behooves everyone to be very careful and only use the diagnosis of psychosomatic backache whenever all possible source of pathology and etiology has been eliminated. Only by being most careful and scrupulous about such a diagnosis is one going to avoid unnecessary harm to everyone in the treatment of backache.

Conclusions

It is hoped that this article will present some of the basic principles in the history taking, the examination, the subsequent study and aftercare of conditions with backache. This paper in no way is meant to be a final analysis and resume of the problem, but is to act as a guide. Everyone who treats patients with backache has many difficulties. Some men are better and more successful in their treatment than others because of training, experience and understanding knowledge of the pathology that exists, and the mechanics of the treatment of this pathology. Others are less successful because they do not understand the problem well. The author does hope that this article in some way has brought out a few pertinent points that may be of value to everyone.

Observations Pertaining to the

PRACTICE *of* CLINICAL PSYCHIATRY

COYNE H. CAMPBELL, M.D.

THE AUTHOR

Coyne H. Campbell, M.D., F.A.C.P., F.A.P.A., Oklahoma City psychiatrist, wrote "A Number of Observations Pertaining to the Practice of Clinical Psychiatry." Doctor Campbell is Professor and Chairman, Department of Psychiatry and Neurology, University of Oklahoma School of Medicine. He was graduated from Rush Medical College.

Physicians acquire many commonplace facts from experience. Often they presume that their confreres already have or soon will acquire the specific knowledge they themselves have; consequently they do not report their observations.

True, many of these seemingly minor observations do not warrant the search into the literature for reference material which makes for a scholarly paper. Nevertheless, from a practical standpoint, these facts are so important that perhaps they should be reported for the benefit of all concerned, much the same, so to speak, as a "household hint."

The observations which follow are of that sort. They are reported with full cognizance that they might be boring and redundant to some but possibly of pre-experiential interest to others.

1. During the past five years, both the front and back doors to the admission unit of our hospital have been unlocked from the outside, but, of course, locked from the inside. This routine has had a profoundly favorable psychological effect upon patients and also upon relatives. The patient's fear of incarceration and repugnance thereto by the accompanying relatives, is of most practical importance in the initial rapport. It is amazing to note that the group relationship between hospital personnel and patients is so powerful that during the day the back doors can be operated in the same fashion. Improved patients serve as aides to prevent escapes by confused patients. Patients in unlocked outbuildings who can at any time enter the locked wards will be most cautious, even without being so instructed, to keep inpatients from going out as outpatients enter through the back door. Our hospital escapes have been remarkably few.

2. For the comfort of the patients on the locked part of the hospital, toilet cubicles

Read at the Mid-Continent Psychiatric Association, Kansas City, Missouri, September 1953.

have thumb locks on the inside to insure privacy. Nervous, tense, and not-too-confused patients appreciate privacy at the toilet. Even if the door is thumb locked, it can always be unlocked from the outside by a master key. The same key that opens the doors from the inside of the hospital also opens the locked toilets. This system obviates the necessity for an extra key.

3. Some psychiatrists have the impression that most psychiatric disorders have no disturbance of intellect but merely a disturbance of emotion and-or behavior. I recently attended a postgraduate conference at which a prominent psychiatrist stressed the point that very few patients suffer from disturbance of intellect. He made this statement, I know, to emphasize that most psychiatric patients do not have overt delusions and hallucinations of the classical type. Yet, this statement could be misleading. I have observed that nearly all psychiatric patients have a serious disturbance of judgment; and to me, judgment is a function of the intellect.

4. Episodic confusions in persons who are middle aged or past middle age quite often are a real milestone to the individual. The event may be the beginning of a psychosis due to cerebral arteriosclerosis. These episodes usually are ominous, and the prognosis must be a guarded one.

5. From clinical experience, without scientific controls, I have observed that insulin coma therapy is generally the treatment of choice in postpartum psychoses.

6. I have observed that if no residual personality change occurs in relationship to a postpartum psychosis, there is no psychia-

tric reason for the patient not to have more pregnancies. On the other hand, if a personality change accompanied by deteriorative symptoms takes place, further pregnancy is inadvisable. Signs of deterioriation include uncleanliness, lack of personal pride, antisocial manifestations, persistent delusions, and other obvious personality changes. A discontinuation of insulin therapy is indicated if any allergic manifestations occur.

7. Prefrontal lobotomy is always an application of "vicarious euthanasia." There are, of course, instances in which the procedure can be justifiably carried out — but then the result is "vicarious euthanasia." In other words, a patient should never be subjected to a prefrontal or trans-orbital lobotomy unless a condition prevails in which "death on earth is preferable to hell on earth" and there is reasonable certainty that the hell on earth will not spontaneously subside before real death takes over.

8. In toxic alcoholism, the medical treatment of choice is eschatin intravenously and large parenteral doses of vitamins. Alcohol, chloral, paraldehyde, barbiturates, and other sedatives, if used, should be administered in rapidly diminishing dosages.

9. When an emotional divorce has occurred in one or both parties, the prognosis for a continuation of marriage is very poor.

10. Marriage counselors have pretty good success because without the counselling the couple probably would have continued their marriage relationship anyway; otherwise, they would have not consulted the counselors.

11. Only after most careful scrutiny of the total situation should a psychiatrist in private practice treat a patient who has ever accepted charity medical care unnecessarily.

12. There is such a phenomenon as the "Neuropsychiatric Industrial Case Syndrome." Its essentials are as follows:
   a. A minor injury with subsequent disabling symptoms.
   b. Examination of the patient by several different physicians.
   c. Return to work by the patient accompanied by exacerbation of symptoms.
   d. Employment of attorney by the "in-

jured."
   e. Further examinations by physicians.
   f. Finally, examination by the neuropsychiatrist at which time the patient is accompanied by the wife, mother, father, and-or other relatives who give the history. (You know the rest: the man with a lame back, a personality change, increased fatigability, "blackouts," indigestion, lots of kids, and a wife.) However, it is most important to remember that such a patient may actually have a very definite serious disability from a psychosis that has arisen out of the accident. If he has, monetary settlement of the case will not restore him to his pre-accident personality status. This is a fact that is to be determined and one that is the responsibility for the psychiatric examiner.

13. A hopeless prognosis for a psychiatric patient is never appropriate, no matter how chronically ill he may be, so long as there remains one single person who is emotionally interested in him.

14. A patient's worry about physiognomy is a malignant symptom.

15. Delusions petaining to the genital organs are usually seriously malignant.

16. Most cases of manifest so-called "psychopathic personality" in adolescents are blessed with biologically determined recovery. Shame, which is latent, usually cures the subject after the antisocial event is brought to the public eye.

17. A psychiatric patient should be admitted to a private hospital with utmost caution if he is brought there under false pretenses. Patients have been brought in the institution by relatives or even sheriffs under pretense that the hospital is a night club, a swank dining place, bowling alley, or museum. A rule has been made that if a patient is brought to our hospital under pretense, then his admission should be most carefully considered.

18. The term "minor psychoses" should be discarded. Psychoneuroses are disorders of stress that are very serious clinical conditions. Most psychoneuroses, by the time that a psychiatrist sees them, are chronic

disorders.

19. Some patients have an expression in their eyes that is pathognomic of a malignant psychiatric illness. It is a physiognomic "strained gazing". It is not a blank stare. It is a *Strained Stare*.

20. "Pathological nostalgia" is a very definite clinical symptom, pathognomic of catatonic personalities. The patient who can say only, "I want to go home — when can I go home" is, of course, a very definite clinical entity! These patients, as a rule, would be classified as catatonic. It is also interesting to observe that regardless of the kind of or intensity of treatment, success cannot be evaluated until after the patient has returned home. Emotional stress will always be manifest as long as the patient is in the hospital. The condition can truly be termed "pathological nostalgia."

21. In bromide psychoses, there is no change in the protein of the spinal fluid. A case without any neurologic lesion was referred by a neurosurgeon who had discovered a spinal fluid protein of more than 100 mgm. percent. The blood bromides test revealed 350 mgm. per cu. mm. The patient had clinical symptoms of a bromide psychosis; and as the bromides were eliminated, he gradually improved and recovered from the psychosis. The high protein in the spinal fluid was never explained. The incident resulted in determinations of spinal fluid protein on the next 25 patients with bromide psychosis. In all, the spinal fluid protein was within normal limits.

22. There is a rather rare clinical phenomenon of echolabia. A simple description is that listener's lips synchronously imitate the speaker's mouth movements. The clinical significance is unknown.

23. The well preserved paranoid personality with psychosis gets along best with a "rest cure" and should be returned, if possible, to the previous environment. No active treatment will be of help. Psychotherapy results only in additional personal problems for the psychotherapist. Shock treatments merely increase the patient's hostility after the effects of electricity and insulin have worn off. The isolation of hospitalization seems to be the therapy of choice.

24. Impactions occur in old folks! One of the first custodial patients in the newly opened sanitarium was an elderly man of considerable prominence, an author of several books. He had delusions of grandeur and spirituality. One day he said, "Doctor, I'm more convinced than ever that I am God, or at least very close to him. I'm really clean. If you'll wait just a bit I'll show you. I'll be right back." He returned shortly with a saucer partially filled with a milky looking substance. "Smell of this," he ordered. It was practically odorless. "What is it" — I just passed that from my anus," he said. even my excrement doesn't stink." On that same day, after examination, a couple of gallons of impacted material were removed. Of course, the delusions persisted, but the fecal impactions were as of the time more important!

25. It is rather precarious to take care of a *wife* without permission of the estranged husband. Quite often, because of the patient's domestic difficulties, relatives will bring an estranged wife to the psychiatrist for treatment. Usually the husband has deserted the wife and children. The relatives assume verbal, written and financial responsibility for the patient. The psychiatrist is confronted with a psychotic individual desperately needing help. Out of sympathy he may thoughtlessly treat the wife without consulting the estranged husband. Look out! The psychiatrist may have to deal not only with an estranged husband but also with relatives who have become estranged toward the psychiatrist!

26. Because common psychiatric disorders have been unrecognized and mis-diagnosed by physicians in the immediate past, a new problem has become manifest. It is one for serious consideration by physicians. Shall the physicians acknowledge their previous ignorance of so-called psychosomatics and begin professional life again with reality as a basis; or shall they make pseudo-atonement by affiliation with the physicians who have become enslaved to freudianism?

This question is proposed sincerely. The awakening to the existence of psychosomatic disorders has somehow put physicians on the defensive. The question to be decided is this: shall physicians accept explanations for psychosomatic disorders made by their freudianly conditioned confreres; or shall

Continued on Page 206

A Doctor's Diagnosis of a Common Ill

ANIMA INFANTIS

C. A. TRAVERSE, M.D.

THE AUTHOR

C. A. Traverse, M.D., author of the special article entitled "Anima Infantis" is a practicing physician in Alva. A general practitioner, he is especially interested in allergy. He was graduated from the University of Oklahoma School of Medicine in 1933 and is immediate past president of Oklahoma State Medical alumni. Doctor Traverse served as a captain in World War II.

Anima Infantis is one of the most disastrous and disabling of the diseases which afflict mankind. Yet you hear nothing of it when the health funds make their annual pleas for funds. Mothers ignore it as they frantically guard their children against contagious diseases, avitaminosis, infectious diseases, and all physical aberrations. Children are shepherded from the orthodontist for their teeth to the opthalmologist for their eyes, the orthopedist for their flat feet, and the pediatrician for all structures in between. Money is carefully husbanded to be spread thinly over the best schools, the best clothes, the best food, and the best entertainment.

Fund raisers and parents alike are overlooking *Anima Infantis*, one of the most debilitating, the most destructive, the most disastrous diseases known to man. This disease has been pandemic throughout the history of man, but it flares into acute form from time to time; and strangely enough, those spurts of virulence seem to come at times of material prosperity. This disease might almost be called the occupational disease of a life of plenty.

Today mankind is like the poor deluded souls of the middle ages who tightly closed their houses to keep out the plague, not knowing that the plague had already crept in on the fleas. Americans in particular strive so hard to protect their children and loved ones from disease and discomfort that they make them susceptible to one of the most disabling diseases of all — *Anima Infantis* (infantile soul) or selfishness.

Show me one child who is crippled by polio and I will show you hundreds leading lives crippled by selfishness, shallowness, and greed. Show me one child incapacitated by a heart condition and I can show you thousands with hearts utterly broken by man's inhumanity to man. Show me one dying from cancer of the bone and I can show you thousands dying from malnutrition while our elevators are so full of grain that men must frantically build to have a place to store next year's crop. Show me one child stumbling down life's path because of cerebral palsy and I can show you thousands stumbling through life with unseeing eyes in the wake of war. Show me one child racked by the cough and fever of tuberculosis and I can show you thousands whose lives are parched and dried because of race hatred, whose breath is drawn in painful gasps of fear because they chance not to belong to the accepted order of society. Show me one person in need of psychiatric care and I will show you thousands crazed by greed, thousands whose lives move in meaningless circles, not because of mental defect, but because they are so self-centered that their whole pathway is a circle around that central stake of "I" to which they are tethered.

Being a physician, I am not, nor could I ever be, opposed to the efforts of modern medicine to bring physical health to the world's population. But each day I am more aware of the need to minister to man's soul, to do something to stimulate some spiritual growth on the part of contemporary man. Individually man has become so engrossed in himself and his own personal problems that he has forgotten the brotherhood of man.

Since diagnosis must precede treatment, I would first consider the etiology of *Anima Infantis* or "infantile soulitis." One of the first noticeable symptoms is crossing of the eyes as they turn inward toward self. There is a convulsive clenching of the fists around all possessions. There is a hunching of the shoulders as the head is lowered to lick the last morsels of pleasure from the plate of life. The knees become ankylosed and stiffened from much standing erect to demonstrate superiority. The toes become flattened and calloused from kicking at those less fortunate who are trying to pull themselves up the ladder.

And what of the treatment? The eyes must first be trained to look away from self and up to God; they must be re-trained to look away from self and see all men as brothers. The fists must be gently pried apart and braced open by deeds of kindness done in the knowledge that "a man takes out of this world in his tightly clenched fists only that which he has given away." Lifting the arms up and holding them out to share will involuntarily cause the shoulders to straighten. The warm moisture of tears shed for the injustices of the world will, dripping on the toes, gradually cause them to soften and return to normal shape and texture. The relaxing of tense muscles in the process of giving and sharing will gradually loosen the knees until the patient will find that he is able to kneel in humility and thank his Maker for renewed spiritual health.

Foolish musing? Possibly, but not half as foolish as the thinking which has brought great segments of humanity to the brink of annihilation where man must decide whether to use his God-given powers to build a bridge across international misunderstandings, jealousies, and callous indifferences, or plunge off into the unknown of a man-made destruction.

During other acute outbreaks of *Anima Infantis* man has been seriously stricken, but never before has he had in his hands the tools for destruction which could cause the sick of soul to bring death to the healthy too.

Yes, let man continue his war against physical ills, but let him also awaken to the fact that a specific cure must be found for *Anima Infantis*, or "infantile soulitis" before it writes the final chapter of man's history on this earth.

Number of Physicians in U.S. Reach All-Time High

The total number of physicians—218,522—licensed to practice in the United States set an all-time record in 1953. Official figures from the 52nd annual report on medical licensure of the AMA's Council on Medical Education and Hospitals indicate that 7,276 persons were added to the medical profession in 1953. During the same period, 3,421 physician deaths reported to the AMA Headquarters gives a net increase of 3,855 in the physician population of the country. In 1952, an increase of 2,987 was reported.

The report shows that 14,434 medical licenses were issued in 1953 by the medical examining boards of the 48 states, the District of Columbia, Alaska, Canal Zone, Guam, Hawaii and Puerto Rico. Of this number, 6,565 were granted after written examination and 7,869 by reciprocity or endorsement of state licenses or the certificate of the National Board of Medical Examiners.

The present high level of medical education in this country is indicated by the fact that of the 5,646 graduates of approved medical schools in the United States to take examinations, only 3.8 per cent failed to pass. In comparison, however, of the 1,463 graduates of foreign medical faculties examined, 45.5 per cent failed.

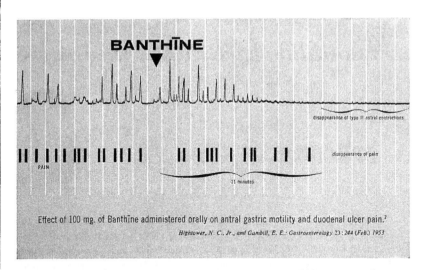

Effect of 100 mg. of Banthīne administered orally on antral gastric motility and duodenal ulcer pain.[2]

Hightower, N. C., Jr., and Gambill, E. E.: Gastroenterology 23:244 (Feb.) 1953

Banthīne® Reduces Hypermotility and Hyperacidity in Peptic Ulcer

A recent evaluation of anticholinergic therapy in peptic ulcer emphasizes the fact that now the profession has at its disposal agents that are "effective in reducing both secretory and motor activity of the stomach."

The effect on motor activity is generally more pronounced and less variable than on secretion; pain relief is usually prompt; a high degree of effectiveness is noted in ambulatory ulcer patients.

Ruffin, J. M.; Texter, E. C., Jr.; Carter, D. D., and Baylin, G. J.: J.A.M.A. 153:1159 (Nov. 28) 1953.

With its proved anticholinergic effectiveness, Banthine has been found extremely useful in the medical management of active peptic ulcer, whether duodenal, gastric or marginal.

The immediate increase in subjective well-being and the simplicity of the Banthine regimen assures patient cooperation. The recommended initial therapeutic dose is 50 or 100 mg. (one or two tablets) every six hours around the clock, with subsequent individual adjustment. The usual measures of diet regulation, rest and relaxation should be followed.

Banthine is effective in other conditions caused by excess parasympathetic stimulation. These include hypertrophic gastritis, acute and chronic pancreatitis, biliary dyskinesia and hyperhidrosis. Banthine is contraindicated in the presence of glaucoma and should be used with caution in the presence of severe cardiac disease or prostatic hypertrophy.

Banthine® bromide (brand of methantheline bromide) is supplied in scored tablets of 50 mg. and in ampuls of 50 mg. It is accepted by the Council on Pharmacy and Chemistry of the American Medical Association. G. D. Searle & Co., Research in the Service of Medicine.

Association Activities

PRESIDENT'S LETTER

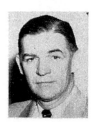

An important and different kind of scientific program was held at the Oklahoma University Medical School, and the Oklahoma Department of Public Safety, Division of Criminal Investigation. It was the first meeting of the Southwestern Homicide Investigators Seminar, and was attended by approximately 100 police officers of Oklahoma and surrounding territory.

During the five day session all phases of homicide investigation were discussed. Papers were given by leaders in various branches of this work. Included in the wide range of subjects covered were such topics as new chemical poisons, abortions, functions of a medical examiner, determination of time of death, errors in homicide investigation, and problems of identifying a body.

The guest speaker at the dinner on May 26th was Doctor LeMoyne Snyder, an internationally known medico-legal consultant. Doctor Snyder's comments bore principally upon the need for an adequate medical examiners law.

At present, Oklahoma, like the majority of states, has a very antiquated system for the investigation of unexplained deaths. It is to be hoped that in the near future the Oklahoma legislature will pass a law that will allow for a scientific investigation by qualified medical examiners of any unexplained death which might occur in Oklahoma. Such a law would be of vital importance for the protection of the family of an individual who might meet an unexplained or violent death, and would certainly be of aid to the members of our profession.

President

Thank you doctor for telling mother about...

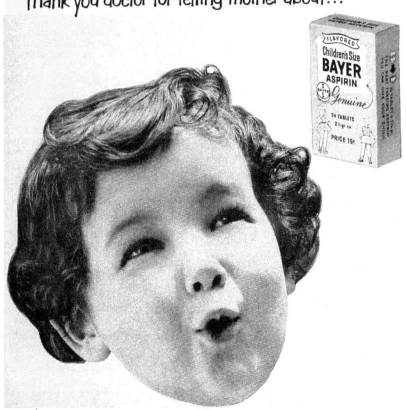

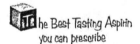 he Best Tasting Aspirin you can prescribe

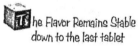 he Flavor Remains Stable down to the last tablet

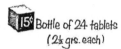 Bottle of 24 tablets (2½ grs. each)

We will be pleased to send samples on request

THE BAYER COMPANY DIVISION of Sterling Drug Inc., 1450 Broadway, New York 18, N. Y.

Golf Tournament Winner Reported

The Oklahoma State Medical Association Golf Tournament held Wednesday, May 12 at Twin Hills Golf and Country Club, Oklahoma City, was very successful, according to P. E. Russo, M.D., Chairman of the Golf Committee. Forty-five physicians entered the tournament and following the dinner, the participants inaugurated plans to make the Tournament a yearly event. James Amspacher, M.D. was named chairman for the next three years and is to appoint four members to work with him, two from Tulsa and two from Oklahoma City, who will cooperate with the local committee on arrangements.

Doctor Amspacher and J. M. Perry, M.D., Oklahoma City tied with a 78 during the tournament. On May 22 they were guests of Hugh Jeter, M.D. at the Oklahoma City Golf and Country Club where the tie was played off with Doctor Amspacher as champion of the Oklahoma State Medical Golf Association. Mel Shaffer of Dallas, representing the Pfizer company, completed the foursome. The Pfizer Company sponsored the tournament, awarded the trophy and many other prizes to the participants.

Practice of Clinical Psychiatry
Continued from Page 200
physicians atone with dignity and have faith that the basic sciences will develop the answers to psychosomatic problems.

27. There are no positive permanent solutions to anything. This point includes everything. Even death may leave relatives to fight over the estate.

Results Reported on X-Ray Screening

As a result of the Roentgen ray screening survey at the Oklahoma State Medical Association's annual meeting held May 10-12 in Oklahoma City, 220 chest films were taken. These were interpreted and were available for viewing by the physicians the day after they were taken. Much interest was manifested in the quality of the films and the detail possible when the small films were enlarged on the viewer which is used by the reader in making the interpretation. The 70 mm film and identifying IBM card with interpretation were later mailed to the individuals at their home addresses.

The results of the interpretation of the 220 screening films were as follows:

Number recommended for 14X17 confirmatory films (for correlation with clinical findings) _____ 9

Number of 70 mm films showing some abnormality _____26

Suspect minimal, arrested, tuberculosis___ 2

Calcifications _____ 2

Old pleurisy _____ 4

Basal fibrosis _____ 8

Elevated diaphragm _____ 2

Chronic emphysema _____ 1

Reserved diagnoses _____ 7

One reason for the State Department of Health's participation in this program was to display the type of equipment recommended for use in x-raying of admissions to general hospitals.

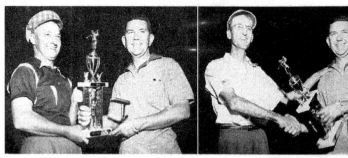

Pictured above are two Oklahoma City physicians, John Perry, M.D. and James Amspacher. Doctors Perry and Amspacher tied for the golf trophy in the tournament the last day of the Annual Meeting, May 12. The tie was played off a week later on a different course with Doctor Amspacher winning the trophy. In the left picture, Doctor Amspacher is shown with Mel Shafer, Dallas, Pfizer district representative.

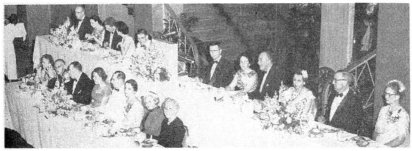

Pictured above is the speaker's table at the dinner-dance held during the Annual Meeting in Oklahoma City in May. Left to right—R. Q. Goodwin, M.D., Oklahoma City, O.S.M.A. President-Elect; Mrs. M. L. Henry, McAlester, outgoing President of the Auxiliary; W. R. Cheatwood, M.D., Duncan; Mrs. Richard Clay; Bruce R. Hinson, M.D., Enid, O.S.M.A. President; Richard A. Clay, M.D., Oklahoma City, master of ceremonies; Mrs. Hinson; John E. McDonald, M.D., Tulsa, outgoing O.S.M.A. President; Mrs. W. R. Cheatwood, incoming Auxiliary President; M. L. Henry, M.D., and Mrs. R. Q. Goodwin.

At the second table left to right—Margaret Lamb, Norman, President of the Oklahoma Hospital Association; Earl Rhodes, Grove, President of the Pharmaceutical Association; Albert E. Bonnell, Jr., D.D.S., Muskogee, President of the Dental Association; Mrs. Bonnell, Muskogee; E. C. Mohler, M.D., Ponca City; Mrs. Mohler, President-elect of the Auxiliary; Nan Green, Executive Secretary of the Nurses' Association and Lucille Terrell, President of the Nurses' Association.

President's Inaugural To Be Televised

Inauguration ceremonies of Walter B. Martin, M.D., new president of the American Medical Association will be televised on the March of Medicine program sponsored by Smith, Kline and French Laboratories. The program will be presented at the time usually devoted to Martin Kane, on 71 NBC stations.

WKY-TV, Oklahoma City, will televise the program Wednesday, July 14 at 10:30 p.m., a 20 day delay from the time of the actual inaugural ceremonies at the AMA San Francisco meeting.

Careful Blood Packaging Urged by Post Office

Information has been received that many doctors offices are mailing blood specimens in glass vials placed in metal screw-topped cardboard tubes to laboratories, and many times the tops are not screwed on securely. The vials often slip from the tubes, are broken, and the blood stains other mail.

The post office urges that an adhesive strip (not scotch tape) be placed across the metal top and down the sides of the container. This will prevent the insecurely screwed tops from comming off.

Physician-Wife Enter Manufacturing Field

Dr. and Mrs. Paul Lingenfelter, Clinton, were recently featured in an article in *Rescourceful Oklahoma*, published by the Oklahoma Planning and Resources Board. Mrs. Lingenfelter is secretary-treasurer of the company founded by her husband and a friend. Plastic picnic beverage coolers and a solution warmer for hospital operating rooms, dentistry tools and equipment and other surgical items are manufactured by the firm. The firm is known as Royal-Mieco. Fred Young is general manager.

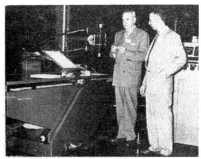

Pictured above with the equipment recommended for use in hospitals for small chest films are R. M. Shepard, M.D., Tulsa; and P. E. Russo, M.D., Oklahoma City. Photograph was made at the x-ray booth sponsored by the Oklahoma State Health Department at the Annual Meeting.

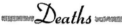 **Deaths**

JOHN H. BEATTY, M.D.
1876-1954

John H. Beatty, M.D., Tonkawa, died April 28, just nine days after his wife's death.

Doctor Beatty was born in Magnolia, Ohio in 1876 and was graduated from medical school in Chicago in 1903. He also attended Hiram College in Ohio.

Doctor Beatty practiced in Canton, Ohio from 1903 to 1918 when he came to Tonkawa. He was a member of several medical organizations and the Catholic church.

MATTHEW KARASEK, M.D.
1874-1954

Matthew Karasek, M.D., Shidler, died May 14 in a Winfield, Kansas hospital.

Doctor Karasek was born in Chicago Sept. 5, 1874 but moved to Tacoma, Wash. when he was 11 years old and received his education there and at Stanford University, Chicago University and the University of Chicago School of Medicine.

He practiced in Chicago and Olney, Ill. before becoming medical representative for the Phillips Petroleum Company at Shidler 30 years ago.

He is survived by the widow of the home, one son, five sisters and one granddaughter.

ROBERT E. LEATHEROCK, M.D.
1872-1954

Robert E. Leatherock, M.D., Cushing, died at his home June 2 after a long illness.

He had practiced in Cushing since 1930, moving there from Drumright. He was born in Indiana and practiced for a short time in Dewey county. His specialty was EENT.

Survivors include the widow of the home, one son, three daughters, a sister and a half brother, and six grand children.

CHARLES B. REESE, M.D.
1879-1954

Charles B. Reese, M.D., Sapulpa, died May 2 at his home. He suffered a fractured hip about eight years ago and had limited his practice since that time.

A native of Hortons, Pa., he graduated from Maryland Medical College in 1912 and moved to Sapulpa two years later. He was a Life Member of the Oklahoma State Medical Association, an Elk and a Mason.

RESOLUTION

WHEREAS, Nesbitt Ludson, Miller, M.D.; Assistant Professor of Medicine, having served on the faculty since September 17, 1931; beginning as an Appointee in the Out-Patient Department, gave of his best for the relief of the suffering of others, and set an example which will long continue to influence and inspire us, died on May 3, 1954, and,

WHEREAS, by the death of Doctor Miller, the Medical Profession, the State, the Faculty of the Oklahoma University School of Medicine, and those who have depended upon him for help and counsel, have a great loss, and,

WHEREAS, we, the members of the Faculty of the Oklahoma School of Medicine, feel a keen sense of loss, both personal and professional, of the passing of our fellow member and desire to convey to the world our appreciation of his devoted service.

THEREFORE, BE IT RESOLVED, that we express to his relatives our sincere sympathy and our desire to share their great loss, and

BE IT FURTHER RESOLVED, that a copy of these resolutions be sent to the relatives of Doctor Miller, a copy spread on the records of the faculty and a copy sent to the *Journal* of the Oklahoma State Medical Association.

Earl D. McBride, M.D.
Resolutions Committee

RESOLUTION

WHEREAS, The Almighty in His wisdom has seen fit to remove our colleague, Dr. E. L. Collins, Panama, Oklahoma, from our midst.

WHEREAS, Doctor Collins because of his genial personality, professional skill, his willingness to help the young physicians in our part of the State, an inspiration to the older physicians, a champion of medical ethics, a gentleman in every respect, was liked by all of us.

WHEREAS, Doctor Collins, born in Alabama in 1874, was a graduate of Memphis Hospital Medical College, now the University of Tennessee School of Medicine in the class of 1894, began the practice of medicine at the age of 21; did his first practice in Wilburton, Oklahoma, and six years later moved to Panama, Oklahoma. Doctor Collins was known throughout the state as an executive and business man of extraordinary ability, and a gentleman of the highest type, was always interested in the progress of the sciences relating to organized medicine, and was a close observer of human nature and abided consistently with the rules of medical ethics. Doctor Collins was a true friend to mankind, a loyal and respected citizen of his community and state. He took post graduate course in medicine in Cook County Hospital, Chicago, Ill.; Mayo Clinic, and Barnes Hospital, St. Louis.

THEREFORE, BE IT RESOLVED, that the LeFlore-Haskell County Medical Society in session assembled on May 3, 1954 in the LeFlore County Medical Hospital, express our appreciation for the fine service Doctor Collins gave to our profession, that a copy of this resolution be spread upon the minutes of our Society, that a copy be given to the members of Doctor Collins' family and a copy be given to the press.

The Resolutions Committee
E. M. Woodson, M.D., Chairman
John H. Harvey, M.D.
C. S. Cunningham, M.D.

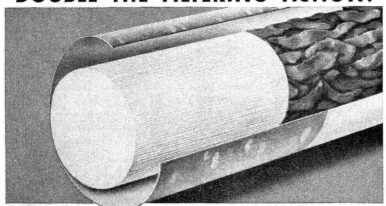

Thank You, Doctor!

To the 64,985 doctors who have visited Viceroy exhibits at medical conventions ... and to the leaders in the medical profession who smoke and recommend Viceroy Filter Tip Cigarettes ... we'd like to say "Thanks." Your approval of Viceroy has helped establish its leadership ... *Viceroy now outsells all other filter tip cigarettes!*

NEW VICEROY GIVES SMOKERS
DOUBLE THE FILTERING ACTION!

1. NEW AMAZING FILTER OF ESTRON MATERIAL
20,000 tiny filter elements in this new-type filter tip, exclusive with VICEROY! Made of Estron—a pure, white cellulose acetate—this non-mineral filter represents the latest development in twenty years of Brown & Williamson filter research. It gives the greatest filtering action possible without impairing flavor or impeding the flow of smoke.

2. PLUS KING-SIZE LENGTH
The smoke is also filtered through Viceroy's extra length of rich, costly tobaccos. Thus Viceroy actually gives smokers *double the filtering action . . .* to double the pleasure and contentment of *tobacco at its best!*

ONLY A PENNY OR TWO MORE THAN CIGARETTES WITHOUT FILTERS

New King-Size
Filter Tip **VICEROY**

OUTSELLS ALL OTHER FILTER TIP CIGARETTES COMBINED

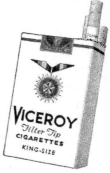

VICEROY
Filter Tip
CIGARETTES
KING-SIZE

Have You Heard?

HAROLD G. SLEEPER, M.D., Oklahoma City, is taking a 14 month postgraduate course at John Sealy Hospital, Galveston.

J. L. WHEELER, M.D., formerly of Oklahoma City, has moved to Texhoma.

THREE ANADARKO PHYSICIANS, J. B. Miles, M.D., E. T. Cook, Jr., M.D. and G. E. Haslam, M.D., are building a new $60,000 clinic annex to the hospital there.

ROBERT A. FURMAN, M.D., Oklahoma City, spoke on "New clues as to how and why the sex hormones influence hardening of the arteries" at a meeting in Atlantic City of the American Federation for Clinical Research.

R. D. WILLIAMS, M.D., Idabel, recently celebrated his 50th anniversary as a practicing physician in McCurtain County.

HARRY E. WILKINS, M.D., Oklahoma City, was recently elected president of the Harvey Cushing Society when it met in Santa Fe, New Mexico. A. C. LISLE, M.D., also of Oklahoma City, became a member of the society at the meeting.

MALCOLM PHELPS, M.D., El Reno, has been named to the Oklahoma Crime Commission.

THE LANGSTON MEDICAL GROUP has moved into its new building at 1214 N. Hudson, Oklahoma City. Physicians associated in the group are Wann Langston, M.D., George N. Barry, M.D., John J. Donnell, M.D., Richard E. Carpenter, M.D., John W. DeVore, M.D., and James K. DeVore, M.D. Practice of the group will be limited to Internal Medicine.

School Health Booklet Available

Health of the School Age Child, a 75 page report of the child annual conference on health of the school age child, has been published by the Oklahoma Advisory Health Council.

Speeches of educators and physicians of the state are briefly summarized in schools of the state are given. Some of the programs described deal with the school recess, mental health, health interests and practices of school-age children, sex instruction, safety, school lunch, and pupil responsibility.

Price of the booklet is 35 cents and it can be purchased from the Oklahoma Advisory Health Council, North Campus, Norman.

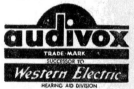
ANNOUNCEMENTS

Sixth International Cancer Congress

July 23-29, Sao Paulo, Brazil. Special pre-Congress and post-Congress tours have been arranged.

Southwestern Surgical Congress

September 20-22, Oklahoma City, Skirvin Hotel. Headquarters office 207 Plaza Court.

North Texas-Southern Oklahoma Fall Clinical Conference

September 22, Wichita Falls Country Club, Wichita Falls, Texas, sponsored by the Wichita County Medical Society. L. N. Simmons, M. D., 1518 10th St., Wichita Falls, is chairman.

Pan-Pacific Surgical Association

Sixth Congress will be held in Honolulu in October, 1954.

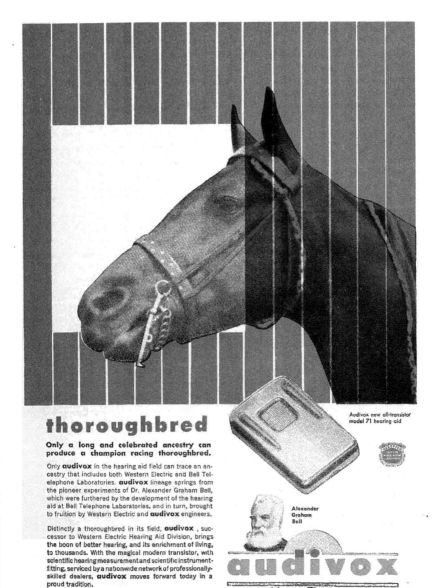

thoroughbred

Only a long and celebrated ancestry can produce a champion racing thoroughbred.

Only **audivox** in the hearing aid field can trace an ancestry that includes both Western Electric and Bell Telephone Laboratories. **audivox** lineage springs from the pioneer experiments of Dr. Alexander Graham Bell, which were furthered by the development of the hearing aid at Bell Telephone Laboratories, and in turn, brought to fruition by Western Electric and **audivox** engineers.

Distinctly a thoroughbred in its field, **audivox** , successor to Western Electric Hearing Aid Division, brings the boon of better hearing, and its enrichment of living, to thousands. With the magical modern transistor, with scientific hearing measurement and scientific instrument-fitting, serviced by a nationwide network of professionally-skilled dealers, **audivox** moves forward today in a proud tradition.

TO THE DOCTOR: Send your patient with a hearing problem to a career Audivox and Micronic dealer, chosen for his interest, integrity and ability. There is such an Audivox dealer in every major city from coast to coast.

Audivox new all-transistor
model 71 hearing aid

Alexander
Graham
Bell

audivox

Successor to *Western Electric* Hearing Aid Division

123 Worcester St., Boston, Mass.

The Thoroughbred Hearing Aid

OFFICIAL PROCEEDINGS OF THE HOUSE OF DELEGATES

of the

OKLAHOMA STATE MEDICAL ASSOCIATION

MAY 9, 1954

Opening Session

The 61st Session of the House of Delegates of the Oklahoma State Medical Association was called to order at 1:00 p.m., Sunday, May 9, 1954, in the Mirror Room of the Municipal Auditorium, Oklahoma City, Oklahoma, by the Vice-Speaker of the House, Keilled Haynie, M.D., Durant.

M. B. Glihman, M.D., Oklahoma City, gave the Invocation.

The Speaker announced that a number of guests were present and would be introduced to the House.

The first guest to be introduced was Mr. Cecil Chamberlin, President of the Oklahoma Chapter of the Student American Medical Association. Mr. Chamberlin expressed the appreciation of his Association for the help and interest shown by the Oklahoma State Medical Association in their activities and introduced the Oklahoma delegates to the Student American Medical Association's House of Delegates, who were Mr. Oliver Patterson and Mr. James Calhoun.

The Speaker introduced Mr. Don Hawkins, representative of the St. Paul Mercury Indemnity Company, sentative of the St. Paul Mercury Indemnity Company, which company carries the Malpractice Master policy of the Association. Mr. Hawkins spoke to the House briefly on the subject of their Malpractice insurance. He praised the State of Oklahoma for their well co-ordinated malpractice policy which he stated was the best working insurance program of its kind in the United States. He advised the doctors that the St. Paul Mercury wanted to work with them and to be partners of the Profesion, and asked their continued cooperation.

The next guest to be introduced was Doctor Charles Kochakian, Director of the Oklahoma Medical Research Foundation, who made a few remarks concerning the work of the Foundation and extended an invitation to the doctors to visit them at the Foundation.

The Speaker introduced Doctor Mark Everett, Dean of the University of Oklahoma School of Medicine. Doctor Everett thanked the d o c t o r s for all the personal things they had done to help the school in many ways and advised them that the School was ·open to all suggestions from the Profession.

Mr. Bill Harkey, Attorney for the State Board of Medical Examiners, was introduced. Mr. Harkey thanked the Association for the invitation to be at the meeting, and advised the Doctors that he would continue to fight their battles in the legislature as he had done in the past.

The next guest was Mr. Glen Leslie, Tulsa, Oklahoma, President of Oklahoma Blue Shield. Mr. Leslie made a few remarks concerning the operation of Blue Shield and stated that he was proud to serve on the Board of Blue Shield.

Hayden Donahue, M.D., Director of the State Department of Mental Health, was introduced. Doctor Donahue thanked the House for the invitation to appear and advised that his department would appreciate any suggestions or criticisms their organization might care to make. He stated they needed all the help they could get from the Profession.

The Speaker introduced James Babcock, Assistant director of the University of Oklahoma Department of Archives, who had been working on the History of Medicine in Oklahoma. Mr. Babcock reported on the progress of the work on the History of Medicine in Oklahoma, thanked the doctors for thenr cooperation, and asked their continued support. ·

Louis Ritzhaupt, M.D., Guthrie, Oklahoma, a candidate for the gubernatorial race in Oklahoma, was next introduced.

As this concluded the introduction of guests, the Speaker proceeded with the business of the meeting.

The first item on the Agenda was the appointment of Reference Committees. Th Speaker appointed the following Committees:

Resolutions Committee

(To meet in Room 2312 Biltmore Hotel, between Sessions.)

H. M. McClure, M.D., Chickasha, Chairman
J. D. Shipp, M.D., Tulsa
Ralph Smith, M.D., Oklahoma City

Committee on Constitution & Bylaws

Wm. Weaver, M.D., Muskogee, Chairman
E. A. McGrew, M.D., Beaxer
E. H. Shuller, M.D., McAlester

Tellers

L. R. Kirby, M.D., Cherokee
H. B. Shorbe, M.D., Oklahoma City
M. O. Hart, M.D., Tulsa

Sergeants at Arms

H. V. Schaff, M.D., Holdenville
L. C. Kuyrkendall, M.D., McAlester
Joe Duer, M.D., Woodward

The Speaker asked the Credentials Committee if a quorum were present. Ned Burleson, M.D., Chairman of the Committee reported that a quorum was present.

Doctor Haynie addressed the House and advised that it was his pleasure to conduct the meeting as they wished it conducted as acting chairman, and to let their wishes be known.

The Speaker asked the pleasure of the House with regard to the reading of the minutes of the last meeting. John McDonald, M.D., Tulsa, moved; "That we dispense with the reading of the minutes, inasmuch as they had been published in the *Journal*." Motion seconded and carried.

Louis Ritzhaupt, M.D., Guthrie, moved; "That we approve the minutes as published". Marshall Hart, M.D., Tulsa, seconded. Motion carried.

At this point the Speaker announced that the Chair would entertain nominations for election of officers for next year. The first office to be filled was that of President-Elect.

Wilkie Hoover, M.D., Tulsa, Oklahoma, nominated R. Q. Goodwin, M.D., Oklahoma City. H. B. Shorbe, M.D., Oklahoma City, seconded the nomination.

L. C. Kuyrkendall, M.D., McAlester, nominated E. H. Shuller, M.D., McAlester, nominated E. H. Shuller, M.D., McAlester. The Speaker recognized Doctor Shuller who addressed the House and advised them that while he felt greatly honored to have his name presented as candidate for President-Elect, he would like to withdraw his name in favor of R. Q. Goodwin, M.D., Oklahoma City.

Doctor Kuyrkendall accepted Doctor Shuller's request and his name was withdrawn.

A. T. Baker, M.D., Durant, moved that the nominations be closed. Motion seconded and carried.

The Speaker called for nominations for Delegate to the American Medical Association for a term of two years. M. B. Glismann, M.D., Oklahoma City, nominated James Stevenson, M.D., Tulsa, for re-election. Hugh Perry, M.D., Tulsa, seconded. Motion carried. I. W. Bollinger, M.D., Henryetta, moved that the nominations cease. Motion seconded and carried.

Nominations were opened for Alternate Delegate to the A.M.A., for a two years term.

L. A. Munding, M.D., Tulsa, nominated E. H. Shuller, M.D., McAlester. Marshal O. Hart, M.D., Tulsa, seconded the motion, and moved the nominations cease. Motion carried.

The House was opened for nominations for Vice-President. Walter Brown, M.D., of Tulsa, nominated Clifford Bassett, M.D., Cushing. D. W. Humphreys, M.D., of Cushing seconded. Doctor Ritzhaupt moved that the nominations cease. Motion seconded and carried.

The Speaker called for nominations for Speaker of the House of Delegates for a term of two years. Frank C. Lattimore, M.D., of Kingfisher, nominated Clinton Gallaher, M.D., Shawnee, James Colvert, M.D., Oklahoma City, seconded. McLain Rogers, M.D., Clinton, moved that the nominations cease. Motion seconded and carried.

The Speaker called for nominations for Vice-Speaker of the House of Delegates for a term of two years. Malcom Phelps, M.D., El Reno, nominated Keiller Haynie, M.D., Durant. John Burton, M.D., seconded the nomination and moved tha tthe nominations cease. Motion carried.

The next order of business was the nomination of councilors and vice-councilors for Districts #2, 5, 8, 11, and 14. The Speaker announced that the nominations of R. Q. Goodwin, M.D., for President-Elect and E. H. Shuller, M.D., as Alternate Delegate to the A.M.A., had created vacancies in Districts #10 and 2, and that these Districts would also have to reelect. A ten minute recess was allowed for these Districts to caucus and decide on their nominations.

The House reconvened and the Speaker called for nominations for Councilor for District #2.

E. H. Arrendall, M.D., Ponca City, nominated E. C. Mohler, M.D., Ponca City, for Councilor. D. W. Humphreys, M.D., Cushing, Seconded the nomination. It was moved, seconded and carried that the nominations cease.

E. H. Arrendall, M.D., Ponca City, nominated Glen McDonald, M.D., Pawhuska, for Vice-Counselor. Cody Ray, M.D., Pawhuska, seconded the motion. Doctor Arrendall moved that the nominations cease. Motion seconded and carried.

The Speaker called for nominations from District #5. Malcom Phelps, M.D., nominated A. L. Johnson, M.D., El Reno, to succeed himself as Councilor. F. R. First, M.D., Checotah, seconded. It was moved seconded and carried that the nominations cease. McLain Rogers, M.D., Clinton, nominated Ross Deputy, M.D., Clinton, as Vice-Councelor. Doctor First Seconded. It was moved, seconded and carried that the nominations cease.

Nominations were opened for District #8. Marshal O. Hart, M.D., nominated Wilkie Hoover, M.D., Tulsa, for Councilor. J. D. Shipp, M.D., Tulsa, seconded and moved that the nominations cease. Earl M. Lusk, M. D., Tulsa, nominated Wendell Smith, M.D., Tulsa for Vice-Councelor. R. W. Goen, M.D., Tulsa, seconded and moved that the nominations cease. Motion seconded and carried.

The Speaker called for nominations from District #10. T. H. McCarley, M.D., McAlester, M.D., nominated Paul Kernek, M.D., Holdenville, for Councilor. E. H. Shuller, M. D., McAlester, seconded, and moved that the nominations Close. Motion seconded and carried. Paul Kernek, M.D., Holdenville, nominated C. D. Lively, M.D., of McAlester for Vice-Councilor. E. H. Shuller seconded and moved that the nominations cease. Motion seconded and carried.

Nominations were called for from District #11. B. B. Coker, M.D., Durant, nominated A. T. Baker, M.D., Durant, as Councilor and nominated Thomas E. Rhea, M.D., Idabel, as Vice-Councilor. E. A. Johnson, M.D., seconded and moved that the nominations cease. Motion seconded and carried.

The Speaker called for nominations from District #14. L. G. Livingston, M.D., Cordell, nominated J. D. Hollis, M.D., of Mangum. R. S. Srigley, M.D., Hollis, seconded and moved that the nominations cease. Motion carried.

L. G. Livingston, M.D., nominated R. R. Hannas, M.D., of Sentinel for Vice-Councilor. Doctor Hollis seconded and moved that the nominations cease. Motion seconded and carried.

Nominations were open for District #6. Ray Balyeat, M.D., Oklahoma City, nominated Elmer Ridgeway M.D., Oklahoma City, for Councilor. James Colver, M.D., seconded and moved that the nominations cease. C. W. McClure, M.D., Oklahoma City, nominated P. E. Russo, M.D., Oklahoma City, for Vice-Councilor. Doctor Colvert seconded the nomination. It was moved, seconded and carried that the nominations cease.

As this completed the nominations for officers, the Speaker proceeded with the next order of business, which was the place and date of the next Annual Meeting. It was decided to postpone this until after the Council Report had been read.

Next on the Agenda was the report of the Officers. The Speaker called on James Stevenson, M.D., Tulsa, Delegate to the A.M.A

Doctor Stevenson advised that inasmuch as the minutes of the last session of the A.M.A. had been published in the Journal, he would report on things coming up. He discussed the Hobby Bill, the proposed extension of Social Security to self-employed persons, and other legislation in which the Profession is interested. Doctor Stevenson concluded his report by advising the doctors that when he returned from the A.M.A. meeting in San Francisco, he would give a complete report to the Council.

The Speaker announced that a degression from the

agenda would be made and that F. Redding Hood, M.D., Oklahoma City, Chairman of the Committee on Military Affairs, would make his report at this time as it was necessary for him to leave. Doctor Hood made the following report.

Report of the Committee on Military Affairs

The Committee on Military Affairs held no meeting during the year, as no business was presented for its consideration.

However, as Chairman of the Oklahoma Voluntary Advisory Committee for Physicians, Dentists, Veterinarians and Allied Specialists, I should like to render a report to this House of Delegates.

As each of you know, the Doctor Draft Law will expire July 1, 1955, unless re-enacted by Congress. At the present time there is no clear indication of what Congress's attitude will be.

Due to cessation of hostilities in Korea, no physicians have been called to active military duty since August of 1953. However, within this past week I have been advised that the Army Air Force will call to active duty their reserve officers who are in Priority I. In Oklahoma we have been notified there are two physicians who fall in this category. In addition to reserve officers the Committee was advised last Wednesday that six Priority I physicians in Oklahoma who have been examined by Selective Service and found physically qualified will be called for induction in June and July, three each month.

Since this call indicates that additional physicians will be called between now and next July 1, County Advisory Committees should be reviewing the medical situations in their counties.

One other piece of information should be understood. From time to time some of you may hear of a physician or dentist being reclassified by his local board. This reclassification is in line with a directive from Natonal Selective Service to all local boards to reconsider the classification of all physicians in Priority 1 and 2 and Priority III physicians who were born after August 31, 1922. As it pertains to dentists, all three priorities irrespective of age.

As further information is received, it will be communicated to the local county advisory committees.

At the conclusion of his written report, Doctor Hood explained to the House the meaning of dual jeopardy as it pertains to the young doctors, who are in danger of being inducted through the regular draft as well as under the Doctor's Draft Law.

The Speaker announced that the Constitution and Bylaws Committee would meet at Room 1059 Skirvin Hotel between session.

Doctor Haynie called on John Burton, M.D., delegate to the A.M.A. for a report. Doctor Burton stated that he believed Doctor Stevenson had covered the matters to be reported pretty thoroughly. He went on to say that the big question as far as the A.M.A. delegates were concerned was the subject of hom they were going to vote on the Osteopathic question at the San Francisco meeting.

Next on the agenda was the report of the Councilors on their Councilor Districts. The Speaker asked if any of the Councilors wished to make an oral report. None were forthcoming.

The next order of business was the Report of the Council. The Speaker called on Doctor John McDonald, Tulsa, Oklahoma, President of the Association. Doctor McDonald prefaced the report with a few remarks expressing his appreciation to the doctors of Oklahoma for their whole-hearted cooperation during the past year, and praised them for their efforts and accomplishments.

Report of the Council

The Council fully realies its responsibility in carrying out the actions and recommendations of the House of Delegates. It is also cognizant of the fact that this report constitutes a record of its stewardship of the Association for the past year and its recommendations for the year ahead.

In its last report an observation was made that with a change in Federal Government leadership, it was the opinion of the Council that sound and conservative consideration would be given, both by Congress and the Executive Branch, to the problems of health and welfare. The Council also pointed out that not withstanding this opinion, the Profession should not assure a feeling of complaceny. Your Council is now of the opinion it might be wrong on its first observation, but is doubly sure it was correct in its second.

While the actions of Congress and the Executive Branch of Government must be given every consideration by the Profession, the fact still remains that medicine must keep foremost in its viewpoint a continuance of rendering to the American Public the highest quality of medical care possible. On this viewpoint your Council endorses the program announced by the President of the American Medical Association, Dr. Edward J. McCormick, at the time of his inauguration, which is as follows:

The expulsion from county medical societies of physicians who are unethical, dishonest and unfair.

The support of the American Medical Education Foundation to assist in the financing and expansion of medical schools and their education program.

The creation by County Medical Societies of emergency and nightcall services.

In 'order that the Council Report may not be too long, the delegates are requested to pay close attention to the Committee Reports which will follow and which will outline many of the problems and programs of the Association.

Membership

The paid membership of the Association on May 1, 1954, was 1412, representing 1290 fully paid members and 122 half due members. At the present time there are 103 Life Members and 47 Honorary Members. Another portion of the Council Report will recommend the approval of 2 Honorary Memberships and 21 Life Memberships which, if aproved by the House of Delegates, will bring the total number of such memberships to 173.

Finances and Budget

The financial structure of the Association remains sound. In addition to $12,000 in Government Bonds, the Association owns $10,000 in Building and Loan through the Ponca City Savings and Loan Association, which is Federally insured. The cash reserve of the Association on December 31, 1953, not counting any 1954 income, was $30,819.39.

As has annually been stated by the Council, the estimating of income and budget expenditures in April or May for the following year is extremely difficult, if not impossible. However, recognizing that such is necessary, the Council submits the following which is predicated on 1953 income from dues and known revenue to be received in 1954 from Annual Meeting income and *Journal* advertising:

Income

Dues	$ 58,000.00
Interest on U. S. Bonds	167.00
Interest Bldg. & Loan	300.00
Comm. from A. M. A.	339.00
Annual Meeting	9,837.00
Journal Advertising	17,392.00
Directory Advertising	1,000.00
Rural Health Conf.	575.00
Total Income	$ 87,608.00

Budget

Office Expense	$ 32,600.00
Journal	24,000.00
Public Policy Committee	3,000.00
Public Health Committee	2,000.00
Legal Expense	1,200.00
Retirement	3,334.00
Annual Meeting	11,000.00
Directory	1,400.00
Travel	6,000.00
Miscellaneous	1,500.00
	$ 86,034.00

Income	$87,608.00
Expenditures	86,034.00
Income over Expenditures	$ 1,574.00

To accomplish this budget, the dues for 1955 must remain at $42.00 and the Council so recommends. The Council further recommends that $10,000 of the Association's cash operating reserve be invested in either Government Bonds or Federally Insured Building and Loan. Ultimate disposition of the reserve funds will be commented on further in the report.

The Cline Committee Report

During early April, Councilor District meetings were held at which meetings 17 different subjects were discussed. The topics so presented will be either in this report or through a Committee.

One subject so presented to the County Societies dealt with recommendations made by the Committee of the A.M.A. headed by Dr. John Cline of San Francisco, a past-president of the A.M.A.

The report has not as yet been adopted by the House of Delegates of the A.M.A., pending a discussion of the report by the State Medical Associations. The Oklahoma delegates to the A.M.A. have requested that they be instructed as to how they should vote on the question at the San Francisco meeting this coming June.

The three basic questions to be resolved by either the adoption or rejection of the report are as follows:

1. Whether or not to consider Osteopathy as a cult.
2. To encourage improvement in undergraduate and postgraduate education of Doctors of Osteopathy. This could include the approval of Doctors of Medicine to teach in schools of Osteopathy.
3. That the relationship between Doctors of Medicine and Osteopathy should be determined at the State level, and that the State Associations should accept this responsibility and that the Committee or a similar Committee should be continued as a permanent body.

Your Council makes no recommendation, but does urge that this House of Delegates give full con-

sideration and discussion to the subject, and that the Oklahoma Delegates to the A.M.A. be instructed by this House of Delegates.

American Medical Education Foundation

In 1951, there was established the National Medical Education Foundation for the purpose of raising money from business and industry to help finance medical education through the medical schools. As one of its counterparts, there was founded the American Medical Education Foundation to raise money for a like proposition from physicians. The money donated to the American Medical Education Foundation by physicians is forwarded to the National Association, which in turn distributes it among the two and four year schools. This distribution is made on the basis of equal amounts to the two year schools and equal amounts to the four year schools. In a few instances special grants are made. The University of Oklahoma School of Medicine has received approximately $60,000. There is some degree of disagreement as to whether State supported schools should receive the same amount of money as privately endowed schools. In Oklahoma there is also the question of support for this program, as well as the Oklahoma Medical Research Foundation.

At a meeting of the Council on March 11, 1954, a report was received from Doctor Joe Duer of Woodward, who had attended a meeting in Chicago of the American Medical Education Foundation. Doctor Duer reported Oklahoma next to the last in contributions. After thorough discussion, the Council voted to endorse the Foundation and now asks the House of Delegates whether it desires to affirm or reject the action of the Council.

Mal-Practice Insurance

This is a continuing subject and program that needs the attention of every county society and its individual nembers. Today over 1,000 members have taken advantage of the Group policy held with the St. Paul-Mercury, and by and large, excellent results have been secured from the individual societies and their members. Since it is extremely difficult for an insurance company to make money on this type of coverage at the premium for which it is offered, it is hoped that the members having St. Paul coverage will consisder giving to this Company their other coverages such as Premises Liability, fire, theft, etc. Attention of all members should also be directed to the limits of insurance they are carrying. On the basis of judgments being given today, limits of $10/30,000 are hardly adequate. Bear in mind that an Oklahoma physician has had a judgment rendered against him in the amount of $60,000.

County Medical Society Committees

Three years ago the State Association, in order to try to expedite the working of its Committees, reduced their number and placed a representative from each Councilor District on the Committees, with the exception of the Public Policy Committee which was divided on the basis of Congressional Districts, with two members from each Congressional District. It is important that the county societies have identical committees, although this does not preclude their appointing any other additional committees to carry on the work of the local society if it is deemed to be more effective.

Secretaries of the County and District Medical Societies have been notified of these Committees of the State Association.

The Journal

Attention is directed to the *Journal* of the Association which has recently undergone a complete renovation, both as to style and type. The Editorial Board is extremely anxious to have individual members give suggestions concerning the *Journal* and to take issue with its Editorial Board if such is indicated. It is extremely difficult to make the *Journal* a readable *Journal* without the cooperation of the County Societies and the individual members. It would be appreciated if the county societies would send to the attention of the Executive Office or the *Journal*, medical or health news of importance that has happened or is happening in their respective communities.

The Council would like to particularly acknowledge its appreciation to the Norman Transcript Co., which is now publishing the *Journal*, for the cooperation it gave in renovating the *Journal*.

Prepaid Voluntary Health Insurance

While this subject will be discussed in the report of the Public Policy Committee, your Council feels that the House of Delegates should know that following the recommendations of the House of Delegates at its last spring session, Blue Cross be asked to offer its coverage to all physicians not covered by their own group, there were less than 75 physicians who enrolled.

Your Council has also been advised that certain resolutions will be introduced before the House of Delegates concerning the extent to which contracts are being written by insurance companies and non-profit hospital and medical care plans whereby hospitals are being paid for certain services that may rightfully be medical services and in some instances when payment for medical services cannot be made to other than full time employees of hospitals. Your Council urges the House of Delegates to give careful consideration to this problem.

Public Public Policy Committee

Your Council has reviewed the report of the Public Policy Committee and urges the delegates to pay close attention to this report. The Council is firmly of the opinion that the work of this Committee between now and the next spring meeting will be an undertaking in which it can succeed only with the cooperation of all of the County and District Societies and each individual member.

Special Memberships

Nominations from the county societies for the various classifications of special memberships have been reviewed by the Council, and the Council recommends their election as follows:

Life Membership Petitions
1954 House of Delegates

Lin Alexander, M.D., Okmulgee, Oklahoma
H. A. Angus, M.D., Lawton, Oklahoma
E. R. Barker, M.D., Healdton, Oklahoma.
Charles E. Calhoun, M.D., Sand Springs, Okla.
Roy F. Cannon, M.D., Miami, Oklahoma
Samuel C. Dean, M.D., Howe, Oklahoma
Edgar Frank Harbison, M.D., Oklahoma City, Okla.
Bunn Harris, M.D., Jenks, Oklahoma
A. E. Hennings, M.D., Tuttle, Oklahoma
Clarence C. Hoke, M.D., Tulsa, Oklahoma
H. L. Johnson, M.D., Woodward, Oklahoma
Powell K. Lewis, M.D., Sapulpa, Oklahoma
Warren T. Mayfield, M.D., Norman, Oklahoma
James W. Rogers, M.D., Tulsa, Oklahoma
R. E. Sawyer, M.D., Durant, Oklahoma
Harry A. Stalker, M.D., Pond Creek, Oklahoma

William J. Trainor, M.D., Tulsa, Oklahoma
I. D. Walker, M.D., Tonkawa, Oklahoma
J. Clay Williams, M.D., Durant, Oklahoma
Divonis Worton, M.D., Pawhuska, Oklahoma
Paul Grosshart, M.D., Tulsa, Oklahoma

Honorary Membership Petitions
1954 House of Delegates

John Evans Heatley, M.D., Oklahoma Ctiy, Okla.
George H. Niemann, M.D., Ponca City, Oklahoma

Associate Membership Petition

Louis Lipnick, M.D., Veterans Hospital, Oklahoma City

Public Health Committee

In connection with the Report of the Public Health Committee, the Council desires to call to the attention of the House of Delegates the Rural Health Conference being sponsored by the Association through the Sub-committee on Rural Health and to urge each County Society to be represented at the next Rural Health Conference which will be held in November or December.

Your Council is most impressed by the apparent lack of interest among the county societies in School Health activities, and would emphasize the committee's attitude that School Health is a most effective means through which the profession may gain sound public relations and improve the health of the people of the state.

Those portions of the report concerning Industrial Health, Blood Banks, and Nutrition require no comment.

The Supplemental Report concerning medical care for indigent Indians is a subject worthy of full consideration by the House of Delegates and the Council urges definite action by the House of Delegates on the recommendations of the Public Committee as contained in the supplemental report.

Educational Committee

As was reported to the House of Delegates at its last session, the Educational Committee of the Association has continued its policy of cooperating fully with the office of postgraduate education of the Medical School of the University of Oklahoma.

It is a belief of the Committee, concurred in by the Council, that the postgraduate courses being offered by the Medical School are fulfilling the need for postgraduate medical education in Oklahoma at the present time and that the courses and material presented have in general been of the highest quality and excellence.

If at any time it appears that the requirements of postgraduate medical education can be better met in some other manner or that the activities of the Medical School should be further supplemented, the Council and the Educational Committee stand ready to take such action as may be indicated.

Grievance Committee

The Council has reviewed the report of the Grievance Committee. In its report the Grievance Committee points out that as a result of consideration of one complaint by the Committee, the physician concerned was suspended from membership for a period of three years by his County Medical Society.

The Council would further urge that the House of Delegates give the most thoughtful consideration to amendments to the Bylaws presented in a subsequent portion of this report which are designed to outline more clearly the duties and responsibilities of the Grievance Committee and to clarify its procedure and relations with the Component medical societies. These amendments have been prepared after consultation with the legal counsel for the Association, Mr. Roy Lytle, and are designed to eliminate some criticism which has been directed toward the manner of operation of the Committee.

Annual Meeting
Your Council has considered the problem of the holding of the Annual Meeting, as it pertains to the cities and dates.

In the past, through custom only the House of Delegates has acted upon invitation extended to it from component societies to hold the Annual Meeting in their particular locality.

In view of the increasing difficulty of scheduling the meeting at given dates in Oklahoma City and Tulsa, your Council recommends that the House of Delegates authorize and approve the rotating of the meeting between Oklahoma City and Tulsa, and that the meeting dates be set up two or more years in advance.

Building Fund
Previously in the Council Report reference was made to the reserve funds of the Association which are in the amount of $22,000, plus an additional $10,000 if the House of Delegates approves the recommendation of the Council that this amount from the cash reserve be placed in reserve, making a total in reserve of $30,000.

The Council at its March 11 meeting discussed at length the advisability of using this reserve to build a headquarters office. The Council approved the appointment of a Committee to make a study of the feasibility of such an action by the Association. The Association is at the present time paying $275.00 a month rent.

This Committee has not yet been appointed, but will be appointed by the incoming president, and will make a progress report at the Fall meeting of the House of Delegates.

Medical Research Foundation
While elsewhere in this report there has been a recommendation that support of the American Medical Education Foundation be approved by this House of Delegates, nevertheless your Council feels that the Profession must not lose sight of the fact that support of the Oklahoma Medical Research Foundation should have the consideration at all times of the Profession.

It should be kept in mind that the creation of this Research Foundation stemmed first from an idea presented by Dr. Tom Lowry, endorsed by a previous House of Delegates, and ultimately placed in the hands of the Alumni Association of the University of Oklahoma School of Medicine.

It is your Council's opinion that the public will support the Foundation in direct ratio to the support given by the Profession.

History of Medicine
This project of the Association, which was approved three years ago, has moved steadily forward through not only the Committee headed by the Editor of the *Journal*, Doctor Lewis J. Moorman, but the Department of Archives of the University of Oklahoma. Field representatives from the Department of Archives have already surveyed approximately 40% of the Counties of the State and researchers have been working in the Archives in Washington, D.C. This field and research work have been financed by past appropriations from the Association, and outside contributions that have been secured by the committee. Your attention is called to the exhibit on this project which will be on display at the meeting.

The Council urges each physician to cooperate in this program, remembering that "The Past is Prologue."

Amendemnts to the By-Laws
Amend Chapter IX, Page 45, by inserting, following the present Section 6, a new Section 7, to read as follows, with remaining Section 7, to be renumbered 'Section 8':

"Section 7, Grievance Committee "

(a) Investigation

The Grievance Committee shall investigate all complaints concerning members of this Association which may be received by the Association when such complaints are received in writing and signed by the individuals making such complaints.

(b) Procedure

The Grievance Committee shall establish its own procedure for handling complaints filed with it, in accordance with these By-Laws, and is authorized to make recommendations to members of this Association complained of and to complainants in an effort, adjust or dispose of cases on a fair and equitable basis for all concerned.

(c) Disposal of Cases

When the Grievance Committee is unable to negotiate the settlement of any case pending before it, as a result of the refusal or neglect of the member of the Association concerned to comply with the recommendations of the Committee, it shall then refer the case directly to the component society of which the physician is a member. In so referring any case to a component society the Committee shall advise the member of such referral and shall provide the component's society with a complete copy of the Committee's file and its recommendations concerning said case.

In any instance in which a case is referred to a component society by the Grievance Committee and in which the component society does not, within thirty (30) days of such referral, initiate action to bring the matter before the component society for hearing, the Grievance Committee may, at its discretion, file formal charges, before the component society, concerning such case and if such charges are not prosecuted as provided in the Constitution and By-Laws of the component society, or within thirty (30) days, the Grievance Committee may then file charges before the Council which shall promptly hear such charges and dispose of the case.

The Council shall hear charges preferred against members of component societies by the Grievance Committee. The Council shall establish its own procedure for hearing such charges, provided, however, that in all instances, the charges against members of component societies shall be reduced to writing and the evidence presented shall be germane to such charges. Copies of the charges shall, in all instances be furnished to the member of the component society against whom the charge has been preferred. The member complained of shall have adequate opportunity to prepare his defense and shall not be required to answer such charge in writing, although he may do so if he desires. The date of hearing shall in no event be less than twenty (20) days from the date copies of the charges are furnished the member complained of. Notice of at least ten (10) days as to the date and place of hearing shall be given the member complained of. The member against whom such charge be preferred shall have the right to be accompanied at the hearing by counsel if he so desires. The Council shall have the right to have present counsel of its choice for advice and assistance during any hearing, but such counsel shall not have any vote.

Amend Chapter IX, Section 1, Page 44, by striking the period at the end of the section and inserting in lieu thereof the following words and figures: "and Grievance Committee."

Amend Chapter IX, Section 2, Page 44, by inserting before the words, "The Committee" on Line 1, the words and figures:

"(a) Committee on Annual Session," and by inserting. following the words "Secretary-Treasurer" on Line 2, the following words and figures:

"(b) Grievance Committee."

The Grievance Committee shall at all times be composed of the last five (5) living Past-Presidents of this Association.

(c) All Other Standing Committees.

Amend Chapter 1, Section 3, Subsection (b), line 13, Page 38, by striking, following the words, "consideration to the," the remaing words and figures in that paragraph and inserting in lieu thereof the following words and figures: "Council and approved by the Council at a meeting prior to the Annual Session."

NOTE: This Amendment eliminates a temporary provision for waiving the five year membership requirement for all applicants whose applications for Honorary Membership were filed before January 1, 1952.

Amend Chapter 1, Section 3, Subsection (c) Page 38, by striking, all of line 17, beginning "Executive Secretary" and the remaining words and figures in that paragraph and inserting in lieu thereof the following words and figures: "Council and approved by the Council at meeting prior to the Annual Session."

NOTE: This Amendment eliminates a temporary provision for waiving the five year membership requirement for all applicants whose applications for Life Membership were filed before January 1, 1952.

Amend Chapter 1, Section 3, Subsection (e) Page 39, Line 9, by striking after the word "Council" and before the word "before," the following words and figures:

"at least ninety (90) days."

Amend Chapter 1, Section 3, Subsection E, Page 39, Line 13, by striking, following the word "Council," the remaining words and figures in that paragraph and inserting in lieu thereof a period.

In conclusion your Council now places the final decisions of the recommendations made in this Council Report in your hands.

Your Council would like further to comment that there are far too many members who have never visited the Executive Offices and herewith invites those of you who may be in a position to visit the offices a sincere invitation to do so. The Executive Offices are located at 1127 Classen Drive, Oklahoma City, Oklahoma.

At the conclusion of the report, Doctor McDonald moved the acceptance of the Report. Doctor First seconded. Motion carried.

The amendments to the Constitution and By-Laws contained in the Council Report were referred to the Committee on Constitution and By-Laws.

The delegates to the A.M.A., Doctors Stevenson and Burton, asked the House for an expression concerning the Cline report.

The Speaker announced that the House would go into Executive Session for a discussion and decision on the Cline Report. All except members of the House of Delegates were asked to leave:

Executive Session

A lengthy discussion was held with regard to the stand the Profession in the State of Oklahoma would take on the Osteopathic question at the San Francisco meeting of the House of Delegates.

It was moved ,duly seconded and carried to adopt the official action taken by the Tulsa County Medical Society on this question, which was as follows:

1. Osteopathy is to be continued to be considered as a cult.
2. The American Medical Association is encouraged to assist in the improvement of the facilities and personnel of osteopathic teaching institutes.
3. The policy governing the relationship of osteopaths to medical doctors is to be considered on a national level, and is *not* to be made a matter for the individual states.

LEWIS J. MOORMAN

FEBRUARY 9, 1875 — AUGUST 2, 1954

A bit of the aristocracy of the old colonial south, Doctor Moorman brought its dignity and its charm to a half century of southwestern medicine. His keen interest in the diseases of the chest enriched his students, his colleagues and the medical literature for many years. His devotion to the task of treating and preventing tuberculosis has been rewarded by the disease's diminishing importance as a factor in our daily lives. His scholarly approach to the total problem of tuberculosis piqued him to study the effect of more time for contemplation on brilliant minds from enforced rest. A portion of these studies he published in *Tuberculosis and Genius*. His intense regard for the history of medicine and its makers led him to write the story of Oklahoma medicine and his own early day experiences in *Pioneer Doctor*. The capacity of the man was truly amazing. For the past fifteen years the *Journal* has been his favorite child and he its omnipresent parent. It is with a frightening sense of inadequacy that the Editorial Board looks to the future.

Editorials

What I Could . . .

Have you done what you could for the *Journal?* Whatever you do to help the editor or the members of the Editorial Board represents a service to the membership of the Association. The *Journal* should be your mouthpiece.

The following quotation from Louis Pasteur was sent in by Gerald Rogers, M.D., Oklahoma City. This counsel to young physicians from Pasteur is worthy of serious consideration by all physicians young or old.

"Whatever your career may be, do not let yourselves become tainted by a deprecating and barren scepticism, do not let yourselves be discouraged by the sadness of certain hours which pass over nations. Live in the serene peace of laboratories and libraries. Say to yourselves first: 'What have I done for my instruction?' and, as you gradually advance, 'What have I done for my country?' until the time comes when you may have the immense happiness of thinking that you have contributed in some way to the progress and to the good of humanity. But, whether our efforts are or not favoured by life, let us be able to say, when we come near the great goal, 'I have done what I could.' "

Such expressions of interest are the Editor's delight.

Sunlight and Cataract

Too much time by the sea may limit one's power to see. Recent investigations on the development of cataract indicates that the ultraviolet rays may be a significant factor. It is well known that sunshine on the beach contains extra ultraviolet rays reflected from the sea. In addition to an almost universal love of the water and the sand, the general effect of these rays may add to the attraction.

Considering our present urge for sunshine and that coveted coat of tan, this new light on the violet ray is discomforting. What good is a seaside vacation if one must worry about the sad day when he cannot see what's on the beach.

Day by day, our knowledge grows and often we learn that nature's way may bring dismay.

One wonders what the outdoor nudists will do sans clothes sans vision.

░░Scientific Articles

The Use of Local Anesthesia

With ALIDASE *For* CERTAIN

Major Surgical Procedures

A. L. BUELL, M. D., F. A. C. S.

The rationale of Hyaluronidase, or Alidase (trade name) is based on the chemistry of the gel-like cement substances of body tissues.

One of these substances is Hyaluronic acid which exists as cement substance in body tissues and acts as a barrier to the diffusion of invasive substances through these tissues. Hyaluronidase is a specific enzyme which hydrolyzes Hyaluronic acid with the resulting lessening of the viscosity of the gel and a consequent reduction in resistance to fluid absorption.

It has been used since 1947, chiefly in pediatrics, as an absorptive agent when giving subcutaneous fluids. Its use has been gradually extended and it is now exployed with intra-muscular antibodies to increase the blood level more rapidly, and with infiltration anesthesia to insure a more profound and more complete local anesthesia.

This paper is concerned with the relative merits of local anesthesia for certain major and minor surgical procedures, since the discovery of Alidase. Our experience with this is limited to the following operations: 1. Inguinal and ventral hernia repairs, 2. Thyroidectomy, 3. Hemorrhoidectomy, 4 Nailing of the fractured femoral neck, 5. Pudental blocks for obstetrical deliveries, and 6. Cesarean sections.

Anesthesia in medical centers is largely handled by highly trained specialists, while in most small towns and cities anesthesia is given by one of the doctors or by a nurse. Occasionally a well trained anesthesiologist is available in small towns. General anesthetics are not without danger even in expert hands.

THE AUTHOR

Doctor Buell, a graduate of the University of Oklahoma School of Medicine, served his internship and residency in Vancouver, British Columbia. He is a Fellow of the American College of Surgeons and practiced in Tennessee and Arkansas before coming to Oklahoma. He served in the Air Force three years.

Discussing some of the dangers: Cyclopropane may cause bronchial constriction and has a tendency to cause cardia arrhythmias. This irritability of the autonomic nervous tissue, if further enhanced by epinephrine or ephedrine to counteract Cyclopropane shock, may result in ventricular fibrillation and death. For that reason Desoxyephedrine or Neosynephrine is recommended always instead of Ephedrine or Adrenalin when Cyclopropane is used. Cyclopropane has often been considered to be the ultimate in anesthetics for poor risk patients, but authorities advise against its use in those patients with cardiac disease or abnormality. Ether is the safest of the general anesthetics and is considered by many to be the agent of choice for heart and chest surgery. It is, however, not without disadvantages; such as its long emergency, gastro-intestinal effects and tendency to cause acidosis. It is contra-indicated in diabetes and is, of course, highly explosive. Sodium Pentothal may cause constriction of bronchioles and is a respiratory depressant. It causes coronary constriction, is contra-indicated in the very young or very old, in the presence of acute or chronic pulmonary disease or asthma, in cardiac changes or decompensation. Anoxia from Sodium Pentothal may cause increased respiration, and if this is interpreted as being due to light anesthesia rather than anoxia, then further administration of Sodium Pentothal to increase depth of anesthesia may cause death.

It is said that no doctor or nurse should administer an anesthetic agent likely to cause respiratory depression unless that anesthetist has the skill and equipment immediately at hand to effectively control the patient's respirations. This refers to Cyclopropane, Pentothal, Curare and even spinal anesthesia. The complcations of spinal anesthesia are hypotension shock, headache, sensory disturbances, impaired bladder and rectal functions and septic meningitis. It is contra-indicated in shock, hemorrhage. debility, in the presence of pre-existing neurospinal diseases such nervous manifestations of pernicious anemia, multiple sclerosis, lues of the central nervous system and mental abnormalities.

These complications are mentioned not only as a reminder of the dangers ever present, but as a talking point in favor of the use of local anesthesia when it can be given with comfort to the patient; and we wish to suggest that this can be accomplished more easily and more often than is generally believed, (especially since Alidase has been employed with Novocain).

In the operations mentioned previously, no complicated nerve blocking technique is required. One may simply inject as the surgery progresses, injecting the skin and subcutaneous tissue to an extent of about two inches on either side of the contemplated incision. The skin and subcutaneous tissues are then incised to the fascial planes. Then one percent Novocain with Alidase is injected with ease and accuracy under the fascial planes. Injection can be carried on as the operation progresses under direct vision. The anesthetic gives almost complete and instantaneous anesthesia. If sensitivity returns, re-injection is simply and quickly done.

Obstetrical anesthesia seems to fall in a class by itself, varying from no anesthetic at all to a continuous spinal or an inhalation anesthetic with several inductions. Vomiting and aspiration deaths seem to be more common in obstetrical anesthesia. During labor the stomach may retain food for 12 hours or more and thus the patient is more susceptible to aspiration of vomitus while in the delivery room or recovery room. *Induc-tion* is a dangerous stage of anesthesia; nevertheless the patient is frequently put through one induction during delivery and another during episiotomy repair. This double induction occasionally results in death. This could have been avoided by the use of local pudental block anesthesia. The obstetrical patient who has a pudental block can lie in comparative comfort while low forceps and episiotomy and repair are accomplished and she may treasure the thought that she was awake when her child was born. In Cesarean sections as soon as the baby is delivered under local anesthesia, the patient is given light sodium pentothal intravenously.

In rectal surgery local infiltration of Novocain with Alidase gives complete anal relaxation. Spinals or inhalation anesthetics are then not necessary for hemorrhoidectomy.

Operations for the repair of hernia, whether inguinal or large upper abdominal, can be performed under this type of local anesthesia without discomfort to the patient. The same may be said of operations on the thyroid gland and there is the added advantage of the patient being able to talk during anesthesia.

Fracture of the neck of the femur is common in elderly, debilitated individuals who are not good risks for general anesthesia. In these cases, after local anesthesia, the incision is made down to the femur, then the periosteum; the capsule and the fracture are injected with one percent Novocain with Alidase. Manipulation and pin and screw insertions can then be made without pain.

Patients who have major surgery under local anesthesia do not suffer from shock; there is no vomiting, no lung irritation, no danger of the many complications previously mentioned.

The possible dangers of Novocain infiltration are: (1) sensitivity to Novocain or Alidase, (2) intravenous injection of too much Novocain, and (3) infection. To prevent or anticipate sensitivity reactions we have the 500 viscosity units of Alidase mixed with the two to four ounces of one percent Novocain, then an intra-dermal skin test is made to test for sensitivity, it is difficult to see how one could cause much harm that way if the needle is kept moving, especially since Novocain is now given intravenously as a medication. Infection is a possibility but we attempt always to prepare the skin well before injection and then in addition given penicillin once daily for the next three days. There have been no infections traceable to local anesthetic in several years of its use.

In conclusion; (1) We believe that local anesthesia is a very useful anesthetic and that its scope and efficiency in major surgery has been greatly increased with the addition of Alidase. (2) Sodium Pentothal drip is a very useful adjunct to local anesthesia. (3) Local anesthesia with Alidase will lower the surgeon's mortality and morbidity rates.

NOTE: Since having presented this paper the author has changed to the use of 1 percent Xylocaine with 1:100,000 Epinephrine rather than the 1 percent Novocaine with Hyaluronidase. This relatively new local anesthetic agent is free from sensitivity reactions. It has the same spreading property as hyaluronidase. It is long lasting (2 hours or more); and a much smaller quantity is necessary to obtain satisfactory anesthesia than with novocaine.

The "Custom-Tailored"

INGUINAL HERNIA REPAIR

MANUEL E. LICHTENSTEIN, M. D.

THE AUTHOR

Doctor Lichtenstein is attending surgeon, Cook County, Michael Reese and Norwegian-American Hospitals in Chicago, and is Professor of Surgery, Cook County Graduate School of Medicine and Associate Professor of Surgery at Northwestern University Medical School. Doctor Lichtenstein delivered his paper on "Custom-Tailored" Hernia Repair at the Oklahoma Academy of General Practice annual meeting held in Tulsa in February.

The "custom-tailored" hernia repair is a surgical technique adapted to the anatomic condition present in the individual patient. A variety of anatomic defects are responsible for the protrusion of abdominal contents in the groin. Many operative procedures have bee described as suitable for their repair. Better results will follow any operative procedure when surgical practice is specifically adapted to the local condition and in addition all of the factors related to wound healing, intra-abdominal pressure, the general condition of the patient and the character of his work are considered. Thus, the emphasis is placed on the patient rather than on the surgeon (Bassini, Halsted, Gerard, Fergusson, Andrews, McVey and many others.)

There are five varieties of hernia that may appear in the groin. Each of these must be specifically sought out and specifically treated.

1. *Indirect Inguinal Hernia.* The indirect inguinal hernia is usually congenital in origin but an acquired sac may occupy the cord structures and simulate the congenital variety. In the former it is an unobliterated vaginal process while in the latter it is a peritoneal fold that prolapses thru an enlarged internal ring, following abdominal wall trauma as seen following appendectomy. The sac may fill with contents at birth, soon thereafter or at any time later. It is called an indirect inguinal hernia because the sac located within the cord structures passes with them indirectly through the abdominal wall. A hernia of short duration results in a slight defect in the fascia at the internal ring but those of long duration produce larger defects.

Repair of such a hernia requires (1.) removal of all of the sac at it's neck within the transversalis fascia and (2.) closure of the internal ring snugly about the cord structures. When examination of the rest of the inguinal region discloses no other defect to be present repair of the abdominal wound is all that is necessary for cure of this type of hernia.

2. *Direct Inguinal Hernia.* The direct inguinal hernia results from a defect in the transversalis fascia at that anatomic site on the abdominal wall that is known as the triangle of Hesselbach. This is the weakest portion of the abdominal wall and it is prone to thin out and even rupture as a result of an increase in intraabdominal pressure. Straining on defection or urination; coughing because of bronchitis, bronchiectasis or a bronchial tumor; obesity; ascites or heavy labor, predispose to rupture of this fascia and necessitate a correction of any of them before hernial repair is undertaken. The patient with the enlarged prostate who as a result of straining on urination develops a large hernia is not likely to have a well repaired hernia for long. It would be better, of course, to repair the hernia after the prostratic condition has been corrected. Repair of the fascia in the triangle of Hesselbach may be made by using the firm fascia that is still present and available for repair and by reenforcing it with fascia from other sources that are in the neighborhood. The external oblique aponeurosis, especially the lower flap of this layer, may well be used to re-enforce the transversalis fascia. In some instances it may be necessary to use fascial sutures or transplants of "free grafts." Extensive defects may require foreign materials such as metal plates, metal mesh or other materials suitable for that purpose.

3. *Pantaloon Hernia.* This is a coexistence of the indirect and the direct hernia and is the type frequently responsible for recurrence. When the inguinal region is exposed, the direct hernia comes into view obviously and receives the most careful attention. Complete repair is accomplished by the method described under 2. However, frequently the indirect inguinal hernial sac is not sought for and is missed. When the patient notices a bulge in the groin following the operative procedure, it is due to persistence of a hernial

sac that was present before surgery was done. Thus, in every patient with a direct hernia it is necessary to examine for an indirect inguinal sac and conversely the patient who has an indirect hernial sac removed must have a careful and thorough inspection of the tissues to make certain that there is no defect in the transversalis fascia in the triangle of Hesselbach. The recognition of a sac in the cord is very important. It is necessary to open the internal spermatic fascia on the antero-medial surface of the cord up to the internal ring. Through this opening inspection of the structures that lie on the inside of the abdomen may be made. There are two positive findings on examination that give a clue as to the presence or absence of a sac. The sac of an indirect hernia lies anterior to the vas deferens and is continous with the peritoneum. When the vas deferens presents itself with no sac lying anterior to it and when it is possible to see the peritoneal fold (infundibulum) with no prolongation extending down the cord no sac is present. Congenital sacs always lie anterior to the vas in the antero-medial quadrant of the cord and when small must be sought for high on the cord lest they be overlooked completely. Acquired sacs and multiple sacs may appear in any quadrant and they too must be sought.

4. *Sliding Hernia.* This hernia is peculiar in that a part of the wall of the sac may be bowel or urinary bladder. On the left side the sigmoid colon frequently participates as part of the wall of the indirect hernial sac, on the right side the cecum may play the same role while in the triangle of Hesselbach the urinary bladder is the organ most commonly involved. The bladder may also participate in the indirect hernia too. Repair of the transversalis fascia is the important element in the cure of the hernia. A thick walled sac in a direct hernia may be returned to the abdomen unopened when bladder is suspected. The transversalis fascia is closed by suture. It is necessary to re-enforce this layer of fascia with such tissues as have been described under 2. In the indirect hernia all redundant sac is removed and the viscus, bowel or bladder returned to the abdomen (within the confines of the transversalis fascia). One must be exceedingly careful that in the ablation of the redundant sac

bowel or bladder is not sutured, punctured, cut off, or ligated. In the obscure case or when a sliding hernia is suspected because of the thickness of the wall of the sac a safe method to expose the lumen of the sac is to open the peritoneum at the internal ring on its anterior surface. Such an opening will not open into the lumen of the bowel, nor will it interfere with the blood supply to the bowel. Through this opening on the anterior wall careful inspection of the lumen of the sac may be made and obliteration of that part of it which is responsible for the herniation of intraperitoneal viscera may be accomplished. Following repair of the transversalis fascia the abdominal wall is repaired to re-enforce the fascial repair.

5. *The Femoral Hernia.* This type must not be overlooked even when an inguinal hernia is also present. The neck of the femoral hernia sac lies lateral to the pubic spine and when noted at the time of surgery should be exposed and removed.

General Considerations

Elimination of all structures which protrude through the transversalis fascia except the cord structures will prevent further protrusion and make certain that the transversalis fascia fits snugly about the cord. The cord must not contain excessive amounts of fat such as lipomas or peritoneal cysts which tend to increase the size of the internal and external rings separated and not opposite each other for the latter anatomic arrangements predispose to bulging and herniation.

Surgical technique must be such that no damage is done to the tissues. The healing process must progress with the least risk of delay. Hemostasis at every point must be carefully accomplished for hematomas interfere with the healing process. The suture of fascia to fascia makes possible strong scar tissue essential to the final healing. The use of muscle tissue for hernial repair is without value. Muscle tissue is only useful when it can exercise its function of contracting. When muscle tissue has been bound down by sutures the muscle atrophies from disuse. Fascial repair gives greater strength than any type of repair using muscle. Suture mat-

erial should not interfere with the healing process. Sutures must remain in the wound to keep the tissues approximated until the healing process runs its course. Catgut sutures frequently lose their tensile strength before the healing process has been completed. The tissues are not held in approximation long enough, the separation delays the healing process and ultimately favors a thin scar. Nonabsorbable sutures have proven their value in hernial repair for they not only hold tissues in approximation long enough but also do this without sufficient reaction to slow the healing process. Too vigorous a repair, multiple sutures placed between the same two parallel fibers of the inquinal ligament or external oblique constitute useless approximations for in the former the tight knot results in a slough while in the latter the tissues separate as do postage stamps along line of perforations.

The "custom tailored" hernia is a procedure which is not only adapted to the region in which the surgical technique is applied for the cure of the hernia but also to the patient as a whole. It requires a careful and detailed anatomic study of the part to determine the total extent of anatomic deficiency or deformity and also the presence of sacs which are not necessary and should be removed. It consists of careful techniques to approximate substantial structures which can hold the sutures and avoid interference with the healing process. It must guarantee no injury to important structures such as nerves or blood vessels.

Systemic conditions that may be a disturbance to the patient must be corrected and the causes for increased intraabdominal pressure must be eliminated if a successful result is to be expected. In the post-operative course the patient must be given advice appropriate to the needs. Some people may return to work following hernia repair in a week or 10 days. Others may have to stay away from work for a period of six to eight weeks. The determing factor is the extent of fascial repair, the amount of intraabdominal pressure and the character of the patient's work. It is more important to adapt the surgery to the condition present in the patient than to adapt the patient to an operative technique.

Special Article

Our PAST PRESIDENT *and* THE PRESS

ALFRED R. SUGG, M. D.

I could begin this discussion with either criticism or praise and make some sort of a case. But if it is worth a public discussion at all it deserves our most thoughtful consideration and frank appraisal—at the very least we should endeavor to resemble emotionally mature people even though we arrive at no wise conclusions.

I am a tolerant critic of editors, for secretly I have always wanted to be one.

I shall reverse the usual procedure and make my conclusions at the beginning:

I believe the newspapers of Oklahoma are doing a good job—both the editorial columns and the news coverage.

They are in close touch with our world and perform miracles in the speed and efficiency with which they serve the public. The reporter seems to arrive at the scene of the murder even before rigor mortis does.

They strive eternally and with some success, to elevate the commonwealth in all fields of endeavor. They labor to enlighten the ignorant; to purify the sinful; to relieve the oppressed; and to expose dens of iniquity.

They extol virtue and magnify patriotism.

They decry crookedness and deceit.

They champion drives and projects for the public good.

They preach reform in taxes, driving habits, and women's clothes.

They excoriate the opposing political party and in general carry the cudgels for every worthwhile activity that affects our lives and fortunes. They even are magnanimous toward rival towns and wish them luck in securing a big industry, but generally with about the same zest that a dowager shakes your hand or a politician kisses the baby along about election time.

THE AUTHOR

Doctor Sugg, a, Past President of the Oklahoma State Medical Association, delivered the special article in this issue at a meeting of the Oklahoma Press Association. An Ada urologist, he graduated from the University of Arkansas. Doctor Sugg is a veteran of World War I, past president of the Ada Kiwanis Club and the Chamber of Commerce.

One thing of which I'm sure: the newspapers in Oklahoma compare most favorably with those in other parts of the country and I believe excel most of them.

They are progressive with out being radical.

They are enthusiastic without being zany.

They are cosmopolitan without losing the common touch. Is there then anything wrong with them? I'm afraid so.

During the war we often heard the bitter criticism, "Too little and too late." That could never be said about our newspapers, but what is worse, "Too much and too soon."

Last year 300 pounds of newsprint per capita were used. That's 24,000,000 tons—and Oklahoma did its share of overproduction. One thousand wire service representatives were at Washington for the President's speech on the State of the Nation. Talk about too much butter! The news market is glutted —we are simply surfeited with news—most of it totally unimportant. The fact that the bride wore a shirred blouse of chartreuse chiffon is probably important to the groom in peg-topped pants but to few other people. Nor would the world suffer from remaining ignorant of the eating habits or the love life of some phony Hollywood character. Halfbaked news, and particularly political news, is comparable to a doughy biscuit, it gives us mental and emotional indigestion. There is a plethora of editorials also. I judge about one good editorial a week would be the average capacity of most writers, (I have learned not to expect that high score from preachers, one a month is excellent going), but they insist on three or four a day. They remind me of a dyspeptic who feels compelled to swallow a bitter pill every night by force of habit.

An extra pair of pruning shears would be my suggestion. To argue that all this drivel is what folks want would be equivalent to my administering a dose of penicillin or a shot of morphine because a customer wanted it.

An editor also should stay within the length of his cable tow. When he bites off more than he can chew, it leaves us frustrated but not informed. After all, an editorial is not a commandment from on High, but only one man's opinion. An analysis of a problem with factual information is a good editorial but a platitude by an uninformed man trying to carry water on both shoulders is a waste of time and a prize piece of asinity.

Editors have made a fetish of freedom of the press—and in as few words as possible. I do not believe in it. (Here is where I come in). Under this revered banner they may go forth to maim and destroy with impunity. I hasten to add that where issues, principles, public officials, government, and even private opinions are concerned, I would shoulder a musket to defend the freedom of the press, for without it we are sunk. But there is too much opportunity and temptation for an editor with a bantam rooster complex to vent his spleen on any one who incurs his displeasure. It's not a fair fight. It's a one way street and libel laws are no protection. He can do more harm by insinuation or innuendo, sarcasm or ridicule, than by frontal assault, and even if he changes his mind and apologizes, it's too late. You can't unscramble eggs nor recover the poison arrow of vituperation.

No, I wouldn't want a law. One that would squelch the unscrupulous editor would hamper the good ones and it isn't worth it. Some one should tell the newspapers that radio and television are here to stay. You simply cannot scoop a storm in Waco or a kidnapping in Kaw City when the customers have been seeing and hearing all about

it for the entire previous day. The effort to do so makes for sorry reading, and much as you might like to retain the status of 10 years ago, you are doomed to failure. You might get some consolation by reading some of your past articles in which you admonish the railroads of the necessity for moving over and sharing at least with the airplane in the name of progress.

Ordinarily I would never have the temerity to offer advice but I have a pocket full of editorials here offering the medical profession pointed advice, so I'll return the compliment.

Most professional people are screened as students, must secure a license, and are subject to laws and regulations—where these do not apply, the Grievance Committee, as in my own profession, helps police the erring brothers and is proving quite effective. I'd suggest you try it and when the editor accepts advertising that is misleading, repulsive, and even dangerous, he should be brought to trial.

A more rigid code of ethics in the matter of reporting would help also. A crackpot pseudo-scientist plus an eager reporter can do harm—never mind if the small print says, "Now this is only in the experimental stage—nothing is really known about it." The headline is the punch line that is remembered. Pills that cure, vitamins that solve the gray hair and wrinkle problem, hormones that bolster sagging vital functions, quacks who can give you a complete examination of liver, lights, melt, and glands, equipped with only a couch and a flashlinght and for three bucks, as advertised in your papers, is bad public relations for you and tragic for gullible people who are at your mercy.

There is a much longer list of gripes, but I'm reminded of a friend of mine who has lost so many of his "marbles" that he needs a guardian. His church gives him a sinecure in the form of janitor work. One day the pastor called him in and suggested that his work could be better and added that some of the parishioners were complaining, to which he replied quick as a flash: "Oh, preacher, that's all right. They are the same crowd that are always finding fault with your preaching. Let's forget 'em."

Amebiasis[1] a "Poorly Reported" Disease

Until serious complications arise,
amebiasis may pass unrecognized and
patients receive only symptomatic treatment.

Although amebiasis is a disease with serious morbidity and mortality, statistics on its incidence[1] are incomplete because its manifestations are not commonly recognized and consequently not reported.

"*Vague symptoms*[2] *referable to the gastrointestinal tract, such as indigestion or indefinite abdominal pains, with or without abnormally formed stools, may result from intestinal amebiasis. Not infrequently in cases in which such symptoms are ascribed to psychoneurosis after extensive x-ray studies have been carried out, complete relief is obtained with antiamebic therapy.*"

To prevent possible development of an incapacitating or even fatal illness and to eliminate a reservoir of infection in the community, diagnosing and treating[3] even seemingly healthy "carriers" and those having mild symptoms of amebiasis is advised.

Early diagnosis[1] is important because infection can be rapidly and completely cleared, with the proper choice of drugs and due consideration for the principles of therapy. For treatment of the bowel phase these authors find Diodoquin "most satisfactory."

For chronic amebic infections, Goodwin[4] finds Diodoquin to be one of the best drugs at present available.

Diodoquin, which does not inconvenience the patient or interfere with his normal activities, may be used in the treatment of acute or latent forms of amebiasis. If extraintestinal lesions require the use of emetine, Diodoquin may be administered concurrently. It is a well tolerated and relatively nontoxic orally administered amebacide, containing 63.9 per cent of iodine.

Diodoquin (diiodohydroxyquinoline), available in 10-grain (650 mg.) tablets, reduces the course of treatment to twenty days (three tablets daily). Treatment may be repeated or prolonged without

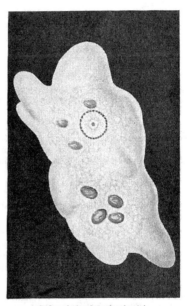

Endamoeba histolytica (trophozoite).

serious toxic effect. It is accepted by the Council on Pharmacy and Chemistry of the American Medical Association. G. D. Searle & Co., Research in the Service of Medicine.

1. Hamilton, H. E., and Zavala, D. C.: Amebiasis in Iowa: Diagnosis and Treatment, J. Iowa M. Soc. *42*:1 (Jan.) 1952.

2. Goldman, M. J.: Less Commonly Recognized Clinical Features of Amebiasis, California Med. *76*:266 (April) 1952.

3. Weingarten, M., and Herzig, W. F.: The Clinical Manifestations of Chronic Amebiasis, Rev. Gastroenterol. *20*.667 (Sept.) 1953.

4. Goodwin, L. G.: Review Article: The Chemotherapy of Tropical Disease: Part I. Protozoal Infections, J. Pharm. & Pharmacol. *4*:153 (March) 1952.

Association Activities

PRESIDENT'S LETTER

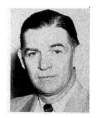

The American Medical Association completed its 103rd annual convention on June 25th in San Francisco. There was a record-breaking attendance of 12,063 doctors, and 30,906 guests, including families, nurses, medical students, and exhibitors. This was a slightly larger attendance than at the meeting in New York last year.

During the opening days of the convention there was much dissatisfaction among the doctors because of the poor housing and the mishandling of hotel reservations by the housing committee. This dissatisfaction was well-founded, and I feel that the American Medical Association itself should deal more directly with the housing problem, and take more responsibility instead of leaving it in charge of any local housing committee of a convention city. The sentiment was strong enough among the delegates that the Oklahoma Medical Association delegates submitted a resolution which will improve this situation in the future, if it is acted upon favorably by the Board of Trustees, to whom it was referred.

Our faithful delegates, Dr. James Stevenson and Dr. John Burton, with their alternates, Dr. E. H. Shuller and Dr. Malcom Phelps had little time to enjoy the cool weather in San Francisco or to attend any of the scientific meetings, because they spent many hours each day the convention was in progress attending sessions of the House of Delegates.

I may be wrong, but to my way of thinking there was very little accomplished by the House of Delegates. Most controversial issues were either pigeonholed indefinitely, referred to the Board of Trustees, or held for further study by the committee. Usually there are one or two issues of importance definitely settled, but I know of none completed at this session. We shall have a full and complete report from our delegates at the mid-winter meeting in Oklahoma in December.

President

P.S. I don't know what doctor won the beautiful Cadillac given away at the convention by White Laboratories.

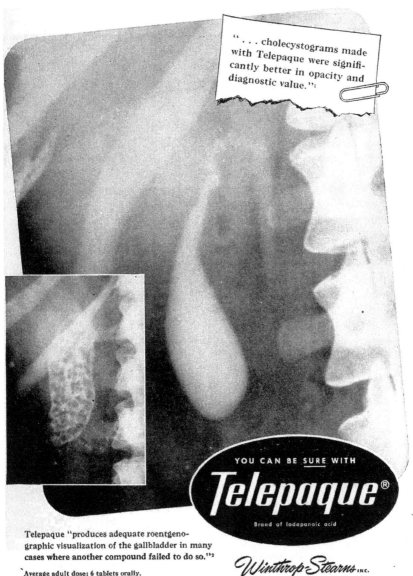

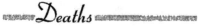# Deaths

HUDSON S. SHELBY, M.D.
1900-1954

Hudson S. Shelby, M.D., Oklahoma City, died early July 14 after suffering a heart attack on the lawn of his home en route to a call he was making around midnight.

Doctor Shelby was born in Tennessee but moved to Prague when he was about a year old. He attended the University of Oklahoma and received a B.S. degree in 1928. In 1932 he received his M.D. He had practiced in Oklahoma City since that time.

LOGAN HERBERT HUFFMAN, M.D.
1873-1954

Logan Herbert Huffman, M.D., pioneer Oklahoma physician, died June 19 after a three year illness.

He was born in Huffman, Ind. and studied at Indiana University and Birmingham, Ala. He received his medical degree in 1903 from the University of the South, Sewanee.

He settled in Indiahoma in 1903 and then became chief surgeon in Mexico for a copper mining company until 1906 when he settled at Hobart. In 1926 he moved to Oklahoma City where he practiced until 1952 when he was forced to retire because of ill health. He served as a captain in the medical corps in World War I.

RICHARD REVEL JOHNSON, M.D.
1881-1954

R. R. Johnson, M.D., Sand Springs, died June 17 at his home after a years illness.

A native of Wolfe County, Ky. he received his medical degree from the University of Kentucky and practiced in Kentucky before moving to Sand Springs in 1920.

Public Relations Meet Set

Circle Sept. 1 and 2 on your calendar right now. That's the time for AMA's third Medical Public Relations Institute to be held at the Drake Hotel in Chicago. Designed primarily for public relations personnel and chairmen of state and county medical societies, this year's informal sessions are designed as an "idea exchange—a public relations seminar"—to stimulate the exchange of ideas in all areas of medical public relations.

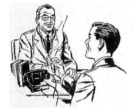
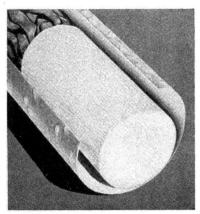
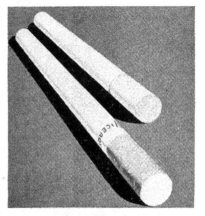

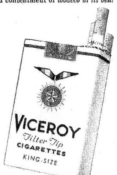

OFFICIAL PROCEEDINGS of the HOUSE OF DELEGATES

of the

OKLAHOMA STATE MEDICAL ASSOCIATION

MAY 9, 1954

Opening Session—Part 2

II.   School Health

The Sub-Committee on School Health has continued its program as outlined in the report of this Committee to the last Session of the House of Delegates.

At that time the issuance of the film, "School Health in Action," produced by the State Health Department with the Public Health Committee as a co-sponsor was announced. The Sub-Committee on School Health was accorded the privilege of almost complete supervision over the content of this film, and the reaction received from the many County Medical Societies which have seen the film has been most satisfactory. "School Health in Action" has been well received by the externely large number of lay groups in the State which have seen it and has in fact attracted nation-wide attention, having been presented at the Fourth National Conference on Physicians and Schools at Highland Park, Illinois. While the Committee has had no part in the sale and distribution of actual prints of the film, it is in a position to know that prints have been purchased by seventeen other State Health Departments and State Medical Associations.

Your Committee is now pleased to r e p o r t the completion of a new film with the same sponsorship entitled, "The Well-Child Examination," which is designed for presentation to professional groups only and which will be presented on the Scientific Program of the Annual Meeting on May 11, 1954 at 4:20 p.m. Your Committee urges that every member of the House of Delegates avail himself of the opportunity of viewing this film at that time, and that he advise his County Society of the availability of the film if he believes it will serve a worthwhile purpose.

The Sub-Committee on School Health has for the past two years again joined in the sponsorship of the Third Annual Conference, "On Better Health for Oklahoma School Children," held in conjunction with the meeting of the Oklahoma Association of School Administrators, at Norman on October 16, 1953. The Sub-Committee assisted in planning the program and supplied as a speaker and consultant, Guy N. Magness, M.D., Director of the Medical Department, University City Public Schools, University City, Missouri, and President of the American School Health Association.

At the present time plans for the Fourth such Conference are being developed and the Sub-Committee on School Health is actively participating in this activity.

As a result of the various School Health Conferences, both State and National, the sub-committee on School Health has been impressed by the fact that neither educators nor physicians who are well versed in the School Health field are satisfied with the type of material contained in the present curricula for teacher training.

The Committee has entered into discussions of this matter with representatives of the Teacher Training Institutions in this State and along with the Oklahoma Advisory Health Council is at this time securing a survey of the teachers of the State in the hope that satisfactory school health curricula may ultimately be developed. It shoud be recognized that this is indeed a long term project and that any progress along this line will not only be slow but difficult. The Committee, nevertheless, is firmly convinced that this is a basic consideration to any satisfactory school health program in the future.

To this end, the first formal conference of representatives from teacher training institutions in the State of Oklahoma on the basic requirements for teacher training in school health was held in Chickasha in April, 1954.

During the last year the Sub-Committee on School Health made every effort to enlist the aid of the individual county societies in evaluation of the County School Health Program and in securing representation of the profession at various School Health Workshops which were conducted in the State by the State Health Department and the schools of the counties. Unfortunately, the response to these efforts was far from enthusiastic. The Committee in that connection · would emphasize that practically every school in the State of Oklahoma is engaged in some way or another in a School Health Program which may be good, bad or indifferent, and that every County Society will find investigation of the School Health Program in the County and the offer of assistance to the School Administrators to be a most effective means of assisting in the development of sound school health policies and the betterment of the health of all the people of this State.

III.   Industrial Health

Due to the predominantly agricultural type of economy existing in this State, the activities of the Sub-Committee on Industrial Health have been somewhat limited. During the past session of the Oklahoma Legislature, this Committee in cooperation with the Public Policy Committee of the Association, followed the progress of a number of bills with industrial health implications. One bill supported by the two committees was "The Oklahoma Occupational Health Act," which was passed by the Legislature and provides for the reporting of occupational disease to the State Health Department when those diseases have been designated as occupational by the State Board of Health. This bill also makes provision for utilization of the facilities of the State Department of Health in the prevention and detection leading to those diseases leading to occupational health hazards.

Amendments to the Oklahoma Workman's Compensation Law to include occupational diseases designated in those amendments were also supported and are now in force as part of the Workmen's Compensation Law.

The Public Health Committee, recognizing that with the increased industrialization of the State of Oklahoma, industrial health will be a growing problem, has authorized the Sub-Committee on Industrial Health to investigate the need for further activities and be prepared to offer means of prevention of those industrial health problems which can be foreseen by the Committee and to enlist in this survey the services of the Council on Industrial Health of the American Medical Association and of such other State Medical Associations which may have had more experience in this field.

IV. Blood Banks

The activities of the Sub-Committee on Blood Banks have been most limited. As a result of a cursory survey by the Committee, it was indicated that local committees in the State through the cooperation of County Medical Societies and other agencies interested in the problem, have been able to formulate their own local plans to meet their own blood needs.

The committee holds itself in readiness at all times to assist any County Society or any community in the State in the organization and development of the type of blood bank which may be suitable to the needs of that community.

V. Nutrition

The Public Health Committee through a temporary Sub-Committee on Nutrition composed of W. T. McCollum, M.D., Turner Bynum, M.D., J. R. Colvert, M.D., William T. Newsome, M.D., and H. V. L. Sapper, M.D., assisted the Oklahoma Dietetic Association in the preparation of the Diet Manual designed for use by the general practitioner and smaller hospitals in the State which do not have available the services of qualified dietitians.

The Public Health Committee wishes at this time to express its appreciation to the members of the Sub-Committee on Nutrition for the valuable services they have performed and to commend them on their part in the preparation of this worthwhile publication.

The results of this work may be seen at the Scientific Exhibit Space Number 13, which has been assigned to the Oklahoma Dietetic Association for the purpose of explaining this Diet Manual and its use to the profession.

Public Health Committee Supplemental Report

During the past year the Public Health Committee has had offered to it for consideration a matter which did not fall within the scope of any of the present committees and was of sufficient importance to be considered by the Committee as a whole.

The Bureau of Indian Affairs has the responsibility of providing medical care for Indians as a result of Indian treaties and Federal Legislation. Up until very recently, the Bureau has provided such medical care through Federal Indian Hospitals throughout the nation. The Bureau is now engaged in a program intended to effect the closing of all Federal Indian Hospitals in those areas in which the hospital facilities and medical personnel available are deemed adequate. Care for indigent Indians would then be provided by local hospitals and private physicians at the expense of the Federal Government on the basis of fee schedules agreed upon with the Bureau.

According to the latest advice received from the Bureau by the Committee, it is contemplated that the first Indian hospitals in Oklahoma to be closed will be those in Pawnee, Clinton and Claremore. In this connection, the House of Delegates should be further advised that as a result of representations by Chambers of Commerce, Indian groups and the Oklahoma Congressional delegation, the closing of the hospitals designated above has been temporarily delayed.

In presenting this matter to the Committee, the Bureau of Indian Affairs did not request the Association to approve or disapprove the plans for the closing of the Indian Hospitals. As a result of the Committee's discussion of the problem with the representatives of the Bureau and its review of fee schedules now in operation in other states in which the Indian Hospitals have been closed, it is the recommendation of the Committee that the House of Delegates approve a plan of cooperation with the Bureau of Indian Affairs in providing medical care for indigent Indians on the basis of a state fee schedule or county fee schedules to be negotiated with the Bureau.

It is further recommended by the Committee that the House of Delegates authorize the appointment of a special Sub-Committee of the Public Health Committee to consist of one representative of each Councilor District, which Committee would be authorized to negotiate with the Bureau concerning the fee schedule for care of indigent Indians if and when the Bureau is prepared to proceed with its plan of closing the Indian Hospitals in the State of Oklahoma.

Respectfully submitted,
R. M. WADSWORTH, M.D., Chairman

* * *

Next on the agenda was the report of the Public Policy Committee. R. Q. Goodwin, M.D., Oklahoma City, Chairman of the Committee made the following report:

Report of the Public Policy Committee

The Public Policy Committee's activities for the past year and the year to come have been to a certain extent outlined for it by the activities of other groups, organizations and agencies of government.

In order that this Report be as concise as possible, it will be divided into three principal parts: (1) Federal Legislation and Related Problems; (2) State Legislation and Related Problems; (3) Inter-professional activities and Prepayment Hospital and Medical Problems.

1. Federal Legislation and Related Problems:

While the A. M. A. Washington Office has reported over sixty bills in Congress in which the Profession is involved, there is in the opinion of your Committee only four that are of major importance at this time. These are as follows:

    a. The Administration's Reinsurance Bill for the subsidizing of Prepaid health insurance coverage—commonly known as The Hobby Bill.

    b. The Reed-Jenkins Bill, formerly known as the Reed-Keogh bill.

    c. Extension of Social Security Benefits on a compulsory basis.

    d. The Bricker Amendment.

In addition to the above, the problem of the care of non-service connected disabilities of veterans in Veterans hospitals will be presented. Each will be discussed separately.

a. The Hobby Bill:

This measure sets up a $25 million federal reinsurance appropriation for commercial and non-profit insurance companies or plans who would qualify. The purpose of the reinsurance feature is an attempt to stimulate companies or plans writing prepaid hospital and medical coverage to increase and/or both their age limit benefits and to perhaps adjust premiums.

By and large the Commercial Insurance Companies have opposed this legislation on the basis that American Free enterprise can accomplish these same ends and without governmental interference. It must be remembered that the Supreme Court of the United States has already held that that which the Federal Government subsidizes, it shall control. The Voluntary Non-Profit Medical Care Plans at their annual conference recently held in New York, of which the Oklahoma Blue Shield plans is a participating plan, adopted the following statement:

"Statement Regarding the Administration Reinsurance Bills"

(HR 8356 and E 3114)

The Annual 1954 Conference of the 78 Blue Shield Plans has studied and endorses the basic objectives of the President's message to Congress on Health insurance matters. It believes in the encouragement of experimentation and expansion in the field of voluntary health insurance.

The Plans recognize and appreciate the sincere intent of President Eisenhower's administration to make comprehensive health coverage available to more people by encouraging and stimulating the expansion of voluntary health programs.

With these premises in mind, the Blue Shield Plans have given careful consideration to the Administration's reinsurance proposal and has come to the conclusion that it may well be unnecessary with respect to Blue Shield Plans for the following reasons:

1. An outstanding characteristic of Blue Shield Plans is that they have experimented and pioneered in a totally new concept of medical protection and have demonstrated their ability to stand on their own feet financially.

2. Since their inception, Blue Shield Plans have been underwritten and hence, in fact, reinsurance by the physicians who sponsor them. Customarily there is either a written or implied agreement that sponsoring physicians will accept a pro rata reduction in fees paid by the Plan should it become necessary for them to do so. Several of the most successful Blue Shield Plans in operation today were subsidized in this manner by their sponsoring physicians during their early days of experimentation in an unexplored field.

3. In but a few short years, Blue Shield Plans have made remarkable progress in both the extension of enrolment and the extension of benefits. At present Blue Shield Plans have an enrolment of over 29 million people. Having come through the early critical period, there is no reason to expect that they will now need to rely upon anything other than their own proven resources as they continue to expand their operations in accordance with the reasonable expectations on the part of the public."

This entire statement has been read to the House of Delegates, due principally to the language of the second paragraph.

The attention of the House of Delegates is drawn to this paragraph due to the fact that this language refers to "Service Type Contracts" of Blue Shield Plans. Your attention is further directed to the fact that the Oklahoma Blue Shield Plan is not a service type contract, but rather an indemnity contract and the adopted statement would not apply to Oklahoma. Your Committee is not attempting to criticize the adoped statement, but more particularly would like to ascertain from this House of Delegates whether or not a committee should be appointed to study the possibility of recommending to the Oklahoma Blue Shield Board of Trustees, the changing of the Oklahoma Blue Shield Plan for an Indemnity type contract to a service type contract in order that Oklahoma physicians could in pure honesty subscribe to paragraph 2, of the statement previously read and endorsed by Oklahoma representatives of the Oklahoma Blue Shield Plan.

While your Committee feels that the proposition presented deserves your careful consideration and action, it will continue to oppose the enactment of such legislation for the reason that in its opinion this legislation is an entering wedge into Federal Control of all insurance programs.

b. Reed-Jenkins Bill:

This measure would provide that self-employed persons would be allowed to create their own retirement programs by being given the privilege on their own request to deduct from their gross earnings $6,500 a year, or 10%, *which ever is the lesser*. This legislation has been proposed and supported by 26 organizations representing self-employed persons, including such organizations as the A. M. A., American Bar Association, American Farm Bureau, etc., and is offered in lieu of compulsory Social Security deductions. Your Committee in the past has supported this legislation and will continue its support unless otherwise directed by the Council or the House of Delegates.

c. Extension of Social Security:

Recently each member of the Association received a questionnaire on this subject from Senator Kerr. Your Committee was advised in advance of the sending out of the questionnaire, but made no effort to influence the answer of the individual physician. Your Committee has not been advised of the results of the survey. Your Committee in the past has opposed this legislation on the basis that at the present time any self-employed person who wishes to avail himself of Social Security may do so, but is not impelled by cumpulsion to enter the program. Your Committee will continue to oppose this legislation unless otherwise directed by the Council or the House of Delegates.

Veterans Administration Care of Non-Service Connected Disabilities

This subject is not new to this House of Delegates. While there is no specific legislation to change the present system, your Committee is of the opinion that the profession must continue to discuss this subject with the Oklahoma representative in Congress. Your Committee would point out that this problem is not solely of the Profession, but involves each and every taxpayer either large or small. Your Committee's attitude on this legislation has been that the Veteran who has a *service* connected disability is entitled to the best medical care available at government expense; on the other hand the veteran with a non-service connected disability should not be cared for by Federal funds, unless he is an indigent veteran or has Tuberculosis or a mental disease and there are no state or local facilities to give him proper care. Your Committee will continue to present this viewpoint to Oklahoma members of Congress unless otherwise directed by the Council or the House of Delegates.

State Legislation and Related Problems

a. Narcotic Legislation
b. Mental Health Legislation
c. Cult Legislation
d. Other Legislation

The above subjects are herewith presented as separate items:

a. Narcotic Legislation

This House of Delegates and the Profession as a whole is well aware of the hearings which were held during the last session of the Oklahoma Legislature on this subject. The House of Delegates is also aware that action was taken by the last House of Delegates whereby the membership of any member of the Oklahoma State Medical Association is automatically cancelled when said member is found guilty of a Narcotic violation by the Oklahoma State Board of Medical Examiners and his narcotic permit is suspended or cancelled by the Bureau of Narcotics.

Your Committee has attended several meetings of legislative Committees of the Oklahoma State Legislative Council since the enactment of the legislation and is convinced that the law must have certain adjustments to give proper authority to the enforcement arm; namely, the Attorney General's office. Your Committee favors any necessary adjustments in the present law to bring about better enforcement, but will continue to oppose the saddling of enforcement costs on to the medical and allied professions, which are involved in this problem. Your Committee is of the opinion that enforcement cost in this field should be no different than the enforcement costs in any other type of crime. It should be distinctly understood that this Committee is in favor of the strengthening of any laws on this subject which do not act to the detriment of the public. Your Committee would like to take this opportunity to express its appreciation to the sub-committee which worked on this legislation; namely, E. Faye Lester, M.D., Oklahoma City, Wm. Gill, M.D., Ada and H. A. Shoemaker, Ph.D., of the University of Oklahoma School of Medicine without whose assistance the end results perhaps would not have been accomplished.

b. Mental Health Legislation

As was stated concerning the Narcotic legislation hearing the House of Delegates remembers the hearings held on Mental Health legislation and the Oklahoma House of Representatives investigation of the Mental Hospitals.

Your Committee has attended several meetings of the Committees of the Oklahoma Legislative Council considering Amendments to the Mental Health Law. At the present time there appear to be two amendments under consideration: one concerning the manner of Commitment of patients and the other, the hospitalization of epileptics.

Your Committee has no specific recomendations to make at this time on these two subjects as it has not as yet seen any actual amendments that have been proposed.

Your Committee would also like to publicly express to the House of Delegates its appreciation for the work done by the Committee appointed by the President at the request of the Oklahoma House of Representatives that made an investigation of Oklahoma's mental hospital. This Committee composed of Dr. J. Hoyle Carlock, Ardmore, Dr. Joe Tyler, Tulsa, and Dr. Maude Masterson of Oklahoma City, did, in the opinion of your Committee, make an outstanding investigation in the interest of professional care for hospitalized mental health patients.

c. Cult Legislation

Discussion of Naturopath and Optometrists bills.

d. Other Legislation

In addition to the previously referred to legislation, your Committee in cooperation with the Public Health Committee has been studying the problems of the Industrial Commission as they apply to medicine.

At the request of the Oklahoma State Legislative Council, your Committee invited the Council on Industrial Health of the A. M. A. to conduct a study of the law under which the Commission is created and works, as well as its internal administration.

The study was made by Mrs. Marjorie Grigsby, who made two trips to Oklahoma for this purpose. Mrs. Grigsby in addition to interviewing physicians, contacted representatives of labor, industry, insurance companies, self insurors, etc.

While the study has been completed, your Committee has not as yet received Mrs. Grigsby's findings. When the final report is received it will be sent the County Medical Societies.

Your Committee is most hopeful that from this study improvements can be made in the Industrial Commission.

Your Committee was indeed pleased by the manner in which Mrs. Grigsby was received by all persons and groups interested in the problems of the Commission.

In addition to problems in the legislative fields your Committee has met with representatives of the Oklahoma State Nurse Association, the Oklahoma State League for Nursing and the Oklahoma State Hospital Association to discuss the advisability of establishing a "Joint Commission for the Improvement of the Care of the Patient." Such a commission has been established at the National level.

Your Committee feels that this is a most worthwhile undertaking and would do much to help work out many mutual problems of the three groups. A progress report will be made to the Council after more discussion between the groups has been held.

Your Committee has also met with the Committees of the Oklahoma State Legislative Council to study the need for a state appropriation for a loan fund to assist medical students to complete their education; these students in turn to obligate themselves upon the completion of their training to locate in small communities in the State of Oklahoma. Counseling with the Committee from the Legislature in addition to this Committee, have been representatives from the University of Oklahoma School of Medicine, its Alumni Association and representatives of the student body of the Medical School.

No definite results have come from these meetings, and it is too early to tell whether or not such legislation will be introduced in the next Legislature.

Physician Placement

Your Committee has had forcibly brought to its attention the matter of communities who feel that they are inadequately cared for and need either a physician or additional physicians. By the same token there has been demonstrated a need for a rather accurate survey of these types of communities for the purposes of informing physicians who are seeking locations of the opportunities that might be available.

In order to attempt to help solve this problem, your Committee is taking a survey by Questionnaire of all communities in the State of Oklahoma under 3500 population to ascertain that community's needs. The survey will develop all phases of the Community's economic, social, educational and religious potential.

In addition to the survey of the Communities, the County Medical Societies will be asked to check the information received and to give their opinions as to the rating the communities should have.

Your Committee would also like to call your attention to a magazine called *Your Doctor* which each each physician and dentist in the State receives complimentary. Your Committee desires to commend Mr. Paul Andres, the publisher of this magazine, for the fine public relations work he is doing for the Profession.

The Committee would also recommend that County Medical Societies or individual members consider subscribing to this publication for the schools, libraries and hospitals in their areas.

In conclusion your Committee knows it is unnecessary to call to your attention that this is an election year in Oklahoma. Your Committee nevertheless reiterates that it is the duty of each physician to interest himself in maintaining good government. Your Committee hopes that the individual physician will consider well the candiates for office and after making its decision as to the candidate he thinks best qualified, to give that candidate his support and to vote on election day."

At the conclusion of this report, Marshall O. Hart, M.D., Tulsa, moved: "That the Report of the Committee be accepted." Motion seconded and carried.

The Speaker called for a report from the Committee on Civilian Defense. Gifford Henry, M.D., Tulsa, Chairman of the Committee, was not present.

The next report to be made was that of the Grievance Committee, in the Absence of C. E. Northcutt, M.D., Ponca City, Chairman of the Committee, L. C. McHenry, M.D., Oklahoma City, made the following report:

Report of the Grievance Committee

In the five years of its existence it has never been possible to estimate the degree of activity of the Grievance Committee by a mere tabulation of the cases considered by the Committee. As has been pointed out in all the Committee Reports preceding this one, the number of complaints actually filed before the Committee remains consistently small.

At the beginning of the past year the Committee had pending in its files from the previous year four cases. During the year 1953-54 fifteen cases were filed and a total of fifteen cases have been closed during the year, leaving a carry over for next year of only four cases.

It will be obvious to all that some carry over of cases from one year to the next is unavoidable in that there are so many factors over which the Committee has no control, that some cases necessarily require a considerable lapse of time and a great deal of correspondence before settlements satisfactory to all concerned can be arrived at. It is likewise obvious that cases filed shortly before the close of the Committee's fiscal year cannot be closed within that year.

While the Committee has never been impressed with attempts to classify the cases as presented to it, it does, however, feel that such classification will be of some interest and perhaps of some assistance in future attempts to evaluate the activities of the Committee on a long term basis.

The fifteen cases filed during 1953-54 are, therefore, classified roughly as follows:

Cases concerning the fee only _____ 4
Cases concerning the service only _____ 6
Cases concerning both fee and service _ _ 5
                                                      ———
                          TOTAL _____15

In every situation in which it is at all possible or practical, the Committee exerts extreme efforts to secure settlements agreed upon between the patient and the physician. During the past year it was found necessary for the Committee to refer two cases to the County Societies of which the physicians concerned were members. As a result of that action in one case a fee adjustment was arranged and in the other the physician was suspended from membership by the County Medical Society for a period of three years.

It will be recalled by the House of Delegates that the Grievance Committee, while established by the House of Delegates, has never been specifically provided for in the By-Laws nor have its powers, responsibilities and procedures been outlined in the By-Laws. This matter has been called to the attention of the Council by a number of members of the Association and has received the consideration of the Council.

In conclusion, your Grievance Committee wishes to emphasize that its experience with both patients and physicians has been most convincing that there is a need for this type of activity on the part of this Association. The Committee is most favorably impressed with the cooperation which it has received from both patients and physicians in all except a few rare instances. It is our firm belief that the very existence of the Committee has created a most favorable impression in the public mind, since it has offered to the public a means through which any misunderstanding or diseagreement with the physician can be negotiated in a fair and impartial manner.

At the conclusion of the report Doctor R. Q. Goodwin moved: "That the report of the Grievance Committee be accepted." Motion seconded and carried.

At this point the speaker informed the House that there were now four colored physicians in the state who were members of the Oklahoma State Medical Association, and that all the colored physicians of the State had been invited to attend the scientific session of the meeting.

Doctor Haynie announced that following the reading of the Necrology Report, the House would be recessed, to reconvene at 7:30 p.m. for the final session. He asked everyone to stand and the following Necrology report was read:

Necrology Report

Since the last Necrology Report in April, 1953, the Almighty, in His Infinite Wisdom has called from our midst 53 of our beloved friends and co-workers. While we bow in sorrow to the will of the Omniscience, we are appreciative of these wonderful men—physicians, scientists, teachers and friends, and their far-reaching influences which will continue to inspire us to carry on their duties to humanity.

THEREFORE, BE IT RESOLVED that the House of Delegates of the Oklahoma State Medical Association recognize the demise of those former fellow physicians and instruct the Secretary to inscribe with honor and regret the following names upon the records of the Association:

Leila E. Andrews, Oklahoma City—April 8, 1954.
Pauline Q. Barker, Guthrie—August, 1953.
J. R. Barry, Picher—April 28, 1953.
Virgil Berry, Okmulgee—March 10, 1954.
Paul R. Brown, Tulsa—March 22, 1954.
J. R. Bryce, Snyder—March 12, 1954.
H. G. Campbell, Tecumseh—October 2, 1953.
P. N. Charbonnet, formerly of Tulsa—March, 1954.
H. C. Cockrill, Mooreland—January 25, 1954.
Robert D. Cody, Centrahoma—February 1, 1954.
E. L. Collins, Panama—March 1, 1954.
F. Maxey Cooper, Oklahoma City—June 16, 1953.
Edward F. Davis, Sulphur—March 15, 1954.
Alberta Webb Dudley, Oklahoma City—June 1, 1953.
James G. Edwards, Okmulgee—May 23, 1953.
H. Lee Farris, Tulsa—April 10, 1953.
Julian Feild, Enid—March 16, 1954.
T. H. Flesher, Edmond—January, 1954.
J. W. Francis, Perry, October, 1953.
L. E. Gee, Broken Bow—July 13, 1953.
Allen G. Gibbs, Oklahoma City—November 27, 1953.
Harry B. Hall, Boise City—May 26, 1953.
J. E. Harbison, Oklahoma City—January 5, 1954.
Walter Hardy, Ardmore—February 16, 1954.
William B. Harned, Walters—January 26, 1954.
G. G. Harris, Helena—September 30, 1953.
J. C. Hooper, Idabel—March 30, 1954.
E. F. Hurlbut, Meeker—April 13, 1954.
L. E. Jacobs, Hanna—August 11, 1954.
Philip Kline, Tulsa—June 16, 1953.
J. B. Lansden, Granite—March 5, 1954.
E. E. Lawson, Medford—January 12, 1954.
Elizabeth E. Lehmer, Vinita—1953.
Charles O. Lively, Pawnee—November 24, 1953.
William C. McClure, Oklahoma City—September 24, 1953.
Ian MacKenzie, Tulsa—October 12, 1953.
H. C. Manning, Cushing—February 8, 1953.
P. H. Mayginnes, Tulsa—January 19, 1954.
Nesbitt L. Miller, Oklahoma City—May 3, 1954.
W. A. Moreland, Idabel—1953.
B. W. Ralston, Commerce—March 26, 1954.
Horace Reed, Oklahoma City—October 7, 1953.
Paul B. Rice, Oklahoma City—March 2, 1953.
Marvin E. Robberson, Wynnewood—June 7, 1953.
D. D. Roberts, Enid—March 2, 1953.
G. W. Scott, Tishomingo—April 1, 1954.
Fred Sheets, Oklahoma City—April 21, 1954.
Carl F. Simpson, Tulsa—June 22, 1954.
Will C. Wait, McAlester—January 19, 1954.
Wendell J. White, Vinita—May 11, 1954.
J. T. B. Widney, Kaw City—April 5, 1954.
Harper Wright, Oklahoma City—May 31, 1953.
Herbert L. Wright, Sasakwa—February 12, 1954.

Minutes of the Second Session will appear in the September issue.

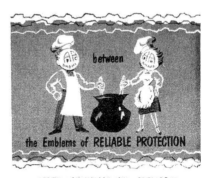
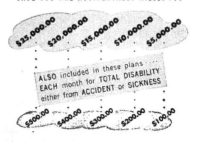

Editorials

The Value of Medical Licensure

The State Board of Medical Examiners was created by the legislature for the purpose of maintaining certain basic standard requirements of those who indulge the privilege of presiding over the health welfare of the people. A part of this duty involves the examining of candidates for licensure and a continuous subscription to the idea that certain basic requirements should be maintained. It is not easy to obtain a license to practice medicine. Only certain individuals are able to qualify.

The value of a license to practice medicine is directly related to the standard of requirements which must be met. All candidates must be qualified according to these standards, whether they seek license by examination in Oklahoma or wish to come to Oklahoma by reciprocity. A part of the value of the license is reflected in the willingness of other states to accept Oklahoma licenses on the basis of reciprocity. The value of medical training and license is also a reflection of the unselfish interest of physicians who have been and are willing to give time to these activities. A part of the heritage of all physicians is the responsibility to pass along to younger men a part of that which has been given to them.

From a purely monetary point of view it is conservatively estimated that the value of a license to practice medicine in this state is worth about $500,000. If the candidate's age is less than 35 years, the value is greater. If he is an old man, the value is less. The interest of health welfare of the people is best sustained by maintaining a relative high value of the licensure. It is reasonable to assume that every physician should take some interest in this matter and, when called upon, or voluntarily, when the occasion arises, each physician should be ready to plow back into his profession something of that which has come to him because of those who have gone before, and passed along the wisdom of experience.

Most readers of the Journal have been familiar with the fact that the Editor of the Journal, the late Lewis J. Moorman, M.D., had during the past 15 years for the most part, borne the responsibility of its editorial columns.

As a result of Doctor Moorman's recent illness and death, the contributors to the Editorial section of this month's Journal are Clinton Gallaher, M.D., Shawnee, Secretary of the Board of Medical Examiners; Rev. Jack E. Sanders, Alva; and Ben H. Nicholson, M.D., Oklahoma City, member of the Editorial Board.

Oklahoma City Clinical Society To Meet October 25, 26, 27, 28

This is addressed to those who are new in this part of the southwest, and to those old ones who forget or who are buried in the rut of imagined indispensability. To the others, this fall conference is part of their plan of professional progress.

The Art of Medicine, 80 per cent of which is letting nature get the patient well, most of us do fairly well. Only occasionally do we thwart her. The Science of Medicine is begot by antiquity and yesterday, grows in the experimental laboratory, is tested by men in clinical research and is finally appraised by men of the caliber of those who are invited to lecture to the Clinical Society.

The whole purpose of the Clinical Society is to put this appraisal, good or bad, into the hands and minds of men and women who are in the field looking after people who are sick or who think they are. This has been done well for 23 years. From the announced program, the twenty-fourth conference will be no exception. The Oklahoma Academy of General Practice accepts this clinical conference and its members will receive credit for the actual hours in attendance toward the 50 hours of formal post graduate study required every three years.

When the Bottom Drops Out

The courage of people who are beset by tragedy is truly amazing. They are, however, not often articulate in expressing the source of that courage and strength.

Since it is the physician's task to give counsel when catastrophe comes, the Editorial Board takes pleasure in reprinting, in part, a sermon by Reverend Jack E. Sanders of Alva about his own s o u r c e of spiritual strength on discovering his only son to be mongoloid:

When hopes crumble into shambles and dearest dreams become terrifying nightmares, can the heart and soul of a man survive? We have found our Christian Faith genuinely tried by little circumstances of life. What, then, is the power of that Faith when the bottom drops out?

Answers to these questions do not come from theory. But as gold by fire is refined, so come our certain conclusions from the hot heat of the suffering soul.

More than 100 years ago a young man named George Matheson entered Glasgow University. He had a keen mind. His hopes were high. Soon he and his fiancee would be married. He dreamed of the future. Then the bottom dropped out! He became totally blind. Because of his misfortune he was rejected by his fiancee. His world crumbled at his feet. Seemingly it was enough to defeat any soul. But this soul had the power of the Christian Faith.

In spite of his blindness he graduated from the university at 19, and entered the ministry of the Church of Scotland. He became one of the greatest preachers of all Scotland, and to this day his devotional books still lend inspiration to troubled hearts.

In this life we must be aware of one truth. It is this: Human tragedy is the common possession of us all. Most every heart has its secret cloister where dark and forbidding memories are kept. For adversity is no respecter of persons, and in a split second of time misfortune can change an entire life.

Our eyes need but look with the speed of a camera shutter at the world about us, and this truth is forever pictured in our minds. Select any newspaper you wish, and you can't turn a page without some human calamity tumbling out. A mother sobs beside a hospital bed because fireworks have blasted away the sight of her son. Parents, their faces distorted by grief, pace a muddy creek bank as firemen drag for the body of a child that has drowned. A mother of four children has an incurable cancer. A promising a t h l e t e has a leg amputated. Polio has stricken three members of the same family. Christmas is celebrated in July for a five year old because he won't be alive in December. One after another these heart breaking catastrophies shatter man's fondest hopes, and day-by-day souls are wrung out until they are limp.

Of course we cannot accept this picture as just another snap-shot; for with troubling intensity comes the hurt soul's quest: "Why this suffering? Why must man's heart be broken constantly by the accidents of the world? Why was the world so created? Why must tragedy come to me and mine? Why? Why? Why?

I shall never forget my father's response when he learned that our baby could never have a normal life. He placed his arm about my shoulders saying, "Son, why you and Pauline?" The only answer I could give was this: "Because we are human, Dad, and being human we live in a world of accidents."

I am aware that for centuries there has been the idea in Christian thought that human tragedy is the direct result of God's Will. This is seemingly a popular conception in our generation. A misfortune occurs, and immediately some will say, "It is God's Will. God is bringing this disaster that thorugh it He might work a greater good." This makes God directly responsible for every calamity that comes to the human family.

We do not and cannot accept this conception of human tragedy. Rather we believe that our Father in Heaven is grieved by our misfortune and stands ever with us to give spiritual strength and courage for our darkest hour. Human tragedy and suffering are not God's Will. But in spite of such human adversity God's will is yet to be done by us with what remains of us.

In life, as in any battle, we must at times withdraw; count our losses, regroup the remaining resources, and with determination once again set out to win.

Whether human tragedy will spell out our defeat or prove to be the beginning of our victory depends on how we respond to the tragedy. When life's calamities strike us down and their haunting memories return again and again, we can respond in one of two ways: We can follow the ill advice of Job's wife, in which event we will "Curse God and die;" or with the Psalmist we can "lift our eyes to the hills" asking "from whence cometh my help?" Then with certainty declare: "My help comes from the Lord who made heaven and earth."

The one response will mean life ripped and torn, battered and ruined by the storm waves of this life. The other response means a life founded on a solid rock in the midst of the angry waves like a lighthouse standing erect as a lone sentinel to give rays of everlasting hope to our fellows t o s s e d on troubled waters.

As you well know, tragedy has recently come to our home, and like a rude, uninvited guest has insisted that he remain. With the birth of our first son our joy broke forth as the morning and our hope was bright as the sun at noonday. But within six weeks our joy turned to bitter sorrow, and our bright hopes were subdued by the blackest night we've ever seen. For we received the news that our boy had not developed mentally. The bottom dropped out! The stars of heaven seemed to crash to earth.

It was so dark. Seemingly no light existed. Then those reassuring rays began shining through. We discovered that our spiritual resources are much the same as the stars of the universe. They are always shining, but we don't see them clearly until it's dark.

We learned that true value does not exist in what we see and touch, but it exists in that which we can neither see nor feel. Real value is found in friendship, loyalty, concern, sympathy, the ever present thoughts and prayers of others, hearts sensitive to another's grief, and love that finds its completeness in humble service. We have learned the importance of people. We have felt the steadfastnses of the Christian faith.

We want you to feel free to speak to us about our son. And never do we want you to feel that you must cease talking about him just because we enter the room. For you see we are not loosers altogether. We know the thrilling joy of having a son. The emotion of telling others he is born—handing out cigars—receiving gifts and congratulations—having friends say, "How's the boy?" and feeling the swelling pride as we answer, "He's the finest boy ever born." Only the loss of memory could ever rob us of this rich experience.

For 10 years, one month and one day our married life was smooth. Then came our first real catastrophe. During the time of our smooth sailing we talked about the Lord: "The Lord is my shepherd . . . He makes me lie down in green pastures . . . He leads me beside still waters . . . He leads me in the paths of righteousness." But when our world crashed in on top of us, we no longer talked about the Lord; we talked to Him: "Even though I walk through the valley of the shadow of death I will fear no evil for Thou art with me. Thy rod and Thy staff they comfort me. Thou preparest a table before me . . . Thou anointest my head with oil." When the bottom really drops out, nothing short of talking to God will meet the need.

As we have talked with God we have not asked that our load be lightened; only that we might have strength and courage to carry it nobly. We asked that we might not whimper, but that with a voice of certainty proclaim what strength and power belong to us human beings who trust in God.

When hopes crumble into shambles and dearest dreams become terrifying nightmares, the heart and soul of man can survive, because God's S p i r i t makes him strong enough to live now and for eternity.

Scientific Articles

Pulmonary Function in the

TREATMENT *of* TUBERCULOSIS

JOHN H. SCHAEFFER, M.D.

THE AUTHOR

John H. Schaeffer, M.D. is associated with the Shawnee Indian Sanatorium in Shawnee, Okla.

This paper will review some important ways in which knowledge of respiratory physiology can affect decisions in treating pulmonary tuberculosis. I will not attempt to compare the effectiveness of the various procedures except with relation to pulmonary function.

Since the present mortality rate of both thoracoplasty and resection is so favorable, the criterion of a successful procedure can no longer be solely the survival of the patient and the control of the disease. One must also include the maximal preservation of cardio-respiratory ability to protect reserves for possible unpredictable future insults. The method of choice must combine the best chance of cure, the minimal risk to the individual, and the least damage to the cardio-respiratory system. The choice of treatment is further complicated because the safer method may not be so promising as to cure. The surgical team, therefore, must interpret the physiologic evidence according to its experience with the particular methods at hand.

The estimate of operative risk is commonly based entirely on clinical judgment, a method we all use but find hard to define. This method includes the appearance of the patient, roentgenographic appearance of the chest, ease of breating, symmetry or asymmetry of breathing, tolerance of exercise, and development of cyanosis. Although many patients undergo successful surgery with no more evaluation than this, unexpected respiratory difficulties are sometimes encountered in patients so appraised. If one believes surgery to be of value in treating tuberculosis, one commonly sees borderline patients who fit the requirements for surgical treatment but who must be rejected because they seem to be excessive operative risks. Since the danger is increased in these patients with apparently poor respiratory reserve, the surgical team must know as much as possible about the preoperative state to extend the benefits of surgery as widely as possible and yet avoid an excessive mortality rate and a number of respiratory cripples. One can measure the many physiologic processes whereby gas is exchanged between the atmosphere and the pulmonary blood and whereby the blood is transported to the tissues. Although these methods are essential to research, not all are desirable for practical preoperative evaluation.

The vital capacity is the most common measurement of pulmonary function but is the least reliable, since it ignores the time necessary to deliver the capacity. I have seen several patients with vital capacity of four liters or more who were dyspneic on the slightest exertion. They had obstructive emphysema and required many seconds to deliver those four liters. While these are extreme examples, tuberculosis often produces bronchial deformity and other damage with prolongation of expiration; as a result, the vital capacity is completely misleading and falsely encouraging.

The timed vital capacity is a definite improvement over the simple vital capacity. The machine records the output in one, two and three seconds as well as the total. The normal person can deliver 75 per cent of his total vital capacity in the first second and more than 95 per cent in three seconds. The time is prolonged in the presence of either localized trapping or diffuse obstructive emphysema. Comparison of the amount delivered in the first second with the normal for one second correlates fairly well with the maximum breathing capacity.

In the test for maximum breathing capacity, the amount of air expired in 15 or 20 seconds with maximal effort is measured and the amount per minute computed. Since this test demands extreme effort, the patient's fatigue and his desire to make a good showing influence the result. Since both ease of fatigue and will to succeed are important in the immediate postoperative period, I believe the M.B.C. to be a little more useful than the preceding tests. Since it measures a large number of breaths, it is also more accurate than the measurement of a single breath.

The M.B.C. varies according to the size, age, and sex of the individual and must be compared with predicted standards or with the normal ventilatory requirement of the individual. This comparison is usually made with the amount of air the patient exhales while walking two miles an hour over a measured course. This activity is comparable to that necessary for normal daily living. The walking ventilation may be divided by the M.B.C. to give the percentage of maximal effort necessary to sustain the body during normal activity, the so called surgical index. If this figure is between .10 and .20, the patient is considered a good surgical risk; if between .20 and .30, a fair risk; and more than .30, a poor risk. Naturally this rating must be interpreted in view of the extent of the intended surgery. As a rule patients exceeding .33 will complain of dyspnea during the exertion.

The fluoroscope is of great use as a "screening tool", when fluoroscopy is performed by a person who has had repeated opportunities to check his judgments against accurate measurements. In functional fluoroscopy, particular attention is given to the degree to which the lungs can be filled and emptied, the speed of filling and particularly of emptying one part of the lungs compared

with the rest. Movement of the ribs and diaphragm are to be noted, and synchrony or lack of synchrony between them observed, particularly in patients with old phrenic paralysis and partially regained function. As is well known, women generally have much less diaphragmatic motion than men. It is therefore important to fluoroscope women in the lateral position to determine the amount of sternal motion and anterior-posterior expansion. Shifting of the mediastinum and cardiac silhouette is very important as it indicates trapping of air or unilateral partial bronchial obstruction. Films taken at the extreme of inspiration and expiration are of value in that they permit a more leisurely examination than fluoroscopy.

If one desires accurate knowledge of the degree to which each lung participated in respiration, he may measure it by bronchospirometry. A double lumened tube is inserted into the main bronchus and is placed so that a side opening connects the second lumen with the opposite bronchus. The two tubes are then connected to twin spirometers, and the respiration of each lung is measured separately. The sum of the two vital capacities so obtained should closely approximate the vital capacity previously measured. The percentage contributed by each lung for M.B.C. type respiration may then be measured and the oxygen consumption determined. In fact, although fluoroscopy gives some information about the bellows function of each lung, and angiograms suggest how much blood flows through the pulmonary arteries, only bronchospirometry can reliably measure the extent to which each lung performs in oxygen uptake.

The timed vital capacity, M.B.C., walking ventilation, and bronchospirometry with measurement of the oxygen uptake are quite useful in evaluating patients for major surgery. Measurement of arterial and alveolar gases are rarely of value. The role of cardiac catheterization in patients with pulmonary disease has not been established. In my limited observation of catheterization studies, they have been of no practical value.

The effect of pneumoperitoneum on pulmonary function is very slight. In some emphysematous patients it permits improved alveolar mixing and increased oxygen uptake by reducing the residual air. It seldom has marked effect on the vital capacity or the M.B.C., although both may be slightly reduced. I see no reason to remove the pneumoperitoneum before conducting function tests preparatory to major surgery.

Therapeutic pneumothorax also has a minimal effect on pulmonary function, although the unpredictable occurrence of pleural thickening may cause great loss of function. Preliminary function studies may be of value in preventing the complication of the unexpandable lobe. Bronchial stenosis accentuated by the distortion of pneumothorax is the usual cause of this complication. Stenosis may be detected by bronchoscopy if it is within the line of vision in the larger bronchi. However, diffuse trapping is usually present within the segment or lobe and is visible by careful fluoroscopy during M.B.C. type of breathing.

Phrenic crush, I believe, should be primarily of historical interest. It is an effective method of destroying about 30 to 40 per cent of the function of a lung. However, it is rarely if ever temporary or completely reversible. I have never seen a patient so treated who did not have some permanent weakness detectable by fluoroscopy. While this weakness is not important if the procedure helps to achieve a permanent cure, it is a great handicap to the patient who must later undergo major surgery. In addition to decreasing the function of the lung, the diaphragmatic dysfunction interferes greatly with the cough reflex and thereby enhances the possibility of such complications as atelectasis, pneumonitis, and the spread of tuberculosis in the immediate postoperative period. I consider it particularly deplorable to paralyze the least involved side in order to clear it and allow surgery on the opposite side. This sort of treatment sometimes reduces the function of the better lung so much that surgery at the site of major involvement is very hazardous or impossible. Although I have no statistical evidence, I believe that the amount of residual damage is likely to be increased when pneumoperitoneum and phrenic crush are used together.

Decortication is a problem in which function studies are of little diagnostic value. Although the studies provide evidence for the loss of function and the need for surgery, they are of no value in predicting the amount of function that may be regained by removing the thick inelastic shell encasing the lung. Much more accurate prediction may be made from careful review of films taken since the onset of the disease. The presence of a large amount of tissue which has never been diseased appears to give the best prognosis. Widespread disease in the past, even though it may have disappeared at the time of surgery, suggests that little improvement will be gained. The length of time the lung has been collapsed or encased has little correlation with the amount of function which may be regained.

Classical thoracoplasty removes the support of the thoracic cage. Without this support a normal lung will hinder proper chest wall motion to some extent. This hindrance to chest wall motion is made more severe when the lung has been made abnormally resistant to distention and collapse by bronchial stenosis, extensive fibrosis or a thick pleural membrane. This accentuated paradoxical chest wall motion is a serious problem which may occur in the immediate postoperative period. If one knows before operation that the lung is abnormally resistant to distention he is warned that the area must be kept small if a soft chest wall must be created. Resection of the anterior ribs should be done with caution since this area has no support after the ribs are removed. Loss of function six to 12 months after conventional thoracoplasty is negligible, provided the operation is confined to the diseased area and severe scoliosis is prevented. A 10 to 15 per cent loss of function is to be anticipated. The large amount of function remaining under a six-rib thoracoplasty is striking. The reasons are several, most important being that most of the motion comes from the lower chest wall and the diaphragm. Since the major source of motion remains intact, the breathing capacity may be unaltered, although the residual volume of the lung may be moderately reduced and the vital capacity also decreased. Since diaphragmatic motion causes much of the function of the lung under a thoracoplasty, one should be doubly cautious in the patient with a partially paralyzed diaphragm.

The advantages of the extraperiosteal plombage thoracoplasty over the conventional type are obvious. This procedure preserves the stability and thus alleviates paradoxical motion. It can be better localized and confined to the diseased area than the classical type. Severe scoliosis may be minimized. There is also the therapeutic consideration, that it gets maximal collapse immediately.

With uncomplicated resection, the thoracic cage is not injured and can soon regain its preoperative motion. The amount of dysfunction is related solely to the amount of healthy tissue removed. One can often find no functional loss after wedge or segmental resection or after removal of a contracted lobe. When more than a lobe is removed, the remaining tissue may be so distended as it fills the space that it exerts sufficient pull to decrease the size of the thorax. As the excessive expansion distorts the balance of power between the muscular chest wall and the elastic lung, the vital capacity and perhaps the M.B.C. will be further reduced. On physiologic grounds one cannot say whether or not a space-correcting procedure should be used. Tailoring thoracoplasty has in my experience usually caused an additional slight drop in function. The possibility that a space will persist is not a physiologic consideration. Whether or not prolonged distention produces obstructive emphysema is a question that needs further observation. Many patients with contracted upper lobes filling practically no space show no signs of true obstructive emphysema, even after many years. A final point often raised in favor of space-correcting procedures is also debatable — that the over-distended lung may have decreased ability to control remaining tuberculosis.

On physiologic grounds there is little to choose between the plombage thoracoplasty and resection. The loss of function from thoracoplasty comes from compression of functioning tissue, further impairment of diaphragmatic motion and the development of scoliosis. With resection it is sometimes possible to conserve more lung, but there is always the possibility of one's being forced for technical reasons to remove excessive tissue. Additional loss of function may be caused by lung leak with delayed expansion, infection, pleural reaction, and hemothorax with subsequent restriction of motion. The possibility of these complications of resection make the plombage thoracoplasty the safer procedure for patients who are poor or fair surgical risks but who have a moderate amount of function in the operative side.

The practical approach to functional evaluation of the tuberculous patient starts with a detailed history and careful physical examination. Before any type of collapse or relaxation therapy is considered, function fluoroscopy should be performed. When considering a patient for major surgery, review of all films is then done, giving attention to the extent of disease at the time of maximal involvement. Particular attention should be paid to the appearance of the other lung, and to other abnormalities such as phrenic paralysis, pneumothorax, and pleural effusion, all of which may limit function more than is apparent on the present film. Fluoroscopy is then performed and an estimate of the function of each lung made.

If the review of films shows a clear or minimally involved contralateral lung and fluoroscopy shows most of the function to be on that side, further tests are not necessary. If both lungs are involved, but most of the function appears to be on the good side, timed vital capacity or M.B.C. is necessary. If moderate or severe reduction of total function is demonstrated and the operative side has any function, then bronchospirometry must be done. If the distribution of disease is such that major surgery offers the best chance of cure, I believe a patient should not be rejected without this amount of study.

Summary

Many patients can undergo surgery without detailed functional studies. To extend the benefits of surgery to as many patients as is safely possible, it is necessary to have accurate methods for measuring the function of the lungs. The more limited a patient's respiratory reserve, the more important it is to know the type and extent of the limitation.

Pulmonary function studies are valuable adjuncts in assessing all patients who need thoracic surgery; they are essential in borderline cases.

Full Term Abdominal Pregnancy
With DELIVERY of LIVING CHILD

GERALD G. DOWNING, M.D.

THE AUTHOR

Gerald G. Downing, M.D., Lawton, graduated from Baylor University in 1933. A navy veteran, he served in the medical department 16 months.

This paper proposes to review a case of abdominal pregnancy in which a living baby was successfully delivered and to review some of the signs and symptoms that may aid in diagnosing the condition.

The records of abdominal pregnancies are constantly growing. Although the condition seems gradually to becoming less of a medical curiosity, it is still something that is difficult to diagnose before surgery but must be kept in mind when surgery is elected.

Symptoms associated with abdominal pregnancies are:

(1) There is a Hofstatter-Cullen-Hillendall's sign caused by the bottled-in intra-abdominally extra-vasated blood through the lymphatics into the neighborhood of the navel (blue navel) and its absorption into the abdominal skin.

(2) In many abdominal pregnancies the abdomen is so tender and rigid that instructive palpation of the fetus is precluded.

(3) Changes in the c e r v i x are, in the first eight to 10 weeks, the same as those in normal pregnancy. However, as a rule, the cervix begins to rise during the third month and is pushed forward. The axis of the uterus is not greatly changed. The inflammatory process begins in the tube; and after rupture or tubal abortion, the cul-de-sac fills with blood and as a result forces the cervix forward. Meanwhile, the growing products of conception tend to draw the cervix upward. The picture is not like the one when a pelvic abscess fills the cul-de-sac and displaces the cervix forward. When there is a pelvic abscess, the inflammatory process usually begins in the connective tissue in the base of one or both broad ligaments and "anchors" the uterus at its initial level.

(4) Nausea and vomiting are not exaggerated but are much more constant and persistent than in normal pregnancy.

Case Report

Mrs. A. C., a 31-year-old small white woman of apparently normal weight was seen for the first time about three and one-half weeks from term on Feb. 19, 1951. She had had one normal pregnancy and delivered six years previously. Her health had always been good.

She said that when she was about three months along in the current pregnancy she was hospitalized because of bleeding and cramping. Bleeding and pains had been intermittent throughout the pregnancy. For the five weeks before I first saw her, she had been in bed most of the time because of weakness and severe pain in the abdomen and back. A marked edema of both lower limbs was present despite a low salt diet. She complained of considerable loss of weight vomiting, and an inability to eat for the past several weeks. She was quite constipated and took milk of magnesia with fair results. One week before admission, she was given a blood transfusion and a roentgenogram was taken. The roentgenogram revealed a normal-appearing fetus in transverse position with the head on the left. She was quite pallid and dyspneic and apparently had severe pain in the back. Her pulse was 120 at rest; blood pressure was 125-75; heart sounds were normal. Moist rales were heard in the bases of both lungs. Her abdomen was extremely distended, tense and tender, and the skin was shiny from stretching. Large veins could be seen through the skin on both sides of the abdomen. It was impossible to feel any fetal parts or elicit any fetal heart tones. The fundus measured 34 cm. in height and 31 cm. in width. External pelvic measurement was within normal limits. Both lower extremities were edematous to the groin. The upper half of the body appeared emaciated.

The patient was hospitalized immediately to permit the membranes to be punctured through the cervix. After the report on her roentgenogram was received, it was decided to remove the fluid through the abdominal wall. I hoped to avoid inducing labor and to be able to convert the position of the baby to a cephalic position. A spinal puncture needle was inserted in the midline just below the umbilicus, a 6000 cc. of fluid which was very dark with old blood (question of being a vein) was drawn off.

Unusual movements of the needle first indicated the presence of a live baby. They resulted when the baby touched the needle in moving. After the fluid was withdrawn, the fetal heart tones were easily heard. The rate was 140 a minute. The patient was able to breathe more easily but still complained of pain in her back. The edema of her lower extremities did not subside during the night as expected from relieving the pressure of polyhydramnios.

Her Hbg. was 55 per cent; and the RBC 3,100,000, WBC 13,100. The urine showed a trace of albumin and numerous white and red blood cells.

The day after admission she was fairly comfortable and an attempt was made to change the position of the baby. During that night the patient began having what was apparently hard labor except there were no contractions. There was a moderate amount of bright vaginal bleeding. At 5:00 a.m. the nurse phoned that the patient was in hard labor but she was unable to feel the cervix by rectal examination. The patient passed a piece of tissue the size of the palm. It resembled placental tissue. Upon rectal examination, nothing could be felt except a "doughy" mass. After a sterile prep, a vaginal examination was done. The cervix could still not be found until a vaginal speculum was inserted. It was found compressed under the pubis on the left and not dilated. The mass below the cervix felt like irregular placental tissue. The baby was moved to the transverse position, with its head on the other side. The change of posi-

tion was verified by roentgenogram. Since normal labor seemed impossible, cesarean section was advised.

The patient was given two transfusions of whole blood before surgery, one during surgery, and five afterwards.

At laparotomy it was difficult to separate the rectus muscle from its posterior sheath. It was also very difficult to separate peritoneum from what was thought to be the uterus. The membranes could be, and were, mistaken for a thinned-out uterine muscle wall because they were of similar color, very vascular, and non-transparent. As an attempt was made to separate the bladder from the lower uterine surface, the membranes were punctured, and approximately two more quarts of very dark fluid were aspirated. The membranes were quickly incised up the midline, and the baby was delivered. The baby appeared discolored and almost macerated. The umbilical cord was so friable that it was difficult to clamp. The baby, a female, weighed 5 lbs. 3 oz. Her heart beat was normal. Dr. Roy Donaghe, pediatrician, who was standing by, took over the care of the baby. After the patient had been resuscitated and a considerable amount of bloody fluid had been aspirated from the stomach, respiraton became established. The membranes were thick enough to be an overstretched uterine wall, but there were no large vessels and remarkably little bleeding. Not until after the baby was delivered did we discover that the pregnancy was extrauterine. On exploration, the uterus was found to be small and flattened against the left anterior pubic ramus and abdominal wall. The placenta was attached to the left and posterior walls of the pelvis. From the upper portion of the amniotic sac, a quart basin full of old clots was removed. The free peritoneal cavity was never entered. When I made a quick attempt to separate the placenta, blood virtually floated my hand from the cavity. The area was quickly packed with four strips of folded gauze, 4 inches wide by one yard long. The ends of these strips were brought out through the incision. The membranes were sutured with chromic, and the abdominal layers closed in the usual manner.

The patient had a rather stormy postoperative course; she suffered distention, vomiting, pain in the back and legs, and weaknesses. The distention was controlled by Prostigmin. Dramamine seemed to be of much value in controlling the vomiting. The patient required a great deal of Demerol and Morphine. The fifth postoperative day, I started pulling the gauze packs out a few inches each day until at the end of the six days they were completely removed. There was profuse sero-sauguinous drainage after the packs were removed, and the sinus had to be reopened almost daily to prevent premature closure.

The patient was released from the hospital four weeks after delivery. She was able to walk with some difficulty and still complained of pain in the back and legs. The incision was healed and the amniotic and placental mass extended well above the umbilicus. The patient had a normal menstruation three and a half weeks after delivery and has menstruated regularly since. Her breasts never became engorged, and there was never any lactation.

The baby, who also had a rather stormy course, lost considerable weight at first and vomited a great deal. At this writing she is well nourished and apparently normal.

The mother has been examined periodically since her release from the hospital. Her pains gradually subsided, and her strength has returned to normal. The placenta gradually decreased in size for about two years, but has remained the same size for the past year. It is firm and non-tender, but it does not give the impression of becoming calcified. Vaginally the mass is the size of an average orange and bulges into the pelvis, but the uterus and cervix are steadily assuming their normal positions. The patient feels fine, has no symptoms referable to the placenta, and does not consider having it removed.

Discussion

The loss of fetuses and the high incidence of congenital anomalies (whether due to ovum defects or subsequent developmental pressure factors) are noteworthy in abdominal pregnancies. The fetal loss runs as high as 76.5 per cent in extrauterine pregnancies of more than five months' gestation: if a living, viable baby is obtained, his chances for survival of eight days or more are rated as only 44.3 to 57.1 per cent. The percentage of reported deformities, moreover, ranges from 10 to 46 per cent. The maternal mortality in recent years has been reduced to about 15 per cent from a previous 35 per cent.

Summary

(1) A case of abdominal pregnancy in which treatment resulted in a living mother and baby has been presented.

(2) Both mother and child are apparently well and healthy to this date.

(3) The case presented some unusual findings which the author hopes will prove beneficial in subsequent cases of this type.

BIBLIOGRAPHY

1. Esau, P.: Abdominal Pregnancy. Blue Navel. Ovarian Pregnancy. Tubal Pregnancy with Monochorconic Twins of First Month, Zentralblatt fur Chirurgie, 61; 620 (March 17, 1934).

2. Mendenhall, A. M. Diagnosis of Advanced Abdominal Pregnancy, The American Journal of Surgery, 18; (November 1932).

3. and 4. McNeile, L. G. Diagnosis of Abdominal Pregnancy, Transactions of Pacific Coast Society of Obstetrics and Gynecology, 6:68, 1936.

5. Full Term Abdominal Pregnancy (a case report); Daniel B. Dooman, M.D., The New England Journal of Medicine; Volume 245, No. 6; (Aug. 9), 1951; pp. 207-210.

ATTEND THE SOUTHWESTERN SURGICAL CONGRESS

Oklahoma City   September 20-21-22

Clinical Aspects of

ENDOMETRIOSIS

ENGENE S. COHEN, M.D.

THE AUTHOR

Eugene S. Cohen, M.D., Tulsa, was graduated from the Universty of Oklahoma School of Medicine in 1946. He previously practiced in Texas and Michigan and served in the army medical corps as a captain in World War II. His specialty is obstetrics and gynecology.

Despite the fact that endometriosis has become a well-established, no longer completely mysterious clinical and pathological entity, it still remains one of the most difficult diagnostic problems confronting the gynecologist. It would seem, from the clearly-defined textbook descriptions of the clinical symptomatology and from the standard illustrations of the typical lesions of this disease, that a high degree of diagnostic accuracy should now prevail. However, this is not the case. There is a large gap between the signs and symptoms and the microscopic and gross pathology of this disorder even many times when the disease is already far advanced. Increasing experience has shown that endometriosis, like syphilis, is a great masquerader and cleverly contrives to conceal its identity in many ways.

During the three years from January, 1950, to January, 1953, a study was made of 102 cases of histologically proved endometriosis treated at St. John's Hospital in Tulsa. In addition, there were larger numbers of suspected endometriosis which were treated medically and still others diagnosed as endometriosis at the time of surgery but not substantiated by histologic evidence. In this study of endometriosis we excluded all of those which could not be established by complete histologic proof.

Incidence

Table I shows the breakdown of our 102 cases of established endometriosis according to age incidence. The age incidence ranged from 20 to 62 years. The average age at the time of operation was 35 years. These figures serve only to emphasize the tragedy of the frequency of endometriosis in young women. The youngest patient, age 20, was operated on for severe dysmenorrhea and the presence of an ovarian cyst. The oldest patient was 62 years of age, and presented the symptoms of vaginal spotting for three months. This patient had undergone a previous fundectomy. During a diagnostic curettage, feces were noted on the curet. A laparotomy revealed the sigmoid to be densely adherent to the cervical stump. It was through this area of the sigmoid that accidental perforation had occurred. The pathological report revealed endometriosis of the ovary and broad ligament. Endometriosis in the adhesions between the cervix and sigmoid could not, however, be proved histologically.

TABLE I

AGE INCIDENCE

Age group	No.	%
20-30	34	33.3
31-40	38	37.2
41-50	28	27.5
51-62	2	1.9

Previous Surgery

Table II shows the types of previous surgery encountered in our series. Sixteen had had appendectomies and fourteen had had adnexal surgery. These two procedures accounted for 86 per cent of the surgery performed previous to the present admissions. The possibility must be borne in mind that some of the previous abdominal surgery was for an earlier, perhaps unrecognized, manifestation of the same endometriosis which later again brought the patient to surgery.

TABLE II

PREVIOUS SURGERY

Type	No.	%
Appendectomy	16	15.7
Adnexal Surgery	14	13.7
Cesarean Section	2	1.9
Hysterectomy	2	1.9
Suspension	1	0.9

Associated Pathology

The association of endometriosis with other pathology has been frequently noted in previous reports, [1, 7]. In our series 33 per cent of the patients had fibromyomas; uterine retrodisplacement occurred in 23 per cent. These two pathological conditions have often been enumerated as possible factors in the etiology of endometriosis. Forty-four per cent had other associated pathology.

Symptoms

The symptoms appearing in this series were similar in many respects to those reported in the literature [1, 2, 7, 8]. See Table III.

TABLE III
SYMPTOMATOLOGY

Symptom	No.	%
Low abdominal pain	47	46.0
Dysmenorrhea	28	27.4
Metrorrhagia	21	20.6
Menorrhagia	15	14.7
Pelvic pressure	10	9.8
Backache	8	7.8
Dyspareunia	7	6.8
Vaginal discharge	5	4.9
Fever	4	3.9
No symptoms	3	2.9

Low abdominal pains and pressure, dysmenorrhea and metrorrhagia were the predominant symptons. Dysmenorrhea was present, however, in only 27.4 per cent of the cases. The absence of dysmenorrhea in a significant number of cases of endometriosis has been noted in previous investigations[8]. In contradistinction to previous reports, dyspareunia and backache occurred relatively infrequently in our series. Four instances of fever occurred in this survey. The importance of this finding has been elaborated on by Forman[4].

It is interesting to note that three patients in our study presented no symptoms. One, a 23-year-old white nullipara, was found to have large ovarian cysts on routine examination. Both cysts proved, histologically, to be endometriomas. The second patient was a 39-year-old multipara who noted only slight irregularity of the menses. She had a history of previous adnexal surgery. Endometriosis of the ovary associated with a large fibromyoma uteri was proved histologically.

The third case, a 44-year-old primipara, was found to have a mass in the cul-de-sac on routine examination. At surgery, endometrial implants in the cul-de-sac were recognized in addition to fibromyoma uteri and an endometrial polyp.

In one of the patients of this series, the symptoms were so indicative of an acute abdominal crisis that the diagnosis of a ruptured ectopic pregnancy was entertained. At laparotomy, free intra-abdominal hemorrhage with clot was present, arising from near the fimbriated end of the oviduct. The pathologist reported, however, only the presence of endometriosis of the mesosalpinx.

One important point was evident from the review of the symptomatology of our study. There was certainly no definite relationship between the frequency and severity of the symptoms and the nature, location and extent of the ectopic endometrium.

Diagnosis

In reviewing our cases, one other important point seems to stand out. This is shown in Table IV. Of the histologically proved instances of endometriosis, only 28 (or 27.4 per cent) were correctly diagnosed pre-operatively. In 74 (or 72.6 per cent) of the patients the diagnosis of endometriosis was completely overlooked in the pre-operative differential diagnosis.

TABLE IV
ACCURACY OF DIAGNOSIS
PRE-OPERATIVE

	No.	%
Diagnosed	28	27.4
Not diagnosed	74	72.6

An error in the gross diagnosis of endometriosis at the time of surgery was also encountered in our series. Table V. Of the 102 cases, only 81 were diagnosed correctly at surgery. Twenty-one (or 20.6 per cent) of the histologically proved cases were not recognized grossly as having endometrial lesions.

TABLE V
ACCURACY OF DIAGNOSIS
SURGICAL

	No.	%
Diagnosed	81	79.4
Not recognized	21	20.6

Most textbooks of gynecology give the impression that the clinical diagnosis of endometriosis is relatively simple. The classic symptoms and pelvic findings are described as being specific for this disease. However, our study and the studies made by Sinclair, Kelley and Schlademan have shown that the correct pre-operative diagnosis is very difficult to make, since not all follow the classic pattern[5, 8].

Undoubtedly, as Crossen points out, "the bedside recognition of pelvic endometriosis is not as easy as might be inferred from the clear cut pathologic changes"[2]. The difficulty in pre-operative diagnosis stems from the fact that extensive endometrial lesions may exist without subjective symptoms, and that the signs and symptoms when present may stimulate other more common diseases.

So closely does the clinical pattern resemble chronic inflammation, or a tumor with inflammation, that such a mistaken diagnosis is usually made. However, if the gynecologist looks beyond the one or two most prominent symptoms, and analyzes critically the remaining features, the true diagnosis will be arrived at more frequently.

The presence of progressively severe acquired dysmenorrhea, premenstrual pain, abnormal uterine bleeding and dyspareunia are certainly significant. The time and character of the pain is somewhat specific in that it begins premenstrually and continues in severity throughout the menstrual flow. The importance of endometriosis in relation to its effect on sterility is well known. Scott and Telinde in a recent review enumerated other varied symptoms which are usually not associated with endometriosis.[11] These were: headaches, swollen ankles, indigestion, flank pain, general fatigue, rectal bleeding and hematuria.

The diagnosis of endometriosis usually rests however, largely on the pelvic findings at the vagino-abdominal and rectovaginal examination. The presence of large adherent ovaries without evidence of pre-existing infection, with fixed retrodisplaced uterus, and with "shotty" nodules in the cul-de-sac is very strongly suggestive of endometriosis. Additional evidence may be the presence of unusual pelvic tenderness out of proportion to the palpable lesion.

Cystoscopic examination is of great value in locating the small blood cysts in the bladder. Proctological and radiographic examination of some patients with implants in the recto vaginal septum or the sigmoid will reveal a narrowing of the lumen of the bowel and congestion of the mucosa. The importance of the digital recto-vaginal examination should not be overlooked. It reveals a lot of information and is a simple clinical diagnostic aid available to all. The pelvic endoscope or cul-de-scope will probably find its most valuable use in the detection and confirmation of endometriosis.

The presence of additional pathology such as fibromyomas and/or infection together with endometriosis certainly precluded or obscured the pre-operative diagnosis in numerous patients of our series, and this alone perhaps accounts for the high percentage of error in diagnosis. If one considers those patients who are treated medically for endometriosis, where the diagnosis often is only presumed, the percentage of error in diagnosis would certainly be even much greater.

One cause for error in gross pathologic diagnosis is the bizarre pattern of the endometrial lesions. The dense adhesions which are formed and the active invasion of the endometrial process into the walls of the involved organs certainly makes the gross diagnosis rather difficult. The most common error in gross surgical diagnosis is the attempt to distinguish various types of hemorrhagic ovarian cysts from endometrial cysts. Mistaken diagnoses of recto-sigmoid carcinoma still persist. Endometriosis is a benign disease with invasion potentialities seen only in cancer.

It is not surprising that in Sinclair's series of 85 cases diagnosed grossly at surgery as endometriosis, only 62 per cent were proved histologically[9]. The reasons for this are two-fold. First, there is much difficulty in identifying endometrial cysts histologically when they are distended with blood, and secondly, the endometrial lesions may become obscured when the gross specimen has been placed in formalin or allowed to dry. The formalin discolors the lesions and the small implants may become hidden in the wrinkled serosal layers. If one expects to obtain histological confirmation of his diagnosis, it is mandatory that one of the smaller areas involved be immediately tagged by a safety pin or suture. If a complete specimen cannot be obtained, a biopsy of the implant should be made and the individual lesion sent to the pathologist. If such a method be adopted, the incidence of confirmatory diagnosis of endometriosis will be greatly increased.

Summary

In summary, 102 cases of proved endometriosis are reviewed. The age incidence, associated pathology, previous surgery, and symptomatology closely correlated that encountered in previously reported series. A high per cent of error of diagnosis both pre-operatively and at the time of surgery has been encountered. It is urged that a higher index of suspicion of endometriosis be cultivated in reviewing the clinical symptomatology of all gynecological problems. Correlation of the gross surgical pathology with the histological findings will be greatly enhanced by close cooperation between the surgeon and the pathologist.

REFERENCES

1. Bennet, E. T. Endometriosis in the older age group; Am. J. Obst. & Gynec. 65:100, 1953.
2. Crossen, H. S., and Crossen, R. J. Diseases of women; St. Louis, 1941, C. V. Mosby Company.
3. Counseller, V. S., and Crenshaw, J. L. A clinical and surgical review of endometriosis; Am. J. Obst. & Gynec. 62:930, 1951.
4. Forman, I. Fever in endometriosis; Am. J. Obst. & Gynec. 63:634, 1952.
5. Kelley, F. J., and Schlademan, K. R. Endometriosis, it's surgical significance, a critical analysis of 179 cases; Surg., Gynec. & Obst. 88:230, 1949.
6. Meigs, J. V. Endometriosis, etiologic role of marriage age and parity; conservative treatment, Obst. & Gynec. 2:46, 1953.
7. Meigs, J. V., and Sturgis, S.H. Progress in Gynecology, New York, 1946, Grune & Stratton.
8. Siegler, S. L., and Bisaccio, J. R. Endometriosis, clinical aspects and therapeutic considerations: Am. J. Obst. & Gynec. 61:99, 1951.
9. Sinclair, M. D. The accuracy of the diagnosis of endometriosis Am. J. Obst. & Gynec. 63:1334, 1952.
10. Te Linde, R. W., and Scott, R. B. Experimental endometriosis Am. J. Obst. & Gynec. 60:1147, 1950.
11. Scott, R. B., and Te Linde, R. W. External endometriosis, the scourge of the private patient: Ann. Surg. 131:697, 1950.

Synopses Requested For Annual Meeting Papers

The dates of the 62nd Annual Meeting of the Oklahoma State Medical Association in Tulsa have been announced for Monday through Wednesday, May 9-11, 1955. All scientific sessions and commercial exhibits will again be at the Cimarron Ballroom. The House of Delegates will meet Sunday, May 8, at the Mayo Hotel in an annual business meeting and election of officers.

Dr. Bruce R. Hinson, President, has appointed Dr. James W. Kelley of Tulsa as General Convention Chairman and Dr. Walter E. Brown of Tulsa as Chairman of the Scientific Work Committee. All arrangements for the 1955 Annual Meeting will be handled through the Executive Offices of the Tulsa County Medical Society.

Doctor Brown last month appealed for papers suitable for presentation on the scientific program. Any member of the Oklahoma State Medical Association interested in presenting a paper at the convention is invited to submit the title and a brief synopsis of the proposed paper to Doctor Brown, c/o B-9 Medical Arts Building, Tulsa. The final date to submit proposed papers will be November 30, 1954.

"It may not be possible to use all papers submitted," Doctor Brown said, "due to limitations of the program schedule, duplication of subject matter, and the necessity of representing most specialties. However, we do hope that every member who has a useful paper will give us the opportunity of considering it for the scientific program."

Although space for scientific exhibits is quite limited, applications for space for this purpose are now being received. The final date for such applications will also be November 30, 1954.

Other members of the Scientific Work Committee, in addition to Doctor Brown, include Dr. E. G. Hyatt, Dr. Thomas J. Hardman, Dr. Earl I. Mulmed, Dr. Wendell L. Smith, and Dr. James B. Thompson, all of Tulsa. Doctor Kelley will announce the personnel of his convention committees in about 30 days.

GRIEVANCE COMMITTEE

Five years after its creation by the House of Delegates of the Oklahoma State Medical Association, the Grievance Committee has been given greater and more inclusive responsibilities than were originally allotted to it by that body. Its powers have been broadened and its method of procedure clarified. In general this would indicate confidence in the accomplishments of the Committee and would appear to acknowledge a need for its continuance. It would, moreover, suggest that the members of this Association are willing to accept and discharge their individual responsibilities in disciplinary matters on the rare occasions when such matters need be considered at the local society level.

As it was set up in the beginning, the Grievance Committee was asked to handle complaints against physicians arising out of questions of fees or services or both. Now it is empowered to consider any complaint involving a member of the Association which is properly presented to the Committee or to the Association.

Your Committee is aware that this step does not have the unanimous approval of the members. It well appreciates that some are naturally hesitant and fearful lest this Committee so constituted, might go beyond its definite responsibilities. Others may feel that it is unfair for any third party to have a part in a controversy involving a physician-patient relationship. To the first group we would say that the Committee was established and its methods of procedure outlined and approved by the House of Delegates to which body the Committee is responsible and before which its actions are subject to review. To that latter group we would say there are many instances in the experience of the Committee where there must be an impartial third party in the negotiations to insure fair consideration and justice for the public and profession alike. Where there is proper physi-

cian-patient relationships, Grievance Committee matters do not occur.

It must be remembered that the Committee has no authority to force any member to take any particular course of action nor to discipline any member. It can only present the evidence revealed by its investigations and make its recommendations.

The Grievance Committee, as you know, is composed of the five living immediate Past-Presidents of the Association. On the average these men have been in the practice of medicine for 25 years. They represent different fields of medical interests and experience and come from various areas of the state. They are acquainted with many physicians and are cognizant of varied community problems. After having given them the highest honor you can bestow, the Presidency of the State Medical Association, you make it obligatory for each of them to serve five years on this Committee. This is a serious responsibility and one that they do not consider lightly. Individually and as a group, their greatest desire is for the practice of medicine in Oklahoma to continue on a high and honorable plane.

Any signed complaint or question coming to the Oklahoma State Medical Association is entitled to consideration and a reply. This is an obligation which the State Association and its individual members owe to the public. Prior to the creation of the Grievance Committee, there was no method of considering, investigating and disposing of complaints.

The recent action of the House of Delegates makes it possible for the Committee to consider in an orderly manner and dispose of problems brought to its attention within a reasonable period of time. Furthermore, it provides that when a request or report of the Grievance Committee is apparently ignored by the local society because of difficulty or embarrassment at the local level, such a report goes automatically to the Council. In fairness to the public and the Profession, these investigations should be handled as speedily as efficient and careful consideration will permit.

An expressed objection to granting the Grievance Committee its present broader field of endeavor was that a physician's reputation or his financial standing might be jeopardized by an inquisitional type of investigation and ruthless action of the Committee. Such jeopardy will NOT be caused by the activity of the Committee, but can only be a result of the behavior of the physician himself whose action originally provoked the complaint. A physician's reputation is NOT to be protected above all things when utter, incompetency, willful neglect, deceit or dishonesty enters into the picture.

Other states are awakening to the rights of the patient and the public, and we can well be proud that Oklahoma was among the first to meet this need by establishing a Grievance Committee. It must not, it cannot fail in its duty. To this end we, the present members of the Grievance Committee, acknowledge that we are sobered by the additional responsibility you have laid upon us, and pledge that our every effort shall be towards a fair and impartial consideration of the problems presented to us. Your cooperation and your understanding will be necessary if this Committee is to serve its purpose in our common efforts.

GEORGE H. GARRISON, M.D.
RALPH A. McGILL, M.D.
L. CHESTER McHENRY, M.D.
A. R. SUGG, M.D.
JOHN E. McDONALD, M.D.

Book Review

A CURRICULUM FOR S C H O O L S OF MEDICAL TECHNOLOGY, edited by Israel Davidson, M.D., and Kurt Stern, M.D., Third Edition, 1953. Published by the Registry of Medical Technologists of the American Society of Clinical Pathologists, Muncie, Indiana, $3.00.

The third edition of the *Curriculum* is of primary interest to those who are responsible for the training of medical technologists. It will be of some use to technologists in preparing for the registry examination. As in previous editions, an attempt has been made to provide standards to which schools of medical technology may be expected to conform in order to insure uniformity and adequacy of their training programs.

Ten of the 15 chapters are devoted to the presentation of a basic curriculum designed to cover the various special fields of laboratory techniques. The remaining chapters include a bibliography, sample examination questions, teaching aids, and laboratory reports (no practical suggestions are offered here).

The emphasis throughout appears to be on the performance and technique of laboratory examinations—necessary but uninspiring to the student who wishes to know why and how as well. As a matter of fact performance and technique improve as the individual is led to a realization of the meaning of laboratory examinations in their proper context of pathology and physiology. This holds true for the practicing technologist as well as the student.

The book will be of some aid to those individuals engaged in teaching medical technology.—*L. L. Conrad, M.D.*

Dramamine's® Effect in Vertigo

*Dramamine has become accepted in the control
of a variety of clinical conditions characterized by
vertigo and is recognized as a standard
for the management of motion sickness.*

Vertigo, according to Swartout, is primarily due*
to a disturbance of those organs of the body that
are responsible for body balance. When the pos-
ture of the head is changed, the gelatinous substance in the semi-circular canals begins to flow.
This flow initiates neural impulses which are
transmitted to the vestibular nuclei. From this
point impulses are sent to different parts of the
body to cause the symptom complex of vertigo.

Some impulses reach the eye muscles and cause
nystagmus; some reach the cerebellum and skeletal muscles and righting of the head results; others
activate the emetic center to result in nausea,
while still others reach the cerebrum making the
person aware of his disturbed equilibrium. *Vertigo
may be caused by a disease or abnormal stimuli of
any of these tissues involved in the transmission of
the vertigo impulse, including the cerebellum and
the end organs.*

A possible explanation of Dramamine's action
is that it depresses the overstimulated labyrinthine structure of the inner ear. Depression,
therefore, takes place at the point at which these
impulses, causing vertigo, nausea and similar disturbances, originate. Some investigators have
suggested that Dramamine may have an additional sedative effect on the central nervous system.

Repeated clinical studies have established
Dramamine as valuable in the control of the
symptoms of Ménière's syndrome, the nausea and
vomiting of pregnancy, radiation sickness, hypertension vertigo, the vertigo of fenestration procedures, labyrinthitis and vestibular dysfunction associated with antibiotic therapy, as well as in
motion sickness.

Any of these conditions in which Dramamine
is effective may be classed as "disease or abnormal stimuli"* of the tissues including the end
organs (gastrointestinal tract, eyes) and their
nerve pathways to the labyrinth.

Dramamine (brand of dimenhydrinate) is supplied in tablets of 50 mg. and liquid (12.5 mg. in
each 4 cc.). It is accepted by the Council on
Pharmacy and Chemistry of the American Medical Association. G. D. Searle & Co., Research
in the Service of Medicine.

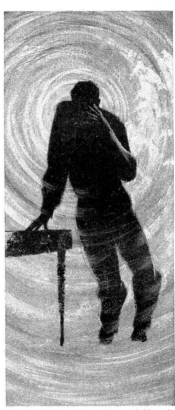

*The site of Dramamine's action is probably in the
labyrinthine structure.*

*Swartout, R., III, and Gunther, K.: "Dizziness:" Ver-
tigo and Syncope, GP 8:35 (Nov.) 1953.

Association Activities

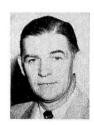

PRESIDENT'S LETTER

The work of the A.M.A. committee headed by Dr. John Cline, former president of the A.M.A., has begun to show results. This was evidenced by an action taken by the House of Delegates of the American Osteopathic Association at its annual session in Toronto on July 15, 1954.

It is well known that after months of extensive and comprehensive study, Dr. Cline submitted his committee's report, with recommendations, to the House of Delegates of the A.M.A. in New York in 1953. Action was deferred and study was continued. In the intervening year the various states publicized and discussed the recommendations. There was, however, no majority opinion, and when the report was again submitted at the 1954 session in San Francisco action was once more deferred.

Most people felt that we should wait for signs of cooperation from the osteopathic organization. This apparently has taken place, for less than a month after the 1954 A.M.A. session the American Osteopathic House of Delegates unanimously agreed that their committee have the authority to negotiate with the A.M.A. for the purpose of instituting on-campus visits by committee members of the A.M.A. The immediate purpose of such visits is to provide information to the A.M.A. committee to assist in its efforts to remove the cultist designation from the osteopathic profession. This, in itself, may not be a terribly important step, but it seems to be one in the right direction.

President

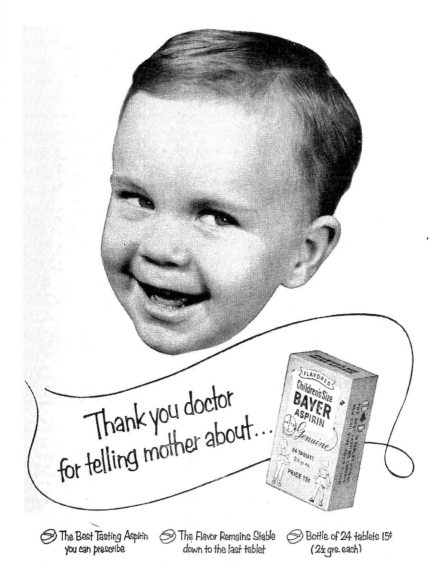

Thank you doctor
for telling mother about...

🖫 The Best Tasting Aspirin   🖫 The Flavor Remains Stable   🖫 Bottle of 24 tablets 15¢
you can prescribe   down to the last tablet   (2½ grs. each)

OFFICIAL PROCEEDINGS of the HOUSE of DELEGATES

of the

OKLAHOMA STATE MEDICAL ASSOCIATION

MAY 9, 1954

Closing Session

The closing session of the 61st Meeting of the House of Delegates of the Oklahoma State Medical Association was called to order by the Vice-Speaker of the House, Keiller Haynie, M.D., Durant, at 7:30 p.m.

C. Riley Strong, M.D., El Reno, Chairman of the Credentials Committee, reported a quorum present.

Wm. N. Weaver, M.D., Muskogee, reported for the Committee on Constitution and By-laws. Dr. Weaver read the following proposed amendment: "Amend Chapter IX, Page 45, by inserting, following the present Section 6, a new Section 7, to read as follows, with remaining Section 7, to be renumbered 'Section 8':

Section 7, Grievance Committee

(a) Investigation

The Grievance Committee shall investigate all complaints concerning members of this Association which may be received by the Association when such complaints are received in writing and signed by the individuals making such complaints.

(b) Procedure

The Grievance Committee shall establish its own procedure for handling complaints filed with it, in accordance with these By-Laws, and is authorized to make recommendations to members of this Association complained of and to complainants in an effort, to adjust or dispose of cases on a fair and equitable basis for all concerned.

(c) Disposal of Cases

When the Grievance Committee is unable to negotiate the settlement of any case pending before it, as a result of the refusal or neglect of the member of the Association concerned to comply with the recommendations of the Committee, it shall then refer the case directly to the component society of which the physician is a member. In so referring any case to a component society the Committee shall advise the member of such referral and shall provide the component society with a complete copy of the Committee's file and its recommendations concerning said case.

In any instance in which a case is referred to a component society by the Grievance Committee and in which the component society does not, within thirty (30) days of such referral, initiate action to bring the matter before the component society for hearing, the Grievance Committee may, at its discretion, file formal charges, before the component society, concerning such case and if such charges are not prosecuted as provided in the Constitution and By-laws of the component society, or within thirty (30) days, the Grievance Committee may then file charges before the Council which shall promptly hear such charges and dispose of the case.

The Council shall hear charges preferred against members of component societies by the Grievance Committee. The Council shall establish its own procedure for hearing such charges, provided, however, that in all instances, the charges against members of component societies shall be reduced to writing and the evidence presented shall be germane to such charges. Copies of the charges shall, in all instances be furnished to the member of the component society against whom the charge has been preferred. The member complained of shall have adequate opportunity to prepare his defense and shall not be required to answer such charge in writing, although he may do so if he desires. The date of hearing shall in no event be less than twenty (20) days from the date copies of the charges are furnished the member complained of. Notice of at least ten (10) days as to the date and place of hearing shall be given the member complained of. The member against whom such charge be preferred shall have the right to be accompanied at the hearing by counsel if he so desires. The Council shall have the right to have present counsel of its choice for advice and assistance during any hearing, but such counsel shall not have any vote.

Amend Chapter IX, section 1, Page 44, by striking the period at the end of the section and inserting in lieu thereof the following words and figures:

"And Grievance Committee."

Amend Chapter IX, Section 2, Page 44, by inserting before the words, "The Committee" on Line 1,, the words and figures: "(a) Committee on Annual Session", and by inserting, following the words "Secretary-Treasurer" on Line 2, the following words and figures: "(b) Grievance Committee.

The Grievance Committee shall at all times be composed of the last five (5) living Past-Presidents of this Association. (c) All other standing committees".

Doctor Weaver moved the adoption of the amendment as read. Motion seconded. There followed a lengthy discussion of the amendment, in which Doctor L. C. McHenry and Dr. George Garrison, members of the Grievance Committee, spoke in defense of the Amendment and explained why it was considered in order. The motion carried and the amendment was adopted.

Doctor Weaver read the following amendment:

"Amend Chapter 1, Section 3, Subsection (b) line 13, Page 38, by striking, following the words, "consideration to the", the remaining words and figures: "Council and approved by the Council at a meeting prior to the Annual Session."

Note: This Amendment eliminates a temporary provision for waiving the five year membership requirement for all applicants whose applications for Honorary Membership were filed before January 1, 1952."

"Amend Chapter 1, Section 3, Subsection (e) Page 39, Line 9, by striking after the word "Council", and before the word "before", the following words and figures:

"at least ninety (90) days."

"Amend Chapter 1, Section 3, Subsection E, page 39, Line 13, by striking, following the word "Council", the remaining words and figures in that paragraph and inserting in lieu there of a period."

Doctor Weaver moved the adoption of these amendments. Motion seconded. The Speaker called for a discussion. Following the discussion the question was voted on, and the motion carried.

This concluded the report of the Committee on Constitution and Bylaws.

Joe Duer, M.D., Woodward, addressed the chair, was recognized and given permission to speak.

Doctor Duer advised that as the Association's representative at the recent meeting of the American Medical Education Foundation, he would like to discuss with the House some of the factors involved. Doctor Duer explained the purpose and the workings of the Foundation as compared with the National Medical Education Foundation, gave information as to what Oklahoma's medical school has received from the Foundation and what our State has contributed. In conclusion Doctor Duer advised that if the recommendation of the Council was adopted, some provision could and should be made to stimulate the contributions.

The Speaker, Doctor Haynie, reread that portion of the Council Report concerning the American Medical Education Foundation. Doctor Haynie asked for a motion to re-affirm or reject this recommendation.

Marshall O. Hart, M.D., moved, "That we reaffirm the Council's recommendation relative to the American Medical Education Foundation." Motion seconded and carried.

The next item of business was the report of the Resolutions Committee

Doctor Malcolm Phelps first read the following Report:

"Your Resolutions Committee has considered four resolutions with regard to the same subject. These four resolutions were presented by the Oklahoma State Radiological Society, the Oklahoma State Association of Pathologists, the Oklahoma Society of Anethesiologists and the Oklahoma County Medical Society.

These four resolutions deal with the legal principles of the practice of medicine by hospitals and or corporations.

Your Committee considered these four resolutions as they pertain to the practice of medicine and prepaid medical care plans including both non-profit and commercial companies. It was your Committee's opinion that predicated on information it had previously received from a report from the Attorney General of the State of Iowa requested by the Iowa State Board of Medical Examiners on this same question, that it is your Committee's recommendation that the Oklahoma State Medical Association request the Oklahoma State Board of Medical Examiners to secure from the Attorney General of the State of Oklahoma an opinion as to whether or not the practice of the specialties of Anesthesiology, Pathology, Radiology or any other branch of medicine wherein a payment is made by a third party, other than to the physician rendering the services, should be considered a violation of the Medical Practice Act of the State of Oklahoma.

Your Committee has also considered the recommendation by the Oklahoma State Associations of Anesthesiology, Pathology, and Radiology, that a Physician Hospital Committee be appointed by the Oklahoma State Medical Association.

Your Committee feels that this Committee should include in addition to the three above named groups the inclusion of representatives of the insurance field.

In view of the above, your Committee recommends to the House of Delegates that the Public Policy Committee c r e a t e as a Sub-Committee a Committee to be known as the Physician-Hospital and Prepaid Insurance Committee.

Your Committee further recommends that the Delegates to the American Medical Association be instructed to re-affirm the previous actions of the American Medical Association with regard to Physician Hospital and Prepaid Insurance Plans."

RESOLUTION
Oklahoma County Medical Society
Oklahoma City, Okla.

WHEREAS, Health insurance has enjoyed acceptance by the public and the medical profession as among the desirable methods of helping defray the costs of health care; and

WHEREAS, the members of the American Medical Association, State and County Medical Societies are bound by the principles and code of ethics of the American Medical Association; and

WHEREAS, the health contracts of the packing industry do not permit free choice of physicians, and

WHEREAS, these contracts distinctly restrict professional services in radiology, pathology, anesthesiology and physiatry, to services only "when rendered by salaried employee of a hospital", and

WHEREAS, these contracts exclude such professional services when rendered by a physician in his office or a physician conducting a private practice of these specialties in a hospital on a fee for service basis, and

WHEREAS, such influences undermine the private practice of medicine and especially of these specialties referred to in these contracts,

THEREFORE, BE IT RESOLVED, that the Oklahoma County Medical Society go on record as being opposed to such restrictions in the practice of these specialties as outlined in the health contracts of the packing industry. And that this resolution be submitted to the meeting of the House of Delegates at the next meeting of the Oklahoma State Medical Association, so that proper opposition to this encroachment on the practice of medicine be formulated to correct the present injustices and prevent future recurrence or spread of such abuses, and

FURTHER BE IT RESOLVED, that our delegates be instructed to bring this matter to the attention of the House of Delegates of the A.M.A. at its next meeting and take whatever steps that may be necessary to curb such practices which infringe on the private practice of medicine."

RESOLUTION

"To the Council:

Be it resolved that the Oklahoma Association of Pathologists in official meeting, March 14, 1954, have unanimously agreed upon certain basic principles concerning the practice of pathology.

1. Since the American Medical Association recognized pathology as the practice of medicine, we request that you initiate action by the American Medical Association to bring

about approval and acceptance of this principle by the American Hospital Association and similar hospital organizations.

2. This acceptance by the hospital association should specifically accord a pathologist all right and privileges extended to other practitioners of medicine.

3. These privileges include the right to render pathology services on a fee-for-service basis. In accordance with the American Medical Association principles regarding consultations and doctor-patient relationship, the fee-for-service should be a direct transaction between the pathologist and the patient.

4. All pre-payment insurance contracts should conform to these principles.

5. For the execution of these principles and for the protection of the entire medical profession, there should be created physician-hospital relationship committees on national, state, and local levels."

James P. Dewar, M.D., Secretary
Oklahoma Association of Pathologists

RESOLUTION

WHEREAS, the practice of radiology, pathology, and anesthesiology has been repeatedly defined as the practice of medicine by the House of Delegates of the American Medical Association; and

WHEREAS, radiologists, pathologists, and anesthesiologists are licensed practitioners of medicine in the State of Oklahoma; and

WHEREAS, radiologists, pathologists, and anesthesiologists are members of their county and state medical societies; and

WHEREAS, as members of these societies they are bound by the same code of ethics as all other physicians who are members of these societies; and

WHEREAS, the Oklahoma State Medical Association has not previously defined pathology and anesthesiology as the practice of medicine;

THEREFORE, BE IT RESOLVED, that the Oklahoma State Medical Association does hereby recognize pathology, radiology, and anesthesiology as the practice of medicine."

Respectfully submitted by
Walter E. Brown, M. D. (Signed)
President
Oklahoma State Radiological Society

Emil E. Palik, M.D. (Signed)
Chairman of Legislative Committee
Oklahoma Association of Pathologists

H. B. Stewart, M.D. (Signed)
Chairman of Legislative Committee
Oklahoma Association of Pathologists

H. B. Stewart, M.D. (Signed)
Chairman of Legislative Committee
Oklahoma Society of Anesthesiologists

RESOLUTION

Requesting the Appointment of a Committee or Subcommittee on Physician-Hospital Relationship

WHEREAS, in the practice of medicine, there are various problems confronting physicians and hospitals in their relations one with another, and

WHEREAS, in an effort to avoid misunderstandings between physicians and hospitals, the American Medical Association has recommended to its component societies that a committee or subcommittee on physician-hospital relationships be appointed, and

WHEREAS, there is need in the State of Oklahoma for such a committee

THEREFORE BE IT RESOLVED, that there be appointed by the Oklahoma State Medical Association or by its officers a committee or subcommittee on physician-hospital relationships, the number of members of which committee and its personnel to be determined by the president in conformity with the provisions of Section 7, Chapter IX of the By-laws.

Respectfully submitted by,
Walter E. Brown, M.D., (Signed)
President
Oklahoma State Radiological Society

Emil E. Palik, M.D., (Signed)
Chairman of Legislative Committee
Oklahoma Association of Pathologists

H. B. Stewart, M.D. (Signed) ·
Chairman of Legislative Committee
Oklahoma Society of Anesthesiologists

Doctor Phelps moved the adoption of this Section of the report. Motion seconded and carried.

Next, Doctor Phelps read a Resolution from the Tulsa County Medical Society. He advised that the Committee recommended the adoption of this Resolution with the following stipulation: "That dues to the A.M.A. must also have been paid by the physician who is reciprocating," and so moved. Motion seconded and carried. The Resolution as adopted was as follows:

RESOLUTION

WHEREAS, it has come to the attention of the Tulsa County Medical Society that the Oklahoma State Medical Association has no provisions whereby physicians transferring their membership from another state membership dues paid during the current year to the state Medical association from which the transferring physician comes, and

WHEREAS, most state medical associations have a reciprocal policy whereby such credit is given,

NOW, THEREFORE BE IT RESOLVED: That any physician transferring to the Oklahoma State Medical Association from another state Medical association, who shall give evidence of having paid his state membership dues in full for the current year to the state medical Association from which he comes, and to the A.M.A., shall not be required to pay dues to the Oklahoma State Medical Association for the balance of the current year, and

BE IT FURTHER RESOLVED: That the Council shall have the authority to make regulations governing the application and enforcement of this resolution as a guide for the Executive Offices.

Respectfully submitted by the Tulsa County Medical Society, May 9, 1954, at the direction of and with the approval of the membership."

Doctor Phelps next read the following section of the Report of the Committee:

"Your Committee considered certain communication sent to the Oklahoma State Medical Association by certain civic organizations with reference to the closing of certain Indian Hospitals in the State.

Your Committee feels that this subject has been adequately covered by previous action of the Council of the Oklahoma State Medical Association."

Doctor Phelps moved that this section of the report be adopted. Motion seconded and carried.

Doctor Phelps moved the adoption of the Report of the Resolutions Committee as a whole. Motion seconded and carried.

The next item of business was the election of Officers. The Speaker read the slate of nominees and called attention to the fact that they had all been nominated without opposition. I. W. Bollinger, M.D., Henryetta, moved: "That all of the nominees be elected by acclamation". Motion seconded and carried: The following officers were elected:

President Elect — R. Q. Goodwin, M.D., Oklahoma City

Delegate to the A.M.A. for two years James Stevenson, M.D., Tulsa

Alternate Delegate to the A.M.A. for two years E. H. Shuller, M.D., McAlester

Vice-President — Clifford Bassett, M.D., Cushing

Speaker of the House of Delegates Clinton Gallaher, M.D., Shawnee

Vice-Speaker of the House of Delegates Keiller Haynie, M.D., Durant

District 2
Councilor—E. C. Mohler, M.D., Ponca City
Vice-Councilor—Glen McDonald, M.D., Pawhuska

District 5
Councilor—A. L. Johnson, M.D., El Reno
Vice-Councilor—Ross Deputy, M.D., Clinton

District 8
Wilkie Hoover, M.D., Tulsa
Vice-Councilor—Wendell L. Smith, Tulsa

District 10
Councilor—Paul Kernek, M.D., Holdenville
Vice-Councilor—C. D. Lively. M.D., McAlester

District 11
Councilor—A. T. Baker, M.D., Durant
Vice-Councilor—Thomas E. Rhea, M.D., Idabel

District 14
Councilor—J. B. Hollis, M.D., Mangum
Vice-Councilor—R. R. Hannas, M.D., Sentinel

District 6
Councilor—Elmer Ridgeway, M.D., Oklahoma City
Vice-Councilor—P. E. Russo, M.D., Oklahoma City

Louis Ritzhaupt, M.D., Guthrie, moved that the Council Report be accepted by the House of Delegates. Motion seconded and carried.

There being no further business, the meeting was adjourned.

Reported By: Mary O'Leary

Film Catalog Available

The revised catalog of medical and health films now available from the American Medical Association's Committee on Medical Motion Pictures may be obtained on request. The booklet gives brief descriptions of more than 100 films.

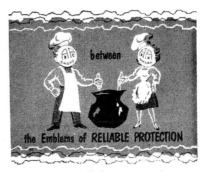
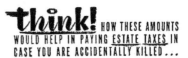
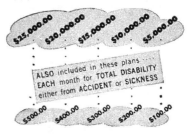

A. M. A. Transactions Reveal State and County
Society Study of Former Controversies

Fee splitting, osteopathy, closed panel medical care plans, veterans' medical care and the training of foreign medical school graduates were among the major subjects of discussion and action during the sessions of the House of Delegates at the 103rd Annual Meeting of the American Medical Association held June 21-25 in San Francisco. Delegates presented formalized opinions showing study of issues by their state and county societies.

Named president-elect was Elmer Hess, M.D., Erie, Pa., who had been serving as a member of the House of Delegates and as Chairman of the Council on Medical Service. Walter B. Martin, M.D., Norfolk, Va., took office as president during the San Francisco meeting.

Summary of the action taken by the House is as follows:

Fee Splitting

" . . . The Judicial Council is still of the opinion that when two or more physicians actually and in person render service to one patient they should render separate bills.

"There are cases, however, where the patient may make a specific request to one of the physicians attending him that one bill be rendered for the entire services. Should this occur it is considered to be ethical if the physician from whom the bill is requested renders an itemized bill setting forth the services rendered by each physician and the fees charged. The amount of the fee charged should be paid directly to the individual physicians who rendered the services in question.

"Under no circumstances shall it be considered ethical for the physician to submit joint bills unless the patient specifically requests it and unless the services were actually rendered by the physicians as set out in the bill."

Osteopathy and Medicine

"The justification or lack of justification of the 'cultist' appellation of modern osteopathic education could be settled with finality and to the satisfaction of most fair-minded individuals by direct on-campus observation and study of osteopathic schools. The Committee, therefore, proposed to the Conference Committee of the American Osteopathic Association that it obtain permission for the Committee for the Study of Relations between Osteopathy and Medicine to

visit schools of osteopathy for this purpose."

Closed Panel Plans

The House of Delegates adopted the report of the reference committee recommending that the House of Delegates request the Judicial Council to . . . investigate the relations of physicians to prepaid medical care plans and render such interpretations of the Principles of Medical Ethics as the Council deems necessary, and report to the House of Delegates not later than the next annual meeting.

Veterans' Medical Care

"It is the opinion of the Committee that the time is at hand when the American Medical Association and its component societies should go all out in preventing the unscientific determination of service-connected disabilities, by legislative presumption, and that we respectfully request that copies of these resolutions be transmitted to the Congress of the United States and other appropriate federal agencies."

Foreign Medical Graduates

Much of the time in the hearings of the Reference Committee on Medical Education and Hospitals was devoted to the evaluation of graduates of foreign medical schools. It was evident that not only the medical school education of many of these graduates is entirely inadequate, but their preliminary and premedical education falls far below the standard of this country. Further study was advised and report is to be made at the 1954 Interim Session.

Registration of Hospitals

The House approved discontinuing Registration by the Council on Medical Education and Hospitals and recommended this service be transferred to the Joint Commission on Accreditation of Hospitals.

Addresses

Edward McCormick, M.D., outgoing President, advised the profession to be realistic in the matter of fees and to adopt average fee schedules in local areas.

Doctor Martin stressed the necessity of increasing the availability of hospital services to a greater number of people by more equitable financing of these services. He advised physicians to take a more active part in civic affairs and in problems affecting public welfare.

Why 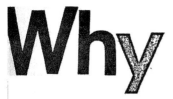 is it, Doctor, that <u>one</u> filter cigarette gives so much more protection than any other?

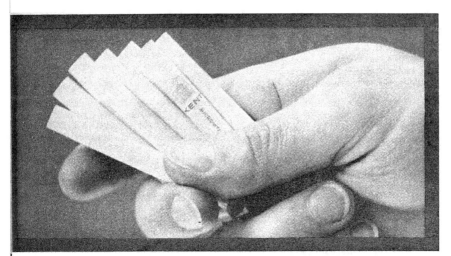

The answer is simply this: Among today's nine brands of filter cigarettes, KENT, and KENT alone, has the *Micronite Filter* ... made of a pure, dust-free material that is so safe, so effective it has been selected to help filter the air in hospital operating rooms.

In continuing and repeated impartial scientific tests, KENT's Micronite Filter consistently proves that it takes out *more* nicotine and tars than *any* other filter cigarette, old or new.

And yet, with all its superior protection, KENT's Micronite Filter lets smokers enjoy the full, satisfying flavor of fine, mellow tobaccos.

For these reasons, Doctor, shouldn't KENT be the choice of those who want the minimum of nicotine and tars in their cigarette smoke?

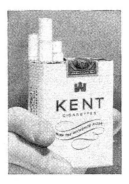

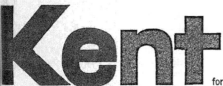

... the <u>only</u> cigarette with the
MICRONITE FILTER

for the greatest protection in cigarette history

T" AND "MICRONITE" ARE REGISTERED TRADEMARKS OF P. LORILLARD COMPANY

Deaths

LEWIS J. MOORMAN, M.D.
1875-1954

Lewis J. Moorman, M. D., Oklahoma City, editor of the *Journal* since 1938, died August 2 in an Oklahoma City hospital.

Because of his long and active service as editor of the *Journal* and many other contributions to the profession, the October issue of the *Journal* will be dedicated to Doctor Moorman and complete biographical information will appear in that issue.

GEORGE W. BAKER, M.D.
1873-1954

George W. Baker, M.D., pioneer Walters physician, died July 15 following an extended illness.

Doctor Baker was born June 10, 1873, at Sneed, Ala. He received his medical education in Atlanta, Georgia, and practiced more than 50 years in Alabama, Oklahoma and Texas.

Survivors include Mrs. Baker and six children.

T. F. RENFROW, M.D.
1871-1954

T. F. Renfrow, M.D., long-time Noble county physician, died July 8 in a Little Rock hospital.

Doctor Renfrow made the run at the opening of the Cherokee Strip September 16, 1893, and homesteaded between Garber and Billings. Later he moved to White Rock but moved back to Billings later. He left Billings about 10 years ago to enter the Arkansas hospital.

H. A. STALKER, M.D.
1871-1954

H. A. Stalker, M.D., Pond Creek physician for 50 years, died July 18 after several months' illness.

Doctor Stalker was born at Durant, Ill., September 14, 1871. After completing his medical education, he practiced for seven years at Fitgerald, Georgia, coming to Pond Creek about 1903.

He was active in medical organizations and in his hobby, trap shooting, in which he had received many local and national honors.

S. W. Surgical Congress
To Meet in Oklahoma City

The Sixth Annual Meeting of the Southwestern Surgical Congress will be held in Oklahoma City September 20-21-22 at the Skirvin Hotel.

Registration will be 1:00-4:00 p.m., Sunday, September 19, and 8:00 a.m. to 5:00 p.m. each day of the meeting.

Twenty-seven scientific papers will be presented. Round table luncheons will be held each day.

Guest speakers will be John M. Waugh, A.B., M.D., M.S., Professor, Mayo Foundation; Staff, St. Mary's and Colonial Hospitals, Rochester, Minn.; Alton Ochsner, B.A., M.D., Sc.D., School of Medicine, Department of Surgery, Tulane University of Louisiana, New Orleans; and Zeph J. R. Hollenbeck, B.A., M.D., Professor of Obstetrics and Gynecology, Ohio State University, Columbus.

Complete information concerning the program may be obtained from the central office of the Congress, 207 Plaza Court Building, Oklahoma City 3, Okla.

C. R. Rountree, M.D., Oklahoma City, is secretary of the Congress.

Annual Seminar Held at McAlester

The annual "Clinical and Cancer Symposium" was held Sunday, August 8, at the McAlester Clinic.

Speakers and their topics were as follows: Thurman Shuller, M.D., "Rectal Bleeding in Infants;" B. T. Galbraith, M.D., "Surgery in Patients with Heart Disease;" F. D. Switzer, M.D., "Retinal Manifestations of Vascular Sclerosis;" S. L. Norman, M.D., "Management of Diabetics;" A. R. Stough, M.D., "Carcinoma of the Prostate;" H. C. Wheeler, M.D., "Pressure Transfusions;" C. K. Holland, M.D., "Demonstration of Gastroscope;" George M. Brown, Jr., M.D., "Carcinoma of the Lower Gastro-intestinal Tract;" and Bruce H. Brown, M.D., "Diagnostic Procedures." The seminar was concluded with a tour of the clinic conducted by John A. Rowland, Business Manager.

VERILOID®

A POTENT, NOTABLY SAFE HYPOTENSIVE

Veriloid, the alkavervir extract of the hypotensive principles fractionated from Veratrum viride, presents these desirable properties in the management of hypertension.

- Uniform potency and constant pharmacologic action assured by biologic assay ..

- Blood pressure lowered by centrally mediated action; no ganglionic or adrenergic blocking, therefore virtually no risk of postural hypotension ..

- Cardiac output not reduced; no tachycardia ..

- Cerebral blood flow not decreased ..

- Renal function unaffected ..

- Tolerance or idiosyncrasy rarely develops; hence Veriloid is well suited to long-term use in severe hypertension ..

- Notably safe ... no dangerous toxic effects ... no deaths attributed to Veriloid have been reported in over five years of broad use in literally hundreds of thousands of patients ..

- Side actions of sialorrhea, substernal burning, nausea and vomiting (due to overdosage) are readily overcome and avoided by dosage adjustment.

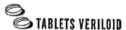

TABLETS VERILOID

Supplied in 2 mg. and 3 mg. slow-dissolving scored tablets, in bottles of 100. Initial daily dosage, 8 or 9 mg., given in divided doses, not less than 4 hours apart, preferably after meals.

SOLUTION INTRAVENOUS

For prompt reduction of critically elevated blood pressure in hypertensive emergencies. Extent of reduction is directly within the physician's control. In boxes of six 5 cc. ampuls with complete instructions.

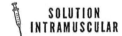

SOLUTION INTRAMUSCULAR

For maintenance of reduced blood pressure in critical instances, and for primary use in less urgent situations. Single dose reaches maximum hypotensive effect in 60 to 90 minutes, lasts 3 to 6 hours. Boxes of six 2 cc. ampuls with complete instructions.

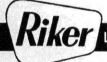

Riker LABORATORIES, INC. Los Angeles 48, California

Have You Heard?

BILL J. SIMON, M.D., Perry, left recently for active duty with the army. He reported to Fort Sam Houston.

ORVILLE HOLT, M.D., has established his practice in Claremore.

BAILEY LEON DIETRICH, M.D., University of Oklahoma School of Medicine graduate, has joined CARL HALLFORD, M.D., in practice in Boise City at the Hall Memorial Clinic.

J. R. HENKE, M.D., formerly of Hydro, has moved to Oklahoma City and is taking a residency at University Hospital.

JAMES T. BOGG, M.D., formerly of Shawnee, and LAWRENCE E. THOMPSON, M.D., a graduate of the University of Oklahoma who has just completed a residency at Ann Arbor, Mich., have joined JACK C. MILEHAM, M.D., in his new clinic at Chandler.

WILLIAM ISHMAEL, M.D. and RICHARD PAYNE, M.D., both of Oklahoma City, presented a symposium "Collagen Disorders, Especially Rheumatoid Arthritis" before the Lubbock-Crosby County Medical Society, Lubbock, Texas, July 6.

ANCEL EARP, JR., M.D., has joined the LeRoy Long Clinic, Oklahoma City.

EMIL PALIK, M.D. and IRON H. NELSON, M.D. announced the opening of the Palik-Nelson Laboratory in Tulsa.

L. I. JACOBS, JR., M.D., 1953 graduate of the University of Oklahoma School of Medicine, has joined the staff of the Henryetta Hospital.

C. W. ROBERTSON, M.D., Chandler, spoke to the Lions club of that city recently on his voyages to South America as ship doctor.

C. B. PINKERTON, M.D., 1953 graduate of the University of Oklahoma School of Medicine, has joined W. R. BYNUM, M.D., in Pryor.

KIEFFER DAVIS, M.D., Bartlesville, will give two papers at the Industrial Health Conference to be held in Houston September 23.

JOHN FLOYD, M.D., has opened his office in Comanche.

LLOYD JUDD, M.D., Pawnee, has joined JOHN G. ROLLINS, M.D., Prague, in the Rollins Clinic.

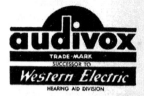
Medicolegal Institute Held

Attendance at the first Medicolegal Institute held at the University of Oklahoma July 8-9 was attended by 169 persons, 31 of whom were physicians.

Members of the Oklahoma State Medical Association appearing on the program were: Hayden H. Donahue, M.D., State Director of Mental Health; Harold B. Witten, M.D., Superintendent, Central State Hospital, Norman; Frank Adelman, M.D., Superintendent; Western State Hospital, Fort Supply; John Meyer, M.D., Director of Research and Education, Central State Hospital, Norman; E. F. Lester, M.D., Oklahoma City; Howard Hopps, M.D., Oklahoma City; R. Q. Goodwin, M.D., Oklahoma City, Sterling T. Crawford, M.D., Oklahoma City; Howard B. Shorbe, M.D., Oklahoma City; and William Schottstaedt, M.D., Oklahoma City.

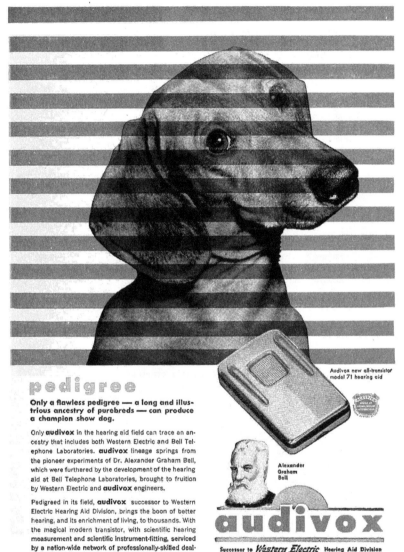

pedigree

Only a flawless pedigree — a long and illustrious ancestry of purebreds — can produce a champion show dog.

Only **audivox** in the hearing aid field can trace an ancestry that includes both Western Electric and Bell Telephone Laboratories. **audivox** lineage springs from the pioneer experiments of Dr. Alexander Graham Bell, which were furthered by the development of the hearing aid at Bell Telephone Laboratories, brought to fruition by Western Electric and **audivox** engineers.

Pedigreed in its field, **audivox** successor to Western Electric Hearing Aid Division, brings the boon of better hearing, and its enrichment of living, to thousands. With the magical modern transistor, with scientific hearing measurement and scientific instrument-fitting, serviced by a nation-wide network of professionally-skilled dealers, **audivox** moves forward today in a proud tradition.

TO THE DOCTOR: Send your patient with a hearing problem to a career Audivox and Micronic dealer, chosen for his interest, integrity and ability. There is such an Audivox dealer in every major city from coast to coast.

Audivox new all-transistor model 71 hearing aid

Alexander Graham Bell

audivox

Successor to *Western Electric* Hearing Aid Division

123 Worcester St., Boston, Mass.
The Pedigreed Hearing Aid

Reprints, Books, Journals Equipment Requested

The Journal has received a letter from Dr. T. K. Thomas, Medical Superintendent of St. George's Mission Hospital, Punalur, P. O., Travancore, S. India, which reads in part as follows:

"The Hospital is a non-profit organization situated in a hilly village and working among the poor labor classes of the locality and its suburbs. As good medical literatures are very few in this part of the world, a small library is started recently, attached to the above Hospital with the idea of collecting used medical journals, books, bulletins, reprints of articles and transactions of medical societies from all available sources in foreign countries so that up-to-date knowledge in medical practice may be obtained.

"Further Ayurvedic and Unani systems of medicine are very troublesome competitors to Allopathic systems here and proper equipment and medical literature are highly essential for the successful management of the Hospital."

Editorials

This Issue

It was the desire of the President of the Association, Bruce Hinson, M.D., that an issue of the *Journal* be dedicated to Lewis J. Moorman, M.D. The editors only regret that they didn't think of the idea first. The enthusiastic willingness of the contributors attests again to the love and respect for him. We wish to thank the Southern Medical Association for permission to reprint "We Owe a Cock to Aesculapius." The editorials below were found in their original draft in pencil in Doctor Moorman's study.

Disease, Disaster, and Achievement

As one studies the history of medicine it is interesting to see how disease in individuals or en masse may change the fate of nations and alter the history of the world. Space will not permit full elaboration of the theme but it is a most intriguing pursuit.

A few examples will reveal its possibilities. Alexander the Great in the latter days of his life developed symptoms attributable to the hypothalamus, hypersomnia and fits of savage anger. In all probability he slept away some of his opportunities to further mold the course of world history. Plutarch indicated that he would sleep from suppertime until noon the next day and sometimes all day. Was Alexander corrupted by Oriental influences or was disease responsible for the change in his character?

Napoleon developed hypothalamic symptoms. In his younger days he thought a few hours sleep quite sufficient and that more sleep represented unpardonable waste of time. By 1813 he had developed symptoms that might have represented disease of the hypothalamus. At the battle of Dresden his indecision converted success into defeat. According to W. R. Bett, M.D., he tarried at Dresden a whole month sleeping most of the time. It is said he was sleeping when a bridge was blown up too early at the battle of Leipzig to consummate his retreat. Fin-

ally, at the battle of Waterloo, he was six hours late because of his own extreme prostration. In this time the Duke of Wellington's army was reinforced and the victory won while Napoleon slept. Bett wonders how history would stand today if he could have had a judicious dose of Benzedrine at the critical time.

Napoleon's early life may have been conditioned by the toxins of his tuberculosis. The autopsy revealed the evidence in the upper lobe of the left lung. While tuberculosis usually spells disaster, it may lead to great achievement. Leaving out of consideration its alleged stimulation of the mind, two or three cases are briefly cited to show how it may shape one's destiny.

Cecil Rhodes leaving Oxford University because of a pulmonary hemorrhage traveled to Africa in search of health, discovered great wealth, changed the course of empire and ultimately gave us the Rhodes Scholarships.

John Hunter working in pathology in London spat blood, thought he should have a change; joined an island military campaign and learned enough to produce his remarkable monograph on "Gunshot Wounds."

William Withering never found time to give the medical world his treatise on foxglove until he had a hemorrhage and was sent to the country 10 years after accumulation of all data on the subject. Fisher Ames, fired by the toxemia of his tuberculosis and urged on by the short shrift of life was able through the pathos of his wasted body and the force of his uninhibited oratory to bring about the passage of the Jay Treaty. Thus our country was saved by ". . . a young lawyer, feeble in health but burning, after the manner of some consumptives, with intellectual and moral fire which strangely belied his slender thread of physical life."

This theme followed through to completion and publication would laden library shelves with learned literature. Who will pursue the intriguing research and place the story on the line?

A Great Showman in a Funny World

According to Homer Croy, Will Rogers appeared on the stage of life a few jumps ahead of the doctor who had been delayed by high water. Croy quotes colored Clement Vann Rogers, then six years of age, who had driven his mother helter-skelter six miles across the plains after receiving the runner's message, "Come quick, Mrs. Clem wants you desperate bad. There's a birth comin'." In the adjoining kitchen with the other colored people, he was one of the wide eyed auditors at Will Rogers first performance and this is what he told Croy many years later. "Finally, there was a terrible screetch and then a lot of little cries like a pig under a gate."

Thus "our own Will Rogers" came upon the stage with humor in his first act. His ever mounting showmanship ultimately covered the world. While his name is on every Oklahoman's lips, the details of his incredible life story are not as well known as they should be. One of the most readable, revealing and rewarding of all the writings about this remarkable personality is this gripping, humorous, *Our Will Rogers*, by Homer Croy. I recommend it to every busy physician, especially to those who think they cannot find time to go fishing.

This story contains the first official account of the extent and character of the injuries sustained by Will Rogers and Wiley Post on their ill fated flight. The details were first given to Croy in an interview with the missionary physician and his wife, a trained nurse, who received the bodies at the little Barrow Missionary Hospital. They worked all night trying to restore the mangled bodies to semblance of the normal and resolved never to reveal the horrible picture. But back in the states, in their home, the doctor conferred with his wife and nurse and decided to place the facts on record.

Apropos our History of Medicine project which includes Indian medicine, it is interesting to note how Indian blood races through our history and how Indian names dominate our geography and dot the pages of our records and our literature.

World traveler Will Rogers, one-quarter Cherokee, born in a log house at Oolagah, Cooweescoowee District, last seen and last heard by the Eskimo Clair Okpeaha at Walakpa Lagoon off the Polar Sea, is now in the simple crypt at the Will Rogers Memorial at Claremore where daily more than a thousand visitors pass and humbly incline their hatless heads. They read this tribute to Will and Wiley and are better for having passed this way.

> *"Oh death—how seldom do you get*
> *Courage and laughter in one net."*
>
> —Ada Jackson

The Committee on the History of Medicine would like to have all available authentic information about the fortunate doctor who arrived in time to announce Will's first appearance on the stage.

As We Knew Him

DICK GRAHAM, *Executive Secretary*

Fifteen years ago in a trip to the southeastern part of Oklahoma, I was privileged to learn in so brief a time a philosophy of life that will stand the test of time. This philosophy was that of a physician who was a scholar and a gentleman, but more particularly a humble man. This philosophy was simple and in my own interpretation could be aptly stated in these words: "Malice towards none."

During the intervening 15 years Doctor Moorman served not only faithfully and well as the Secretary-Editor of the Oklahoma State Medical Association, but more particularly shared the joys and sorrows of those with whom he worked with in the Executive Office. Rare was the day that he did not have a cheery word or an interesting anecdote to relate to all of us.

Others have written of his scientific accomplishments, his literary works, his teachings and his honors, but to those of us who knew him so intimately, he never wore these accomplishments. He only wore the spirit of friendship and understanding.

Lewis Jefferson Moorman, M.D., met the measure of Teddy Roosevelt's expression that every man owed some of his time to the profession to which he belonged. Had Teddy Roosevelt extended his saying to include his fellowman, it would have been more aptly applicable to this distinguished physician to w h o m this edition of the *Journal* is dedicated.

"We Owe a Cock
to AESCULAPIUS . . . "

LEWIS J. MOORMAN, M.D.

By way of introduction, may I call your attention to Walter Moxon's beautiful tribute to truth:

"A golden thread has run throughout the history of the world, consecutive and continuous, the work of the best men in successive ages. From point to point it still runs, and when near, you feel it as the clear and bright and searchingly irresistible light which Truth throws forth when great minds conceive it."

While we may look upon scientific medicine as the child of our own times, a searching retrospective study with reference to its origin leads us far along the path of the golden thread. Though startled by the light of recent achievements, we follow on through the still glowing period of the Renaissance into the shadowy stretches of the Dark Ages, to emerge in the bright light of the glorious Hellenic period where Greek culture sprang like magic from Aegean shores. It was here under the favorable influence of the rare Greek genius with its peculiar racial and environmental factors that scientific medicine found its germination. Through their frank intellectualism and their insatiate yearning for truth, with a level gaze focused on the course of nature, the people of this unprecedented age added an unwonted glow to the golden thread of truth. Brightest among their contributions are the time-resisting fibers which medicine spun from the outworn fabric of magic and religious dogma.

In the Fifth Century, B.C., Thucydides, the first scientific historian, the first constructive critic, had spurned the credulity of Herodotus and was subjecting everything to the test of truth. Pericles proclaimed the cause of Justice with majesty and gravity, excelling "the course of ordinary orators." Euripides, Aeschylus, Aristophanes and Sophocles, the world's first great dramatists, had departed from the epic and lyric poe-

"We Owe a Cock to Aesculapius" was the President's address at the general session of the Southern Medical Association, November 15-18, 1932, Birmingham, Alabama, and is reprinted from the *Journal of the Southern Medical Association*, Vol. XXV, No. 12, Pages 1197-1202, December, 1932.

try and were presenting the bare truths of life with simple and impressive directness. Democritus, philosopher and founder of the atomic theory, succinctly expressed the theme of the Hellenic race when he said: "Wealth of thought, not wealth of learning, is the thing to be coveted." According to current rumor he had contemplated the destruction of his own sight in order that he might become better acquainted with his reason.

Socrates, the world's greatest philosopher, the incarnation of the genius of reason, was walking and teaching in the market place, logically solving the social, moral and political problems of his day, giving comfort to all who sought his advice. Was it not time for medicine to throw off the veil of mystery and submit to the law of reason? Evidently the Greek passion for truth found an abiding place in the mind of Hippocrates. Though the break with magic, religion and philosophy must have required much courage, the psychological moment had arrived. Hippocrates, the father of medicine, stood ready to receive and sustain the hardiest among the promising offspring of the youthful and prolific spirit of reason.

Democritus, the spiritual descendant of Thales, the advocate of the atomic theory, the student of cosmology, wrote: "O Hippocrates, to know the art of medicine—is at once a fine thing and useful in life." Hippocrates must have been greatly encouraged by the teaching and methods of Socrates, and when this great champion of the freedom of reason met the supreme test of the true scientist, sacrificing life for principle and achieving immortality through courageous submission to death, it is comforting to know that he employed his last words to exclaim: "Crito, we owe a cock to Aesculapius. Will you see that it is paid?" Whether we consider this the recognition of a personal obligation or as a final tribute to the virtue of medicine, it is nevertheless significant, coming from this great exponent of justice and virtue at a time in the world's history when the ideal of community service reached its highest level.

Socrates' logical thinking, his analytical approach to the moral and psychological problems of those who sought his advice, and his direct remedial methods may have had much to do with the bold departure of Hippocrates from the domination of religion, philosophy and magic. Certainly he accepted Socrates' simple teaching that "behind every living form there is the divine reality of life itself," with the added consciousness of life's legitimate demands upon the science of medicine.

In the words of William Osler:

> "Everywhere one finds a strong, clear common sense which refuses to be entangled either in theological or philosophical speculations. What Socrates did for philosophy, Hippocrates may be said to have done for medicine. As Socrates devoted himself to ethics and the application of right thinking to good conduct, so Hippocrates insisted upon the practical nature of the art, and in placing his highest good in the benefit of the patient. Empiricism, experience, the collection of facts, the evidence of the senses, the avoidance of philosophical speculations, were the distinguishing features of Hippocratic medicine."

Not only did Hippocrates lay a secure foundation for the science of medicine but he established for all time, within that science, the essential principles of moral and ethical conduct. Unfortunately the historians of the world have given little thought to medicine's luminous contributions to the golden thread of truth. However, we must credit Gomperz in his comprehensive work, "The Greek Thinkers," for referring to the Hippocratic oath as a "monument of the highest rank in the history of civilization." The recorded evidence of his wisdom is not limited to the immortal Hippocratic oath,

but we find it dominating the current of his aphorisms and other writings, mingling with contemporary streams of thought to participate in a world heritage, enriching the literature of all races. Striking evidence of this is found in his famous aphorism, "Life is short and Art is long; the occasion fleeting, experience fallacious, and judgment difficult," or in the following: "There are, in effect, two things to know, and to believe one knows; to know is science; to believe one knows is ignorance."

In the words of Euripides, medicine should be proud of an illustrious birth and its accompanying rank; and while with Plato we accept the renown of ancestors as a precious treasure, for our idealism we should return to the fountainhead and humbly receive from Homer the startling challenge: "We honor our name by becoming greater than our fathers."

In the Fourth Century, B.C., Aristotle, son of a physician, tracing his ancestry through Machaon to Aesculapius, became the world's first apostle of natural history and the rightful progenitor of all the positive sciences. At his famous school in the grove of Apollo, favorite haunt of Socrates, Aristotle established the first of the world's great libraries. Here he also founded the first museum of natural history and the first zoological gardens. Alexander the Great supported his studies in natural history and placed at his disposal eight hundred talents, the first recorded voluntary contribution for the sake of science. Aristotle mentions five hundred different kinds of animals and reports having dissected at least fifty. There is also evidence of his having dissected the human embryo.

He was far ahead of his day in many phases of natural science, including those which bear directly upon medicine, displaying an extraordinary knowledge of embryology, anatomy and physiology; also an amazing sense of sanitary science. After cautioning Alexander the Great against idleness or overwork on the part of his soldiers, he makes this astounding statement:

> "Do not let your men drink out of stagnant pools—Athenians, city born, know no better; and when you carry water on the desert marches, it should be first boiled to prevent its getting sour."

Though this advice was given twenty-three hundred years before the day of typhoid vaccine, it might have averted our national catastrophe at Chickamauga.

Aristotle helped to stabilize the teachings of Hippocrates and added the fundamental principles of scientific research. He was a voluminous writer and his works, like those of Hippocrates, were of sufficient interest and importance to carry through the centuries, penetrating the Dark Ages, participating in the revival of learning and guiding the early progress of science. Voltaire considered Aristotle's studies of animal life the best book of antiquity. In Darwin's "Life and Letter" we find the following:

"Linnaeus and Cuvier have been my two gods, but they were mere boys to old Aristotle."

The Third Century, B.C., is unique in the history of medicine because of the Alexandrian school. Here we have the world's first great university. There were four research schools, medicine, literature, mathematics, and astronomy; also a library with four hundred thousand volumes, one of the wonders of the world. All this came largely through Aristotle's influence over Alexander the Great. For five hundred years medical students from all parts of the world made their pilgrimages to the Alexandrian school. It is said that Galen traveled from Pergamus to Alexandria in order to see a skeleton. The founders of this school, Herophilus and Erasistratus, were perhaps the first to dissect the human body. Though we consider Vesalius of the Sixteenth Century the true father of human anatomy, in the words of Dr. W. W. Keen,

"If we wish to see its starting-point we must retrace our steps to the Third Century, B. C., and transfer ourselves from the Amphitheatre of Padua to that of Alexandria to discover the bold innovators who first forced the dead body to disclose its secrets for the benefit of the living."

After the First Century of the Alexandrian period there was no known dissection of the human body for at least twelve hundred years. However, the golden thread of truth received many distinct accretions during this period of Alexandrian supremacy.

We now turn to the first epoch-making Greek physician after Hippocrates. Galen.

the famous Pergamite, was born 130 A.D. He was an omnivorous observer with a knack for recording what he observed. He championed the teaching of Hippocrates and could not identify himself with any of the post-Hippocratic schools. In fact, he was often at daggers' points with the devotees of these various sects. While he considered Hippocrates his master, it is said he called slaves those who followed any man and that he reserved the right to choose the good wherever he found it.

Two of the most important periods of his life were spent in Rome. Though Rome conquered the world, Greek learning is said to have conquered Rome, and Galen was one of the chief participants in this conquest. Galen traveled widely and studied at all of the best schools, including Alexandria. Unfortunately the dissection of the human body had passed with Herophilus and Erasistratus. His limitations in this respect were a source of constant irritation. His anatomic conceptions were based upon the dissection of animals, chiefly pigs and apes. He and his students gathered bones from neglected graves and his followers were advised to go to Alexandria, where two skeletons were still intact. Naturally his osteology was much better than his visceral anatomy.

Though Harvey is considered the father of physiology, Galen was the first ardent student of this subject. He carried out extensive experiments, proving the function of the laryngeal nerves and the motor and sensory functions of the spinal nerves. His experiments included section and hemisection of the spinal cord. He proved that the arteries contain blood and not air; he observed the action of the heart; the function of the heart valves; the pulsation of the arteries under the force of the heart muscle, and he came astonishingly near the discovery of the circulation of the blood.

Though not endowed with the poise, simplicity and modesty which characterized the life of Hippocrates, Galen possessed a dominating personality. This, coupled with his comprehensive store of knowledge, not only enabled him to fix the standards for his own day but for fifteen hundred years to follow. His animal anatomy remained inviolate until Leonardo da Vinci's beautiful anatomic drawings served as a forerunner of Vesalius, who carefully studied the human body and gave to the world his "fabrica." Galen's laudable pus, though challenged by Paracelsus and Paré, remained laudable until the work of Lord Lister shattered the last claims of Galenism. The death of Galen marks the end of the creative period of Greek medicine. That the works of Hippocrates, Aristotle and Galen constitute the greatest legacy bequeathed to the world by ancient Greece is a fact that has never, even to our own day, been fully appreciatd.

It seems well to dwell upon this period, not only to show that scientific medicine had its origin here, but that it witnessed also the crystallization of a consciousness that science can thrive only in an atmosphere where the human mind is free to pursue its uncharted course. Here was distilled the choice nectar which gives added zest to every scientific adventure. With this in mind we pass hurriedly to consider epoch-making events and personalities in the succeeding history of medicine.

Athenian, Alexandrian and Roman culture withered under the blighting conquest of the barbarians. One wonders if Christianity may not have placed unwarranted emphasis upon the importance of death, judgment, heaven and hell. Only the base flesh of a corrupt body intercepted man's search for redemption. The Greek ideal of physical strength and beauty maintained by the science of medicine found little encouragement in the medieval period. Fortunately the teaching that the body is the temple of the soul was recognized by some of the clerics, especially the Benedictines. Their cloisters became the repositories of ancient medical literature and the study of medicine constituted a legitimate part of their intellectual pursuits.

Although we pass hurriedly through the desert of the Dark Ages, we should also acknowledge our indebtedness to South Italian schools. The language employed in these schools was Greek, and here medicine found its refuge through the Middle Ages, and medical students were taught under the authority of Hippocrates and Galen. We also give credit to Byzantine and Arabian medicine, where the current of Greek thought and teaching supplied and preserved many valuable manuscripts on medicine, later to be cast upon the shores of the Renaissance, the most famous addition being the work of Avicenna, Eleventh Century, A.D.

In the Thirteenth Century, the rise of the universities helped to collect, assimilate and preserve the existing knowledge of medicine. Here we have the first faint glimmer of light which in the Fifteenth Century ultimately emerged from the medieval period with a steadily increasing glow. It has been said that "Greece arose from the dead with the New Testament in one hand and Aristotle in the other." Aristotle, Hippocrates and Galen furnished the foundation for medical teaching. The leaders of medicine in the Sixteenth Century were steeped in the knowledge of the old humanities, translating and editing the works of Hippocrates, Aristotle and Galen; many of them teaching Greek and Latin and otherwise enriching the world through their erudition.

The arrogant Paracelsus, living in the first part of the Sixteenth Century, possessing the spirit of intellectual freedom, deserves credit for having the courage to break away from the dogmatic dominion of the schools of his day with their fixed teachings of fifteen centuries and for his valuable contributions in practical chemistry and pharmacy. No doubt the independence of Paracelsus prepared the way for the next great nonconformist who has been designated the father of anatomy.

Vesalius, who came from Belgium, was elected to the chair of anatomy in Padua in the year 1537. Here he found freedom of thought and action such as he had not been permitted to exercise in Louvain or Paris. As we have noted, for many centuries following the Alexandrian period the human body had not been dissected. Immediately prior to the time of Vesalius, dissections must have been only occasional. The anatomy taught was atrocious. The great teachers of anatomy were Galenists, and they dared not depart from his teaching, even though their eyes revealed the fact that his descriptions failed to conform to nature as exhibited in the human body.

Vesalius had been a fellow student under Sylvius with the ill-fated Servetus, who was burned alive at Geneva because he discovered the lesser circulation and made bold to declare it. Inspired by a desire to familiarize himself with the structure of the human body, encouraged by the tardy but growing tolerance of his contemporaries and the unprecedented wealth of material, Vesalius industriously pursued his purposes with the "Fabrica" as the ultimate result. He boldly corrected and supplemented the work of Galen and finally, when only twenty-eight years of age, after five years of untiring effort, his manuscripts were ready and plans for the publication of one of the world's greatest books were under way. He gave up his routine work in order to devote himself wholly to the consuming desire to give to the world an accurate, artistic and lasting description of the entire anatomy of the human body. His estimate of the importance of this great work has been fully justified by the results. It is of interest to note that Montanus, who first taught medicine at the bedside, was his colleague and may have been indebted to Vesalius for his topographical anatomy.

Approximately fifty years after Vesalius had completed his work at Padua, we find William Harvey receiving his degree after four years' work in the same school. We can imagine Harvey assisting his famous teacher, Fabricius, with his dissections for the purpose of demonstrating the valves in the veins. The position of these valves later caused Harvey to undertake his monumental investigation which led to the discovery of the circulation and fixed him in the history of medicine as the father of physiology. Harvey's work on the circulation of the blood represents the first great well ordered bit of experimental research for the purpose of determining the function of an important organ of the body. The modern spirit of investigation was perfected as Harvey uncovered the mystery which had troubled Aristotle two thousand years before and which barely escaped Galen in the Second Century, A.D. It would be difficult to estimate the influence of Harvey's work in the progress of medicine; suffice it to say in his own words he has taught that "nature herself must be our adviser; the path she

walks must be our walk," and that we should blush "to credit other men's traditions only."

It is said that the first chemical laboratory in Europe was established at Leyden by Franciscus Sylvius, who, in addition, seems to have perfected bedside teaching. In 1664 he gave the following account of his clinical methods:

> "I have led my pupils by the hand to medical practice, using a method unknown at Leyden, or perhaps elsewhere, i. e., taking them daily to visit the sick at the public hospital. There I have put the symptoms of disease before their eyes; have let them hear the complaints of the patients, and have asked them their opinions as to the causes and rational treatment of each case, and the reasons for those opinions. Then I have given my own judgment on every point. Together with me they have seen the happy results of treatment when God has granted to our cases a restoration of health; or they have assisted in examining the body when the patient has paid the inevitable tribute to death."

With anatomy and physiology supporting this type of clinical investigations, the rise of modern medicine was assured. At this period Morgagni reenforced the foundation by adding morbid anatomy. Sydenham, through his teaching that "all disease could be described as natural history," shielded medicine of his day from many errors, false theories and mischievous prejudices. Boerhaave, the Dutch Hippocrates, following the lead of Sylvius, Morgagni and Sydenham, made a great contribution through a galaxy of well trained and widely scattered pupils, among whom were the founders of the Vienna school. John Hunter not only embodied the spirit of these great teachers, but he introduced experimental pathology and laid the foundation for all medical museums and pathological collections. He materially influenced the course of medicine in Europe and had much to do with the early history of medicine in America.

In the year 1798, Edward Jenner, to whom John Hunter had said, "Don't think, try!" published his experiments on vaccination for protection against smallpox. As a result, burying grounds became less popular, war less pestilential, and the sight of friends less painful as pitted faces became a thing of the past.

In the first quarter of the Nineteenth Century, the French school, through clinical pathological studies, materially advanced clinical medicine. Corvisart, Bichat, Laennec and Louis were supplementing Morgagni's principles with a more enlightened bedside study. Percussion was perfected and auscultation with the stethoscope added. Many new signs were elicited, distinct clinical entities discovered and recorded. Virchow advanced from Bichat's tissue pathology to cellular pathology. The microscope had revealed new anatomic secrets. Virchow had laid the foundation for many advances in diagnosis, pathology and therapeutics.

In 1842, Crawford W. Long first employed ether for surgical anesthesia, thus initiating medicine's greatest boon to suffering humanity, "the death of pain," through the birth of temporary oblivion. In the wake of anesthesia came the discovery of bacteria, a demonstration of their part in the causation of disease, the establishment of laboratories and the dawn of antiseptic surgery with asepsis near at hand. Though we pass hurriedly over this period, we must pay homage to such men as Pasteur, Robert Kock, Lister, Cohnheim, Metchnikoff, Ludwig, Weigert and Claude Bernard.

This brings us to the dawn of our own day. Many who are now within the reach of my voice recall the rosy tints of this scientific morning; the rapid diffusion of light and the ultimate glow of midday. As may be seen by this brief recital, the golden thread of truth has literally run consecutively and continuously from point to point through the history of medicine.

With few exceptions, the world's historians have failed to realize that "the history of medicine, in a sense, is the history of civilization." H. G. Wells, though not a scientist, writes as follows:

"When the intellectual history of this time comes to be written, nothing, I think, will stand out more strikingly than the empty gulf in quality between the superb and richly fruitful scientific investigations that are going on and the general thought of other educated sections of the community. I do not mean that scientific men are, as a whole, a class of supermen, dealing and thinking about everything in a way altogether better than the common run of humanity, but in their field they think and work with an intensity and integrity, a breadth, a boldness, patience, thoroughness, fruitfulness, excepting only a few artists, which puts their work out of all comparison with any other human activity. In these particular directions the human mind has achieved a new and higher quality of attitude and gesture, a veracity, a self-detachment and self-abrogating vigor of criticism that tends to spread out and must ultimately spread to every other human affair."

Pasteur, a true scientist, wrote:

"In our Century science is the soul of the prosperity of nations and the living source of all progress. Undoubtedly the tiring discussions of politics seem to be our guide—empty appearances! What really leads us forward is a few scientific discoveries and their application."

Voltaire, the friend of scientific medicine and the avowed enemy of charlatans, says:

"Men who are occupied in the restoration of health to other men by the joint exertion of skill and humanity, are above all the great of the earth. They even partake of divinity, since to preserve and renew is almost as noble as to create."

While we are busily engaged in the quiet, relentless, absorbing pursuit of truth, or in the "joint exertion of skill and humanity" in its application, we should find a historian who will give the annals of medicine their rightful place in the general history of the world. The people at large must be made to realize that medicine, through innumerable channels leading to prevention and cure, has saved more lives than have been lost through war, through natural and industrial catastrophe and the ravages of disease; that medicine has succeeded in reclaiming the waste places of the earth where money, man power and machinery have utterly failed; that the building and occupancy of great cities would be impossible if it were not for sanitary engineering; that the world's significant social and moral reforms would have been improbable without the contributions of medical science; that the progress of industry is to a great extent contingent upon the efficacy of public health and sanitation and that in the ultimate, the sum total of human happiness is largely dependent upon the progress of medical science.

In the rapid progess of this mechanistic age, few people realize how adequately medicine has met the exacting demands. If medical and sanitary science had not outstripped progress in other lines of endeavor, we should have been wiped from the face of the earth through improved transportation resulting in the sudden intermingling of all nations of the world with their varied diseases and their racial susceptibilities.

If our professional interests seem to be seriously threatened for the moment, may this not be largely due to our cherished altruistic traditions, our superficial methods of education and the present public absorbing interest in the general theme? Obviously a little learning is a dangerous thing. If we hope to retain public approval, and at the same time preserve our coveted independence, our necessary initiative, our individuality and our self-respect, we must teach the public the history of medicine, the heroic and sacrificial pursuit of pure science, the modest and conscientious application of its revealed truths.

Once the progress of medical science and its application to the needs of humanity are adequately appreciated, the best philosophers of our own day may be led to exclaim with Socrates, the father of them all: "We owe a cock to Aesculapius."

OSLER, *the Man*

LEWIS J. MOORMAN, M.D.

"Osler, the Man" was presented by Doctor Moorman before The Osler Club at the Royal College of Surgeons, London, July 12, 1949, commemorating Sir William Osler's hundredth birthday.

Without taking time adequately to acknowledge the unmerited honor this occasion confers upon me, I hasten to say that one hundred years ago on one of your far flung frontiers a strange, intangible force came into being. It was highly potential, creative, acquisitive, vitalizing, scintillating, contagious force; it was called William Osler; it became Osler the Man and ultimately the medical mentor for all mankind.

Though never having had the privilege of personal contact with Sir William Osler, through his writings, his pupils, his patients, his relatives and friends, I have achieved a spiritual intimacy with him which continues to grow.

When Mrs. Moorman and I were in London in 1909, I carried a letter of introduction from his student and admirer, Dr. Henry A. Christian of Harvard, but an emergency clipped our plans and opportunity passed forever.

I am proud to stand here as a representative of my country, one of the three in which Osler lived and worked and moved toward world wide influence and acclaim. Fortunately, the citizenry of these three countries, sharing a possessive interest were fused in the same crucible, speak the same language and live and die by the same ideals which reached a high tide in Sir William Osler, — the man.

Having been a doctor on horseback in a log cabin community, a horse and buggy doctor on the uncharted plains and finally a city practitioner where ultimately I walked the wards with colleagues and students I can claim a comprehensive appreciation of what Osler has meant to the American physician in all walks of life.

My association with Osler through the channels I have mentioned, was unusually close because it came through the gift of loneliness.

It began with the third edition of the

Principles and Practice of Medicine in 1899. This textbook well launched on its remarkable career turned the century with me, set the pattern for my country practice and remained my chief council and companion; it introduced me to Hippocrates and Plato and stirred strange new aspirations which were fanned into flame by his successive historical and cultural writings.

It was Osler who rode with me on the lonely trails and accompanied me into the cabin, the dugout, the sod house and the windswept prairie shack. It was he who sat with me at the bedside in attendance upon the sick. It was he who followed me to the city and became my mentor as physician, philosopher and teacher. It was he who taught me to exercise the heart equally with the head and to treat the purse as a secondary consideration.

It was he who gave me "The Leaven of Science", "The Master Word", "Unity, Peace, and Concord", "A Way of Life", and finally, "Equanimatas". It was Osler, the Man, who taught me to strive for something above the common level.

While conveying the art and science of medicine to his pupils he was giving comfort, health and life to his patients and yet he was living in the mystic realm "of the shadowland" always on guard for "Glimpses that might make us less forlorn". He knew that "the hopes and fears which make us men are inseparable" and bravely he trod the "wine press of doubt" that others might not be afraid. The things that created Osler, the Man, became the criteria for the young who came under his power and experienced love of youth.

In a recent meeting of the American Association of the History of Medicine at a great dinner session devoted to the theme we now pursue, I heard some of these one-time young men tell of this love. I had the honor of sitting with Mrs. Abbott, Sir William's niece, the cousin of W. H. Francis who last read to him and forged the final link between the man and his books and suggested this valedictory, "He prayeth best who loveth best all things both great and small." In addition to Mrs. Abbott's gracious response to the President's invitation, I was favored with intimate flashes from her memory. One of these is sufficient partially to explain Osler's intellectual ascendancy. At a gay informal dinner party he whispered in her ear, "Please excuse me, I have an appointment with Plato."

His facility for friendship, his personal charm, his magnetic appeal, his spontaneous mirth, his unmatched erudition, his artless exhibition of rare gifts and his unbounded generosity captivated all who came. Unlike Atlas, he never stooped to shoulder the world, but always kept his arms around it.

According to his own record he left Canada rich in the goods "which neither rust nor moth have been able to corrupt".

He left America saying truly:

"I have loved no darkness,
    sophisticated no truth,
    nursed no delusion,
    allowed no fear."

He left England with the last verses of "The Ancient Mariner" in his mind and a simple, affectionate "nighty-night" on his tongue. No doubt he had an appointment with the Master, perhaps with Plato, Thomas Brown, Robert Burton, Francis Adams, John Locke or Sydenham and not irreverently, we can imagine him whispering to one of these, "Excuse me, I have an appointment with Isaac Walton Junior (his son, Revere, killed in World War I) where enchanting trout streams flow in rhythmic beauty through Elysian Fields."

What You Should Know

ABOUT MEDICINE

LEWIS J. MOORMAN, M.D.

"What You Should About Medicine" was a
Special Article by Doctor Moorman that appeared in the May, 1950, issue of the *Journal of
the Oklahoma State Medical Association,* Vol.
43, No. 5.

Medicine was not sired by government.
On the contrary it found its birth in "The
primal sympathy of man for man". Thus
it became one of the most sacred of all
human relationships, ranking with the Divine right of worship. When this relationship is interferred with, medicine's highest
function is lost.

Modern medicine has reached its present
state of efficiency through an evolutionary
process. It is not the result of government
planning and like religion and freedom of
speech, it cannot survive government control. Through new discoveries, sanitary engineering and preventive measures it has
kept abreast with progress in other fields
of endeavor and made it possible for us
to survive the coming of "one world" and
the intermingling of the nations with their
varied racial diseases and susceptibilities.
Medicine has followed the course of nature
not the mandates of government. It has
met the needs of mankind as they have
arisen.

The function of medicine has been stifled
wherever government control has arisen. Experience in other countries shows that the
cost of government medicine rises as the
quality falls. There is no such thing as free
medicine except that voluntarily tendered
by the patient's private physician, at his
own expense, according to his present privilege as a free agent. The sum total of
this free service if paid for by the government would reach deep into the taxpayer's
pocketbook and rob the physician of the
chastening influence of this voluntary service.

Without exception nationalization of
medicine has been associated with national
decline. Only in small countries with homo-
genous socio-economic conditions has socialized medicine attained seeming success. But
it has been observed that the people from
these countries live longer when transplant-
ed to the U. S. where they have the benefit
of voluntary medical service under our system of free enterprise. The United States
is the most heterogenous nation in the
world and its citizenry the most independent, therefore, the least adaptable to any
form of socialized medicine. It is well
known that nationalized medicine, like other functions of the welfare state, destroys
individual initiative, honor and integrity,
discourages thrift and lessens the will to
produce. Thus the socialistic trend now
threatening the integrity of free enterprise
in the United States will reverse the character building principles upon which our
republican form of government was founded. From a medical standpoint this is important because successful medical care is
part of both patient and physician.

The hue and cry about the shortage of
physicians is largely a result of political
propaganda. The United States has more
physicians in proportion to population than
any other country in the world except Palestine where the profession is surcharged
with refugee doctors. We have the best
system of medical education and the most
nearly adequate medical school facilities in
the world for the training of physicians.
The fear of a serious shortage of physicians in the future is obviously unfounded
unless we enter another national emergency. The Federal Security Agency's bulletin recently published under the title,
"Health Service Areas" ostensibly to forecast the alleged shortage of doctors by 1960
is founded on false premises. It is inac-

curate in its local appraisals and estimates, and as has been suggested, it seems to have been molded to fit "assumed conclusions". This is significant in that the survey has cost the taxpayers a lot of money and its false conclusions are being employed to mislead the people and to highpower medical schools into Federal subsidy and the accompanying danger of control. Also the report unjustly becomes a part of the Federal Security Agency propaganda for compulsory health insurance. The same agency and socialistically minded politicians are overplaying the need of doctors in rural communities. This propaganda has penetrated the public mind and needs to be analyzed and counteracted by fair presentation of the facts. In Great Britain soon after the Health Act went into effect it was realized that the strain on the treasury, the profession and on the nursing service might be eased "quite as much by reducing the number of patients as by increasing the number of nurses and other services." This is an example of what the cold, impersonal hand of bureaucracy can do to people once they come under the rule of the welfare state.

Those who think doctors have deliberately limited the number of medical graduates should know that the number is determined by physical limitations of teaching facilities and not by the doctors engaged in medical education. The required buildings, laboratory equipment and hospital beds are the necessary facilities. This should come from local sources, either through appropriations by state legislatures or public philanthropy. During the past few years according to an editorial in the New England Medical Journal, seven four year medical schools have been added to those already in operation and five more are contemplated.

There are good reasons why doctors are not locating at the crossroads in rural communities as they did 50 years ago. Before the turn of the century the country doctor could make à living on typhoid fever, diphtheria, pneumonia and summer complaints. Immunity measures provided by medical discoveries have virtually eliminated typhoid and diphtheria. Sulfonamides, penicillin and aureomycin and other new drugs, have ren-

dered pneumonia much less ominous for the patient and much less profitable to the doctor. Refrigeration, sanitation, and improved medication have almost eliminated summer complaints. Improved roads, automobiles, and transportation by air, plus education with reference to clinics and hospitalization tend to whisk the patient by the country doctor while he is being penalized by the new medical publicity and motorized psychology. Considering modern transportation the country patient 50 to 100 miles from the nearest city relatively speaking is much closer to medical care than the patient living 10 miles from his country doctor fifty years ago. Under these circumstances, it is hardly fair to expect the well trained young doctor to invest 30 to 50 thousand dollars for sufficient modern facilities to stop the motored marathon toward city doctors. Are the people and the trend of the times to blame or must the medical profession be held responsible for the dearth of country doctors.

The communities in need of good doctors and desirous of scientific medical care should consider the feasibility of providing modern facilities for the well trained young doctor when one is available. Many of the medical schools are now encouraging students to consider the need of general practitioners in rural locations. Our own medical school is now stimulating interest in country practice by placing senior students with selected general practitioners in rural communities for valuable experience and training.

Apropos the alleged shortage of doctors it seems reasonable to consider the health and physical competency of the nation in the calculation. The population of the U.S. has been doubled since 1900. Average longevity is increasing at a rapid rate. At the turn of the century the lowest maternal mortality rate was 4.3. In 1947 the highest rate was 2.6. At the present time the whole national socio-economic status is being seriously upset by the increased birth rate, (sign of physical competency) the saving of life in infancy and the pyramiding of the old age group. Already the burden of old age pensions may be charged to the doctors. Certainly physicians are largely accountable for the above mentioned gains, whether they be considered national credits or debits. But the government gives no credit for these advances and paradoxically cries out for better medicine. The bureaucrats might do well to shoulder the responsibility of finding a better way of life for the ever increasing number of people who because of good medical care live longer and move faster than ever before. Must the people and the physicians accept a system of medical care which will rob them of the scientific, moral and spiritual values which have been responsible for the best medical service in the world. With the known inaccuracies of government bureau surveys and investigations and the administrative incompetency so flagrantly displayed from time to time and the susceptibility to political expediency does it seem reasonable to place our health and our lives in the cold impersonal hands of a government agency.

Our own Indian medical service supplies a shocking example of government failure. Though better managed and more adequately financed the medical department of the Veterans Administration has many shortcomings. Every effort has been made to bring it as nearly in line with civilian practices as government red tape allows and yet many a well meaning VA physician is still struggling through time consuming paper work toward patient welfare. These medical services should have careful study before compulsory health insurance is considered.

Forgetting medicine except as the administration's proposed beachhead for the conquest of all independent industry, should not every loyal citizen take his stand on the question of free enterprise based as it is on the sound principles laid down by our Founding Fathers.

Think of Jefferson, who wrote the Declaration of Independence and championed the constitution of the United States. Think of Washington, who with modesty matching his valor, declared his reluctance to accept the presidency because of the responsibility of building a republican form of government designed to keep alive the "sacred fire of liberty" and forever furnish a haven of safety from "oppression and misrule." Think of John Marshall who sought to safeguard these principles in the conduct of the supreme court. And finally of Lincoln who left so many burning words mounted on the imperishable wings of truth. Is it not time to listen while this great champion of liberty speaks? "You cannot strengthen the weak by weakening the strong." . . . "You cannot help the poor by tearing down the rich." "You cannot keep out of trouble by spending more than your income." "You cannot built character and courage by taking away a man's initiative and independence." "You cannot help men permanently by doing for them what they could and should do for themselves." This might well be considered the citizens Bible brought from polyglot jargon and political parleying into plain English. If these principles are put into practice they will afford full protection against the threat of socialized medicine and give a free people their only remaining chance to successfully defend themselves against the catastrophy of the welfare state.

In addition to medicine's routine care of the sick, rich and poor, it has voluntarily become "the guardian of health and life itself." Through the sleepless critical pursuit of scientific research it has thwarted disease, minimized suffering, stayed the hand of death and doubled average longevity. Its phenomenal discoveries, once proven beneficial to humanity, have been made available without thought of commercial gain.

Through scientific advances, medicine has provided the principles for progress in public health and social medicine and has pointed the way for government participation. Finally, it may be said that the medical profession in the United States, conscious of the changing socio-economic picture is actively encouraging all voluntary insurance programs in an effort to help meet economic emergencies ever arising on account of illness in the lower income groups. Approximately one-fourth of the people in the U.S. now have Blue Cross hospitalization insurance. Approximately 15,000,000 are protected against surgical emergencies by Blue Shield and many others are protected by voluntary plans offered by the nation's great free enterprise insurance industry. In the last analysis, our souls, our health, our hopes are dependent upon free enterprise.

In Memoriam,

LEWIS JEFFERSON MOORMAN

LEA A. RIELY, M.D., New Canaan, Conn.

"Who broke our fair companionship
And spread this mantle hard and cold
And wrapt thee formless in the fold
And dull'd the murmur of thy lip.

And bore thee where I could not see
Nor follow, tho' I walk in haste,
And think that somewhere in the east
Thy shadow sits and waits for me?"

THE AUTHOR

Lea A. Riely, M.D., one of the first professors of Epworth Medical College, was Emeritus Professor of Clinical Medicine on retirement from the faculty of the University of Oklahoma. A close personal friend of Doctor Moorman, he continued in private practice until 1951 when he moved to Connecticut to retire completely and be near his daughter and her family.

History is merely the summation of individual biographies, yet I believe, Clio, the Muse of History, is most deified. It, history, depicts the lives and doings of various individuals of a particular time, the things they had to combat in raising themselves from youth through the hard and strenuous, and often rocky roads, on to the 'lengthening shadows of their eventide. The chronicle of the individual, his biography, is colored of course by the history of his civilization (the *mores* and *penates)*, by the status of religion, of politics, of economics, and of medicine during the time through which he sailed on the sea of life. Ontogeny recapitulates phylogeny, as we all know, and if a people has struggled upward it is because high minded individuals have struggled upward and led the way. The chronicle of such an individual's struggle becomes an inspiration when the man concerned is of high purpose and character—a man of ideals, yet humble and kind.

The story of Lewis Jefferson Moorman, physician, begins in a mining area in Kentucky where he practiced between terms at the University of Louisville. With pill bags flapping at his horse's flanks, he studied the "simple annals of the poor first hand." After graduation and two years of postgraduate training in New York he began his practice at Jet and his habit of contemplation behind a team of ponies, the three

of them serving the community well until he came to Oklahoma City in 1907.

After a year in Vienna, then the mecca for post graduate work, he limited his practice to internal medicine. In time his medical interest narrowed to diseases of the chest and he started the first tuberculosis sanatorium in Oklahoma in 1913. At the same time a broadening of Moorman, the man, made him acutely sensitive to the impact of the disease on society and on the individual. Considering the first of these, he became interested in the Oklahoma State Tuberculosis Association of which he served as president from 1917 to 1946; the National Tuberculosis Association of which he became a director in 1927 and president for 1944; the Trudeau Society, being 'president in 1940; the American Sanatorium Association of which he was vice-president in 1937. The second, the effect of tuberculosis on the individual, interested him greatly and he began early to collect biographical data, a portion of which he published in *Tuberculosis and Genius*[1].

His absorption in the problem of tuberculosis did not disturb his interest in medicine in general and medical education in particular. He was a member of the American Clinical and Climatological Association, a fellow of the American College of Physicians, a licentiate of the American Board of Internal Medicine, and his presidential address to the Southern Medical Association

1. *Tuberculosis and Genius.* Lewis J. Moorman, M.D., University of Chicago, Press. 1940.

appears elsewhere in this issue. While Lewis was not one of the founders of Epworth Medical College which later became the medical department of the University of Oklahoma, he joined the faculty soon after coming to Oklahoma City and held a chair (or settee, as Oliver Wendell Holmes called it) in the department of medicine. He became Dean of the School of Medicine in 1931 and shepherded the school through the depression but was forced to resign in 1935 rather than bow to expediency and sacrifice principles, an impossibility for him. He continued, however, to lecture to the students on the history of medicine, an appreciation of which is expressed in this issue by Lawrence McHenry, a senior student.

The thirst for knowledge of the history of medicine is just another facet of this extraordinary man. We had only a few Boswells or Pepys to chronicle events of doing in Oklahoma. Records then were few and secretaries none too good at saving their notes, so Lewis set about to have a book on the early medical history of Oklahoma. He first made fast the interest of the Oklahoma State Medical Association and then that of the University of Oklahoma. This work was well under way at the time of his death and must some way be completed. His own experiences, humorous and pathetic, he has related in *Pioneer Doctor*[2].

In 1941 he became editor of the *Journal*. His yen to write was a valuable asset to the State Association, and under his leadership, the *Journal* became a shining star in the galaxy of state medical journals. His usually placid disposition boiled over on the editorial pages when he considered the degradation of medicine in America that must follow socialization.

May I parallel another biography which he so oft quoted. It was that of Daniel Drake, also a Kentuckian, of Mays Lick, a farm boy who had an obsession to study

2. *Pioneer Doctor*. Lewis J. Moorman, M.D., University of Oklahoma Press. 1951.

medicine. He read medicine in Cincinnati, then to the University of Pennsylvania, then back to Cincinnati, where he grew in stature as a physician. He held seven different chairs as professor of medicine, a prolific pioneer writer of his many observations which he collected oft times while touring the country on foot. He wrote the *Diseases of the Mississippi Valley* and many other books. He started and edited the first medical journal in the north central states and Cincinnati. His polemics against unscrupulous and unethical adversaries was most pungent and satirical. Osler considered him the most advanced of any doctor of his time.

I first met Lewis at a medical meeting in El Reno in 1901 and our friendship from the very beginning remained unsullied and increased over a half century. He married Mary Christian in 1909 and the year in Vienna was their honeymoon. After their three children no longer required her presence at home, she became as imporant as he as ambassabor for Oklahoma to medical society meetings here and abroad, but when at home nothing pleased them more than having a coterie of friends around. Mrs. Riely and I numbered ourselves among them and this association is one of the things we have missed most since leaving Oklahoma City. This personal and intimate relationship has furnished me the data and enabled me to write this tribute, a commission which I so gladly accepted. It is to be printed in the State *Journal*, to which he gave his heart and soul as Skipper for 13 years.

The deciduous tree (my friends) was full of healthy leaves at the turn of the century. They have fallen one by one as spring time has turned to summer and summer to autumn. It is winter now and all of them not yet fallen, but even those who have are still with me.

"To lose a friend is the greatest of all evils, but endeavor to enjoy that you have possessed them rather than to mourn their loss."—Seneca.

Association Activities

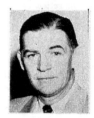

PRESIDENT'S LETTER

The Oklahoma Medical Association could choose no more fitting medium for a memorial to Dr. Lewis J. Moorman than the *Journal*, to which he contributed 15 years as editor in the same high purpose that characterized his life and practice.

Since his pioneering service in pre-statehood days he compiled an impressive number of firsts, in research, legislation and general advancement of the profession.

His tremendous personal contribution to tuberculosis research and education is a matter of record. Doctor Moorman reflected tribute on the state and the state association through his unselfish efforts in behalf of worthy organizations, serving in countless unsalaried positions.

Always in demand as a speaker at medical association meetings throughout the United States, he made appearances at international conventions in London and Athens, contributing to understanding and good will.

Members of the profession and laymen alike who were personally acquainted with Doctor Moorman felt more than impersonal respect for the dean of Oklahoma physicians. His warm, friendly manner won him as many friends personally as his experience and competence won him admirers professionally.

I feel Doctor Moorman's loss personally. I enjoyed him as much as a hunting companion and friend as I respected him as the foremost representative of our profession. His high ideals and selfless work form a solid foundation for a lasting tribute, an inspiring statement of the highest purposes of the practice of medicine.

President

Roentgenographic pattern of colon mass propulsion:[1]

(1) Ascending colon filled.

(2) Unsegmented mass propelled through transverse colon.

(3) Propulsive force follows mass through descending colon.

(4) Pelvic colon reservoir filled.

Reestablishing Bowel Reflexes with Metamucil®

Nervous fatigue, tension, injudicious diet, failure to establish regularity, too little exercise, excessive use of cathartics—all factors which contribute to constipation.[2]

Sufficient bulk and sufficient fluid form the basic rationale of treatment of constipation with Metamucil.

Metamucil (the mucilloid of Plantago ovata) produces a bland, smooth bulk when mixed with the intestinal contents. This bulk, through its mass alone, stimulates the peristaltic reflex and thus initiates the desire to evacuate, even in patients in whom postoperative hesitancy exists.

Factors Contributing to Chronic Constipation

Such gentle stimulation is of distinct advantage in reeducating and reestablishing those reflexes which control bowel evacuation. Many factors may pervert the normal reflexes, causing finally chronic constipation. Among them are: nervous fatigue and tension, improper intake of fluid, improper dietary habits, failure to respond to the call to stool, lack of physical exercise and abuse of the intestinal tract through excessive use of laxatives.[2]

Correction of constipation logically, therefore, lies in the suitable adjustment of these factors. The characteristics of Metamucil permit the correction of most of these factors: it provides bulk; it demands adequate intake of fluids (one glass with Metamucil powder, one glass after each dose); it increases the physiologic demand to evacuate; and it does not establish a laxative "habit." Metamucil, in addition, is inert, and also nonirritating and nonallergenic.

Dosage Considerations

The average adult dose is one rounded teaspoonful of Metamucil powder in a glass of cool water, milk or fruit juice, followed by an additional glass of fluid if indicated.

Metamucil is the highly refined mucilloid of Plantago ovata (50%), a seed of the psyllium group, combined with dextrose (50%) as a dispersing agent. It is supplied in containers of 4, 8 and 16 ounces. Metamucil is accepted by the Council on Pharmacy and Chemistry of the American Medical Association. G. D. Searle & Co., Research in the Service of Medicine.

1. Best, C. H., and Taylor, N. B.: The Physiological Basis of Medical Practice: A Text in Applied Physiology, ed. 5, Baltimore, The Williams & Wilkins Company, 1950, pp. 579-583.

2. Bargen, J. A.: A Method of Improving Function of the Bowel, Gastroenterology *13*:275 (Oct.) 1949.

A GENTLEMAN *of the* OLD SCHOOL

SAVOIE LOTTINVILLE

Dr. Lewis Jefferson Moorman had given so much to his adopted state of Oklahoma by the time of his death on August 2, at the age of 79, that, for a just assessment of his contributions, a book would be necessary. He will be remembered in the history of medicine, obviously, for the immense work and thought he gave to the problems of tuberculosis. In this field he was one of America's most distinguished scientists and writers.

As a human being he had that inestimable endowment, a genuine interest in and affection for his fellow mortals—patients, professional associates, acquaintances whom he had met in America, Europe, and even the Near East. For like Robert Browning's "great mind who knows the power of gentleness," he made himself at home instantly, wherever he was, and explored with zest the small things and large that interested or troubled or motivated people.

He joined with this great quality an immense fund of geniality. His sense of humor and his story-telling ability were highly developed and nicely balanced. One had the feeling of listening to a man who had explored human nature thoroughly in literature, from the time of the Greeks to the present, and even more thoroughly at first hand. He had escaped any of the cynicism expressed by Mark Twain in the latter's well-known phrase about "the damned human race." People were to Doctor Moorman the world's most enjoyable resource.

Evidently from an early age he had derived great personal delight from being a wayfarer on the highways and byways of world literature. His personal library was large and well-chosen. And the delight he found in great books, he transmitted to his friends and acquaintances. There was an aptness and easy pertinence to his literary and historical references, both in conversation and in writing. To call this "humanism" doubtless would have struck him as odd, for in spite of his obvious intellectual qualities, he probably

THE AUTHOR

Savoie Lottinville, author of "A Gentleman of the Old School," is Director of the University of Oklahoma Press. At Doctor Moorman's invitation, he was one of the guest speakers at the 1953 meeting of the American Medical Writers' Association. A previous article of his, "Dealing with Medicine Historically," appeared in the June, 1953, issue, Vol. 46, No. 6, page 153.

never thought of his literary interests as anything but having a good time.

Applied to his own calling, this curiosity about the past led, over a period of half a century, to a large and accurate understanding of medical history. The technique he applied here, not only for his own satisfaction but for the benefit of the students he subsequently taught at the University of Oklahoma Medical School, was much more than merely factual. His mind was philosophical as well as scientific: he wished to know, in the broadest possible terms, *how* a medical advance had been brought about, as well as *when* and by *whom*.

There is a natural tendency to speak of Doctor Moorman as "a gentleman of the old school." Taken for what it usually means in its most complimentary sense, this still doesn't say enough. It means, really, that he had exploited intellectual and cultural resources rarely undertaken by busy human beings today. But he had gone even further: he was as current in his thinking as the most advanced among his younger contemporaries.

Nowhere is this more evident than in his occasional and more extended writings. The changing structure of medical service, coming requirements in medical education, the status of the community doctor, ends and means in medicine and surgery—to all of these he applied powers of critical analysis which mark him as one of the most forward-looking professional men of his age.

Writing recently on the enormous gains that modern medicine had made in prolonging life and easing pain, he made the following very sage observation:

"Admitting all this and noting that we have minimized the vastness of continents and the breadth of intervening seas, we cannot escape this disturbing query: Can we be sure we are not soaring on wings of wax? In this age of atomic energy it is well to remember that in the last analysis these achievements are relatively unimportant. Even longevity is not the measure of life. Deeds not days determine our usefulness and our satisfactions. Amiel says, 'Life has been lent to us, and we owe it to our traveling companions to let them see what use we make of it to the end.' "

During the fortnight before his death, he was thinking and planning for the history of medicine in Oklahoma. Although he was confined to his bed and in considerable pain, he took the trouble to write me some ideas that he had developed for this large project. He had been able to secure, he said, some remarkably good materials on the early history of medicine in Oklahoma and was commissioning more research. Here was a last manifestation of that profound sense of responsibility which had imbued his professional life.

What he thought and said and did during a long lifetime, from his Kentucky boyhood through the 53 years of his career in Oklahoma, need not be conjectured. He wrote about these things in a modest, absorbing way in *Pioneer Doctor*, published in 1951 by the University of Oklahoma Press. At the end of the book he set down in a single short paragraph the answer that all men seek to the largest question of their existence. He had recently returned with Mrs. Moorman from a medical congress in London at which he had delivered an address:

"Once more in my own home among the things I love, I contemplate the strange new world; and while scanning my remembrance book, I thank God for what has gone before, and knowing that Nature, the mother of us all, will wipe the world's tears away, I am content to say with Virgil, 'Fortunate old man, here among familiar rivers and these sacred founts shalt thou take the shadowy coolness.' "

Chairman Requests Resume' of Papers

Walter. Brown, M.D., Tulsa, chairman of the Scientific Work Committee for the 1955 annual meeting has again requested that physicians who would like to present papers, send a synopsis of the paper to him before November 30.

Dates of the Annual Meeting are May 9-11, 1955. All scientific sessions and commercial exhibits will again be held at the Cimarron Ballroom. A resumé of the paper to be presented should be sent to Doctor Brown, c/o B-9 Medical Arts Building, Tulsa, *not* to the Oklahoma State Medical Association Executive office.

"It may not be possible to use all papers submitted," Doctor Brown said, "due to limitations of the program schedule, duplication of subject matter, and the necessity of representing most specialties. However, we do hope that every member who has a useful paper will give us the opportunity of considering it for the scientific program."

Although space for scientific exhibits is quite limited, applications for space for this purpose are now being received. The final date for such applications will also be November 30, 1954.

Other members of the Scientific Work Committee, in addition to Doctor Brown, include Dr. E. G. Hyatt, Dr. Thomas J. Hardman, Dr. Earl I. Mulmed, Dr. Wendell L. Smith, and Dr. James B. Thompson, all of Tulsa.

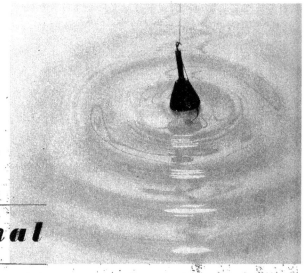

minimal

side

effects

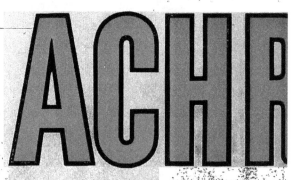

ACHR

LEDERLE LABORATORIES DIVISION *AMERICAN Cyanamid COM*

One of the notable qualities of ACHROMYCIN, the Lederle brand of Tetracycline, is its advantage of minimal side effects. Furthermore, this true broad-spectrum antibiotic is well-tolerated by all age groups.

In each of its various dosage forms, ACHROMYCIN provides more rapid diffusion for prompt control of infection. In solution, it is more soluble and more stable than certain other antibiotics.

ACHROMYCIN has proved effective against a wide variety of infections caused by gram-positive and gram-negative bacteria, rickettsia, and certain virus-like and protozoan organisms.

ACHROMYCIN ranks with the truly great therapeutic agents.

OMYCIN*

HYDROCHLORIDE
Tetracycline HCl Lederle

arl River, New York

He Was My FRIEND and TEACHER

LAWRENCE McHENRY

THE AUTHOR

Lawrence McHenry, senior student at the University of Oklahoma School of Medicine, wrote "He Was My Friend and Teacher." A past president of the Oklahoma Chapter of the Student American Medical Association, he was also a guest speaker at the 1953 meeting of the American Medical Writers' Association.

Four years ago during my freshman year of medical school, Dr. Moorman gave his last series of lectures on the history of medicine. Our class was new to the medical field and did not know the meaning of the art of medicine. We had only been inspired by the volume of work which had recently become our responsibility until Dr. Moorman gave his last lecture. In this he spoke at random, not using his notes. With his fine, strong voice he mentioned the old-fashioned family, and the old-fashioned family doctor, the creeping paralysis of false security, the idea of living each day at a time with the preservation of equilibrium, and to cling to those things that are good and worthy. As he finished a spontaneous applause filled the classroom. I had been fixed in awe at his words, but only then did I suddenly realize, he was indeed an inspiration to all the students. From then until his last appearance before the students when he introduced Dr. Douglas Guthrie, he has been a living symbol of the profession to his students. His aphorisms have been included with those of Hippocrates and Osler in our Yearbook. When we are told of Francis Adams, we feel little for we can not comprehend such a dim past, but when we had before us this great physician whom we all knew, we felt that perhaps there was something greater to our profession than merely writing a prescription.

Before he introduced Dr. Guthrie, he requested, "that we dedicate this hour to the history of medicine, without which we could not hope to maintain the traditional culture of our profession, and, without this culture we could not have a satisfactory patient - physician relationship, and without this relationship, we could not hope to fulfill our mission in the field of human weal." After the talk many of my classmates told me that they felt true wisdom in his words as he spoke to us for the last time. So, my friends, he was not only a leader of your State Medical Association, but he was also our living strength and pride in the medical profession.

Dr. Moorman came to Oklahoma in the early 1900's when our forefathers were founding their homes and lives on the new territory. He began on horseback as a pioneer doctor, and over the past fifty years, he had seen and lived the growth of this state, and its medical profession. He was a leader, a participant, and an observer. We can say that not only was his life a parallel in the history of Oklahoma medicine, but it was the epitome.

To his fellow men and students he is a great loss, but we gladly give him up, for we know that in his new life he will walk among the great of history. He has gone to join his colleagues, Osler, Adams, and Trudeau, in the gardens of Aesculapius. By now he has met Hippocrates, and has taken his place in the timeless where the past and future are combined into the eternal infinite present. He will enjoy talking to Ebstein and Lawrence Fick about tuberculosis and with Keats and Moliere. St. Francis and he will walk among the flowers beneath the music of the birds. Plato and Socrates, I am sure, will give a warm welcome to their student. In Virgil's words, "Fortunate old man, here among familiar rivers and these sacred founts shalt thou take the shadowy coolness."

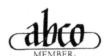

CLASSIFIED ADS

FOR SALE: 1948 Watpler cold cautery scalpel. Slightly used. Forty per cent of cost. Write Key E, care of the *Journal*.

WANTED: General Practitioner—Excellent set up for recent graduate or older man seeking relief from rigorous practice. Regular hours—comfortable living. Family maintenance at nominal cost. Oklahoma license. Veteran preferred. Oklahoma State Veterans Hospital, Sulphur, Oklahoma.

FOR SALE: Eye, Ear, Nose and Throat surgical instruments, diagnostic equipment, 64 medical books and miscellaneous office furniture. Will sell individual or as a group. Contact Mrs. R. E. Leatherock, 603 E. Oak, Cushing, Oklahoma. Phone 596.

SITUATION WANTED: Technician, Reg. A.M.T., six years experience laboratory, four years experience x-ray. References furnished. Write Key G., care of the *Journal*.

FOR SALE: Excellent physician's table, chair, instrument cabinet by physician retired from practice. Phone JA 5-1600, Oklahoma City or write Key A, care of the *Journal* or write c/o 1521 N. Shartel, Oklahoma City.

PRACTICE FOR SALE: Good sized town. Excellent, hospital; industries. 100ma X-Ray, diathermy, many other items. Will sell some equipment separate. Specializing. Write Key R, care of the *Journal*.

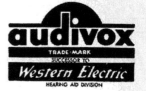

PATRONIZE JOURNAL ADVERTISERS

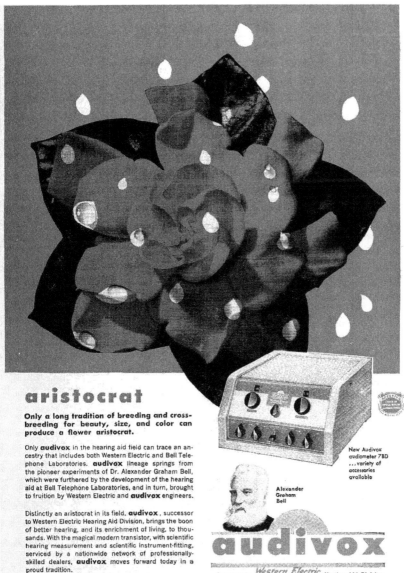

Officers and Councilors

OKLAHOMA STATE MEDICAL ASSOCIATION

President—Bruce R. Hinson, M.D., Enid.

President-Elect—R. Q. Goodwin, M.D., Oklahoma City

Vice-President—Clifford Bassett, M.D., Cushing

Secretary-Treasurer—W. W. Rucks, Jr., M.D. Oklahoma City

Delegates to the A.M.A.—John F. Burton, M.D., Oklahoma City; James Stevenson, M.D., Tulsa

Alternate Delegates to the A.M.A.—Malcom Phelps, M.D., El Reno; Ned Burleson, M.D., Prague

Speaker of the House of Delegates—Clinton Gallaher, M.D., Shawnee

Vice-Speaker of the House of Delegates—Keiller Haynie, M.D., Durant

District No. 1: Craig, Delaware, Mayes, Nowata, Ottawa, Rogers, Washington
Councilor (1956)_____F. S. Etter, M. D., Bartlesville
Vice-Councilor (1956)____J. E. Highland, M. D., Miami

District No. 2: Kay, Noble, Osage, Pawnee, Payne
Councilor (1957) _____ E. C. Mohler, M. D., Ponca City
Vice-Councilor (1957)_____
_____ Glen McDonald, M. D., Pawhuska

District No. 3: Garfield, Grant, Kingfisher, Logan
Councilor (1955)____C. M. Hodgson, M. D., Kingfisher
Vice-Councilor (1955)____Wm. P. Neilson, M. D., Enid ,

District No. 4: Alfalfa, Beaver, Cimarron, Ellis, Harper, Major, Texas, Woods, Woodward
Councilor (1956)_____L. R. Kirby, M. D., Cherokee
Vice-Councilor (1956)___Joe L. Duer, M. D., Woodward

District No. 5: Beckham, Blaine, Canadian, Custer, Dewey, Roger Mills
Councilor (1957)_____A. L. Johnson, M. D., El Reno
Vice-Councilor (1957)____Ross Deputy, M. D., Clinton

District No. 6: Oklahoma
Councilor (1955)_____
_____Elmer Ridgeway Jr., M. D., Oklahoma City
Vice-Councilor (1955)_____
_____P. E. Russo, M. D., Oklahoma City

District No. 7: Cleveland, Creek, Lincoln, Okfuskee, Pottawatomie, Seminole
Councilor (1956) _____Paul Gallaher, M. D., Shawnee
Vice-Councilor (1956)_____
_____Charles A. Smith, M. D., Norman

District No. 8: Tulsa
Councilor (1957)_____Wilkie Hoover, M. D., Tulsa
Vice-Councilor (1957)__Wendell L. Smith, M. D., Tulsa

District No. 9: Adair, Cherokee, McIntosh, Muskogee, Okmulgee, Sequoyah, Wagoner
Councilor (1955)__ ___ F. R. First, Jr., M. D., Checotah
Vice-Councilor (1955)__ ____
_____ I. W. Bollinger, M. D., Henryetta

District No. 10: Haskell, Hughes, Latimer, LeFlore, Pittsburg
Councilor (1956)____Paul Kernek, M. D., Holdenville
Vice-Councilor (1956)__C. D. Lively, M. D., McAlester

District No. 11: Atoka, Bryan, Choctaw, Coal, McCurtain, Pushmataha
Councilor (1957)_____A. T. Baker, M. D., Durant
Vice-Councilor (1957)_____T. E. Rhea, M. D., Idabel

District No. 12: Carter, Garvin, Johnston, Love, Marshall, McClain, Murray, Pontotoc
Councilor (1955) _____J. H. Veazey, M. D., Ardmore
Vice-Councilor (1955)_____W. T. Gill, M. D., Ada

District No. 13: Caddo, Comanche, Cotton, Grady, Jefferson, Stephens
Councilor (1956)____H. M. McClure, M. D., Chickasha
Vice-Councilor (1956)____J. B. Miles, M. D., Anadarko

District No. 14: Greer, Harmon, Jackson, Kiowa, Tillman, Washita
Councilor (1957) ___ _____ J. B. Hollis, M. D., Mangum
Vice-Councilor (1957)__R. R. Hannas, M. D., Sentinel

1954 County Medical Society Officers

Society	President	Secretary-Treasurer
Alfalfa	Nova L. Morgan, M.D., Cherokee	George A. Hart, M.D., Cherokee
Atoka-Bryan-Coal	A. C. Fina, M.D., Atoka	Seals L. Whitely, M.D., Durant
Beckham	Phil J. Devanney, M.D., Sayre	Donald Lehman, M.D., Elk City
Blaine	Kenneth Godfrey, M.D., Okeene	Virginia O. Curtin, M.D., Watonga
Caddo	E. T. Cook, Jr., M.D., Anadarko	B. E. Stone, M.D., Anadarko
Canadian	C. Riley Strong, M.D., El Reno	James P. Jobe, M.D., El Reno
Carter-Love-Marshall	John Pollock, M.D., Ardmore	
Cherokee-Adair	P. H. Medearis, M.D., Tahlequah	G. W. Buffington, M.D., Tahlequah
Cleveland-McClain	George A. Wiley, M.D., Norman	F. C. Buffington, M.D., Norman
Comanche-Cotton	W. F. Lewis, M.D., Lawton	G. G. Downing, M.D., Lawton
Creek	Louis A. Martin, M.D., Sapulpa	Thomas D. Burnett, M.D., Sapulpa
Custer	C. J. Alexander, M.D., Clinton	Glenn P. Dewberry, M D., Clinton
East Central	D. Evelyn Miller, M.D., Muskogee	Maurice C. Gephardt, M.D., Muskogee
(Muskogee, Sequoyah, Wagoner, McIntosh)		
Garfield-Kingfisher	John R. Taylor, M.D., Kingfisher	Roscoe C. Baker, M.D., Enid
Garvin	W. H. Smith, M.D., Lindsay	Hugh H. Monroe, M.D., Pauls Valley
Grady	B. B. McDougal, M.D., Chickasha	Arnold G. Nelson, M.D., Chickasha
Grant	R. W. Choice, M.D., Wakita	F. P. Robinson, M.D., Pond Creek
Greer	Dwight D. Pierson, M.D., Mangum	J. B. Hollis, M.D., Mangum
Hughes-Seminole	W. E. Jones, Jr., M.D., Seminole	Andy N. Deaton, M.D., Wewoka
Jackson	E. A. Abernethy, M.D., Altus	E. W. Mabry, M.D., Altus
Jefferson	Jose Abelarde, M.D., Waurika	Lee Pullen, M.D., Waurika
Kay-Noble	E. H. Arrendell, M.D., Ponca City	John Gilbert, M.D., Ponca City
		C. D. Northcutt, Exec. Secty., Ponca City
Kiowa-Washita	J. B. Tolbert, M.D., Mountain View	M. Wilson Mahone, M.D., Hobart
LeFlore-Haskell	C. S. Cunningham, M.D., Poteau	G. J. Womack, M.D., Wister
Lincoln	Harold T. Baugh, M.D., Meeker	Ned Burleson, M.D., Prague
Logan	Webber Merrell, M.D., Guthrie	J. E. Souter, M.D., Guthrie
Northwestern	M. K. Braly, M.D., Woodward	M. C. England, M.D., Woodward
(Beaver, Dewey, Ellis, Harper, Woodward)		
Okfuskee	N. E. Gissler, M.D., Okemah	M. L. Whitney, M.D., Okemah
Oklahoma	Henry G. Bennett, Jr., M.D., Oklahoma City	Elmer Ridgeway, Jr., M.D., Oklahoma City
		Alma O'Donnell, Exec. Secty., Medical Arts Bldg., Oklahoma City
Okmulgee	A. L. Buell, M.D., Okmulgee	S. B. Leslie, Jr., M.D., Okmulgee
Osage	P. H. Haralson, M.D., Fairfax	W. A. Geiger, Jr., M.D., Fairfax
Ottawa-Craig	J. M. McMillan, M.D., Vinita	John E. Highland, M.D., Miami
Payne-Pawnee	Harold Sanders, M.D., Stillwater	C. W. Moore, M.D., Stillwater
Pittsburg	Ben T. Galbraith, M.D., McAlester	Sam Dakil, M. D.,McAlester
Pontotoc	Orange Miller Welborn, M.D., Ada	David Cozzens Ramsay, M.D., Ada
Pottawatomie	John R. Hayes, M.D., Shawnee	Clinton Gallaher, M.D., Shawnee
Rogers-Mayes	Bert Morrow, M.D., Salina	William Bynum, M.D., Pryor
Stephens	Jack Gregston, M.D., Marlow	W. R. Cheatwood, M.D., Duncan
Texas-Cimarron	Not Reported	James E. Morgan, M.D., Guymon
Tillman	R. L. Fisher, M.D., Frederick	O. G. Bacon, M.D., Frederick
Tri-County	A. E. Hale, M.D., Idabel	Thomas E. Rhea, M.D., Idabel
(Choctaw, McCurtain, Pushmataha)		
Tulsa	Wilkie D. Hoover, M.D., Tulsa	Charles G. Stuard, M.D., Tulsa
		Jack Spears, Exec. Secty., Medical Arts Bldg., Tulsa
Washington-Nowata	H. E. Denyer, M.D., Bartlesville	J. H. Lindsay, M.D., Dewey
Woods	Not Reported	T. D. Benjegerdes, M.D., Alva

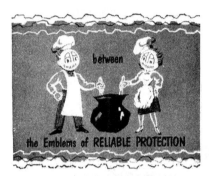
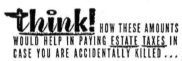
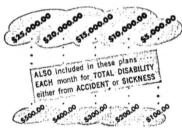

Editorials

Home Office Building For Blue Cross-Blue Shield

The formal dedication of the Blue Cross-Blue Shield home office building points up a mark of stability that every home owner recognizes. Any uneasiness that these service organizations are getting too big and too powerful will be allayed if one considers their purpose, their past history, their structure and their competition.

Their purpose is to offer a means of allowing the people of the state to pool their resources in advance and with this fund to take care of each other's families in event of serious sickness. From the beginning, the emphasis has been on the family and not just the employed person. This concept of community service, though not at the outset considered actuarily sound, was secured by the hospitals who guaranteed the service promised by the Blue Cross Plan.

The past history of these service plans indicates that they are anxious to go as far as is financially possible toward increasing their services to the contract holders, and their payments to hospitals and to doctors. They have repeatedly made alterations in these directions as their financial position has improved. Two galling points have been treated as well as could be: (1) a set of rules for inclusion under the contract is necessary since participants must be equally benefited; and, (2) inequalities of payments to hospitals are in some measure unavoidable since there is a great difference in costs due to the variation in the number of services offered by the different hospitals. Blue Cross is going all the way in helping a committee of hospital people try to solve these inequities.

The structure of these organizations is such that no one makes any profit from them. All income not required for operation and for discharging obligations under the contracts is set aside for future benefits to contract holders. At the beginning it took most of the income to pay for the cost of operation alone. This early period was managed with borrowed capital. It now requires only about seven per cent of the income for all operational costs — the balance is used to pay for the participants' hospital and medical care or is placed in reserve. All personnel in the employment of the plans receive salaries. None receives a percentage of income from the sale of contracts. This all means that the total cost of medical care for people covered under the contract is increased very little by paying for the service in advance in small monthly payments.

While most of us believe that the family who has a Blue Cross-Blue Shield contract has the best that can be obtained, nevertheless, there are many good commercial companies in the field. This competition is healthy for both, and as long as it exists, neither can become too dictatorial.

The building of a Blue Cross-Blue Shield home office is a landmark of stable development. The large sum that has been necessary for rental space can now be left in reserve. With so many fly by night companies around it will be reassuring for people to look at the home office building and realize that Blue Cross and Blue Shield are here to stay.

Hospital Personnel Shortage

A recent brochure on this subject released by the Health Resources Advisory Committee on the Office of Defense Mobilization points out many of the problems and suggests steps to help in solving them.

While the shortage of personnel is not limited to that of nurses, an increase in their number is urgently needed. The family doctor is often asked his opinion of nursing as a vocation. Every young girl should learn how to make a living. There is no better field for this than nursing. There is a tremendous inner satisfaction that comes from the work itself in all its many phases, and it offers superb training for future family life if a career in nursing is set aside for marriage. Nursing education today means the development of mature, educated young women who have the skills peculiar to the nursing profession. The family doctor can advise his young inquirer that she, with a nursing certificate or degree, can always be proud, useful, independent and secure. She could not ask for more.

The Search For Hidden Diabetes

The protean specter of diabetes mellitus haunts the consulting room of every practicing physician. It lurks behind the folliculitis, furunculosis, and pruritus ani in the office of the dermatologist. It peers out from retinal microaneurysms, pigmentation, hemorrhages, and retinitis profiferans at the ophthalmologist. It hides behind altered sensation and reflexes in the clinic of the neurologist, and leers through an albuminous cloud in the test tube of the urologist. It troubles the sleep of the surgeon concerned about ketosis and wound healing; and of the obstetrician vacillating between forceps and cesarean. It hides behind the cough of the phthisical, and the elevated T-wave on the cardiogram. It complicates the peaceful diagnostic life of practitioner and specialist alike.

It is the responsibility of medical men to be wary of this dissimulator; it is also the responsibility of the profession to discover diabetes as early as possible and to institute proper management. Poor control of diabetes usually results in a high incidence of complications: infection, acidosis, retinitis, nephropathy, vascular calcifications, and neuropathy. Good control reduces the incidence of these complications and increases longevity in the diabetic.

For the early detection of diabetes, each physician-practitioner and specialist alike must perform a screening test, even though it be only a urine test for glucose one hour after a high carbohydrate meal, on every patient he sees.

Each of us owes it to the community to cooperate with the intensive campaign of diabetes detection and education; but let us not forget that this is a year round program. — Milton R. Weed, M.D., in the Detroit Medical News, Nov. 16, 1953.

Scientific Articles

Routine Operative

CHOLANGIOGRAPHY

BRUCE H. BROWN, M.D. and GEORGE M. BROWN, JR., M.D.

The idea and technique of operative cholangiography is not new, being reported by Cotte in 1929 and Mirizzi in 1932. It has enjoyed increased usage by those doing biliary tract surgery during the past 15 years, though both surgeons and radiologists have been reticent to adopt its general use. This reluctance stems from misconceptions regarding time element, expense of equipment, and patient safety. Unfortunately, in some instances, there is also false pride regarding ability to do satisfactory common duct exploration.

This presentation includes 150 consecutive cases of biliary tract surgery in which approximately 200 series of operative cholangiograms have been done at time of surgery.

THE AUTHORS

Bruce H. Brown, M.D., and George M. Brown, M.D., staff members of the McAlester Clinic, are joint authors of "Routine Operative Cholangiography. Both are graduates of the University of Oklahoma School of Medicine. Doctor Bruce Brown specializes in radiology and served his internships and residency at St. Anthony, Mercy and University Hospitals, Oklahoma City. Doctor George Brown specializes in general surgery and proctology. He interned at the U. S. Navy Hospital, Bainbridge, Maryland, and served his residency at the Cleveland Clinic.

In this group there have been no operative deaths, and as far as the authors have been able to determine, there has been no increased morbidity or sequela from the use of radio-opaque media injected into the biliary tract. The surgical and radiological facilities for doing this group of cases have been divided between two 65 bed hospitals in a town of 20,000 population.

The indications for common duct exploration have been handed down through the years as a precise dogma, and we do not feel that operative cholangiography in any way should replace good surgical judgment. However, it is quite apparent that even today common duct exploration, alone, leaves something to be desired in view of the great number of techniques, types of probes, etc., designed to prevent overlooking stones in the common duct. When there has been any question of accuracy of the cholangiograms in this series of cases, we have done common duct exploration. Correlation of positive and negative radiologic findings with surgical findings has been excellent (98 per cent). This further emphasizes the value of routine cholangiography as an adjunct to common duct exploration.

Therefore we present this group of cases, together with details of technique, and pitfalls of interpretation. We shall briefly discuss, with case presentation, the clinical usages and valuable information we have obtained from routine operative cholangiography.

Technique

A. *Radiology:* The time involved in carrying out the x-ray technique of routine operative cholangiography is relatively short in comparison to the operative procedure, nevertheless, the x-ray technique is very important and vital to its success. The average time involved in this group of cases has been 7-10 minutes. The actual x-ray technique is best considered under three headings; namely: equipment, position and factors. Equipment consists of (1) a portable x-ray machine, preferably 30 M.A., (2) a portable Bucky, (3) three 10" x 12" casettes, and (4) 70 per cent urokon sodium as contrast media. The patient is in the usual supine position for gallbladder surgery with the portable Bucky and casette in place between the folded pads on the table and centered under the right upper quadrant of the patient. The tube is centered over the casette aided by the surgeon in localizing the junction of the cystic and common duct. Factors consist of (1) distance — 25 inches, (2) Ma. — 30,

(3) KV—70, (4) time — three seconds. These are composite averages which must be varied depending on the weight and size of the patient.

B. *Surgery:* From the standpoint of surgical technique operative cholangiography may be classed into three types.

1. Needle cholangiography. Either the cystic duct, the common duct or•the gallbladder itself may be needled directly. A single injection of radio-opaque material is introduced into the biliary system. In this series, the first group of 44 cases were of this type. As we gained experience we found this procedure unsatisfactory in about 20 per cent of cases, for the following reasons: a. The introduction of a needle into the common duct or cystic duct without penetration of the posterior wall was quite difficult. b. The leakage of dye around the ductal system was often quite pronounced resulting in inaccurate interpretation of films. c. Any movement of the patient, unuusual depth of the wound, or poor exposure greatly increased the possibility of error. Because of these difficulties the second type of cholangiography has been used in the last 106 cases.

2. Catheter cholangiography. A Touhy continuous spinal catheter or comparable polyethylene catheter is introduced into the cystic duct for fractional instillation of radio-opaque material. The cystic duct, common duct, and cystic artery are dissected out completely. The cystic artery is divided between clamps and ligated. This clears the area at the junction of the cystic and common ducts. A loose ligature is then placed around the cystic duct. With the duct under tension a small nick is made transversely near its junction with the gallbladder. The catheter is readily inserted into the cystic duct for a distance of 2 cm. and ligature tightened, fastening the catheter securely. Such access to the ductal system then allows fractional injection of the radio-opaque media.

3. Terminal cholangiography. This type is done through the T-tube while the abdomen is still open and after common duct exploration has been completed. With watertight closure of the common duct obtained about the T-tube, the T-tube is flushed and filled with sterile water. The long limb of the T-tube is then needled, the radio-opaque media

injected, fractionally, and serial films exposed. This type of cholangiography is probably the most effective of all. With attention paid to small details and cooperation of both surgeon and radiologist, films should be obtained which are completely satisfactory to determine continued presence or absence of intra-biliary tract pathosis.

In taking serial films, 3 cc. of urokon sodium 70 per cent are injected immediately prior to exposing each of three films. All air bubbles, stones which may be covered up with excessive radio-opaque media, structures intra-biliary tract tumors, etc., can then be readily detected since one has three separate films for study.

C. Miscellaneous: 1. Controlled respiration. The patient must not breathe during the time of film exposure. With spinal anesthesia the patient may voluntarily cease respiration. Under general anesthesia, the respiration may be stopped by pressure on the anesthesia bag. We have not found it necessary to resort to drugs to produce momentary apnea.

2. Removal of instruments. All instruments, retractors, etc., must be removed prior to the exposure of the films so that portions of the biliary tract will not be obscured.

3. Removal of radio-opaque sponges. Sponges and tapes with radio-opaque markers contained within them must likewise be removed to prevent obscuring any portion of the biliary tree.

4. Elimination of media spillage. Contrast media outside the biliary tree gives a distorted picture which handicaps accurate interpretation. This can be eliminated by proper placement of the needle or catheter prior to the exposure of the films. In those instances where the gallbladder is removed prior to the exposure of the films, closure of the liver bed will eliminate spillage coming from the occasional accessory biliary duct emptying into the liver bed.

5. Catharsis. Adequate removal of all barium is necessary in patients who have had concurrent preoperative gastrointestinal tract studies.

6. Stomach decompression. A Levine tube should be inserted into the stomach routinely. This not only facilitates adequate exposure by keeping the stomach decompressed, but likewise eliminates troublesome shadows overlying the biliary tree.

7. Spasm. Spasm of the ampulla of Vater may present diagnostic difficulties. This is believed to be largely initiated by the rapid injection of large amounts of radio-opaque media under pressure. The incidence of spasm with 3 cc. injections of the urokon sodium 70 per cent has been negligible in this series. Those few cases have been readily relieved by the patient's inhaling a small amount of amyl nitrite. Repeat films may then be necessary.

Clinical Usage With Case Discussions

The stimulus for doing operative cholangiography has stemmed, by and large, from the necessity of determining the presence or absence of common duct calculi. However, with excellent visualization of the biliary tree, the true anatomical picture of both the extra-hepatic and intra-hepatic systems is readily visualized. This makes routine operative cholangiography a proven diagnostic aid in many conditions involving the biliary ductal system.

I. Normal anatomical variation
II. Common duct stones
   A. Suspected cases
   B. Non-suspected cases
III. Hepatic duct stones
IV. Cases which are found normal with the aid of cholangiography in which common duct exploration would have to be done otherwise.
V. Strictures
   A. Common duct
   B. Hepatic duct
VI. Tumors
   A. Intra-hepatic
   B. Biliary tract
   C. Ampullary
VII. Cases of common duct reconstruction
VIII. Biliary atresia and other anomalies

The following are representative cases of both calculous and non-calculous lesions selected from this series. The diagnosis and final decisions were made during surgery on the basis of routine operative cholangiography.

No. 1: Mrs. M. A. This 71-year-old white woman had repeated episodes of biliary colic. Physical examination revealed marked right upper quadrant tenderness and an icteric

Illustrated below are four representative films showing a few of the normal variations of the biliary system.

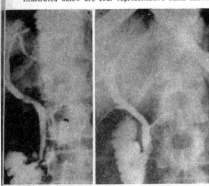 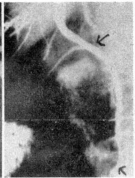 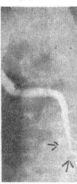

Fig. 1   Fig. 2   Fig. 3   Fig. 4

1. Small diverticulum of the distal common duct.
2. Several pancreatic ducts emptying separately into the duodenum.
3. Unusually long common duct.
4. The common duct crossing the midline and emptying into the duodenum on the left side by three separate small branches of the distal common duct.

tint to the sclera. The serum bilirubin was 4.5 mgm. per cent with a direct positive Vandenburg and urine positive for bile. At surgery a thick walled, acutely inflammed gallbladder containing numerous stones was found. The common duct was moderately enlarged. Cholangiography revealed normal filling of the hepatic radicals with common duct moderately dilated and containing several non-opaque stones. One non-opaque stone was partially blocking the distal common duct, however, there was dye in the duodenum. Following common duct exploration and removal of the stones, terminal T-tube cholangiogram revealed normal filling of the biliary tree and normal emptying of the dye into the duodenum. (See Fig. 5 and 6.)

No. 2: Mrs. O. P. This 24-year-old white female had biliary colic, jaundice and a serum bilirubin of 3.7 mgm. per cent. Surgery revealed an empyema of the gallbladder and also many biliary stones. The cystic and common ducts were moderately dilated with a marked amount of induration of the head of the pancreas present. Cholangiography revealed a dilated common duct and hepatic tree with an obstruction by a non-opaque calculus measuring approximately 5 mm. in diameter. Common duct exploration was done, and by transduodenal approach,

the stone was teased through the ampulla of Vater, with delivery into the duodenum. Following this, terminal T-tube cholangiograms revealed a perfectly normal duct. (See Fig. 7 and 8).

Comment: These are typical cases in which the decision to do common duct exploration was clear. However, in many instances such decision is not clear. In those instances routine operative cholangiography plays a most important role. No one can question the increased morbidity and mortality

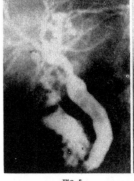 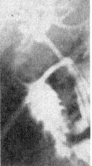

Fig. 5   Fig. 6

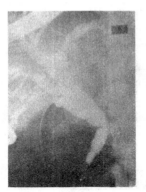

Fig. 7

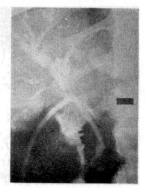

Fig. 8

associated with common duct exploration. Likewise further increase is present when secondary operations are necessary for removal of common duct stones which have been overlooked. Terminal cholangiography prevents a secondary operation from becoming a necessity.

No. 3: Mrs. R. D. This 20-year-old obese white female had food dyscrasias, right upper quadrant pain, nausea and vomiting, but no chills, fever or jaundice. Physical examination and laboratory findings were normal. Preoperative x-ray studies showed stones in the ballbladder with a normal upper gastrointestinal tract. At surgery a distended thick-walled gallbladder containing numerous stones was found. Multiple anomalies of the cystic artery with three short branches from the right hepatic artery were present. The common duct was of apparent normal size. However, operative cholangiography revealed slight dilation of the common duct and hepatic radicals with a single, round 1 cm. non-opaque stone in the center of the common duct. The dye emptied readily into the duodenum. Following exploration of the common duct and removal of the stone, terminal cholangiograms were normal. (See Fig. 9).

No. 4: Mr. J. W. This 70-year-old male had repeated bouts of right upper quadrant pain but no other positive history of biliary tract disease. Physical examination revealed tenderness in the right upper quadrant and

a palpable mass. Laboratory findings were entirely normal. At surgery an acutely inflammed, thick-walled gallbladder containing multiple stones was found. The ducts appeared normal. Operative cholangiograms revealed a normal size biliary tree with three small non-opaque stones present in the distal common duct. On serial films, with additional injection of radio-opaque media, these were impacted at the ampulla of Vater. With the stones removed, terminal cholangiograms were normal. (See Fig. 10 and 11)

Comment: These cases further emphasize the benefits of routine operative cholangiography. Repeatedly, cases of cholecystitis with cholelithiasis have no previous history of jaundice. At operation the ductal system

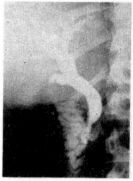

Fig. 9

300

appears normal in size, and palpation shows no evidence of intraductal pathology. The size of the patient, the amount of periductal inflammatory reaction, and induration in the head of the pancreas all affect palpation of the ductal system. These points emphasize that the usual criteria for common duct exploration are inadequate for determining intrabiliary tract pathology.

No. 5: Mr. E. W. This 69-year-old white male had intermittent abdominal pain, increased flatulence, occasional nausea and vomiting and associated weight loss. Physical examination was normal except for tenderness in the right upper quadrant. No jaundice was present and laboratory studies were normal. Preoperative films showed non-visualization of the gallbladder. At surgery the right upper quadrant was filled with dense adhesions from a previously ruptured gallbladder, and scarring was present about the common and cystic ducts. Operative cholangiography showed a slight dilation of the left hepatic and common hepatic ducts with an oval 1 cm. stone present in the left hepatic radical. An unusual anomaly of the cystic duct was present, emptying into the distal common duct from behind and on the left side. The stone was removed and terminal cholangiograms, which clearly outlined this anomaly, were otherwise normal. (See Fig. 12, 13 and 14.)

Comment: Examination of the serial films revealed that the stone present in the common duct moved into the hepatic radical fol-

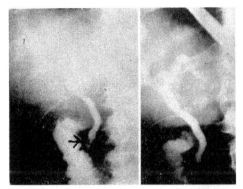

Fig. 10   Fig. 11

lowing fractional injection of urokon sodium. With common duct exploration and the vigorous irrigations advocated by some, many stones may similarly be displaced upward into the hepatic radicals. These later block the common duct and necessitate a secondary operation. Too often the liver is then falsely blamed for reformation of stones.

No. 6: Mr. C. B. This 73-year-old white male had right upper quadrant pain, nausea and vomiting, with a rising white count and serum bilirubin level. Previous cholecystostomy with removal of stones, and more recently sump drainage for a ruptured gallbladder, had been done. Physical examination revealed an acutely ill elderly white male with electrocardiographic findings of coron-

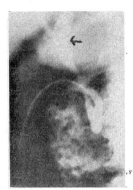 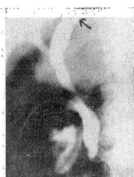 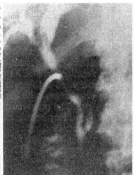

Fig. 12   Fig. 13   Fig. 14

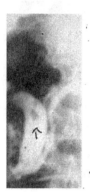
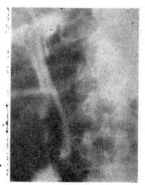

Fig. 15   Fig. 16

ary insufficiency. At operation the gallbladder was tremendously thickened with a massive inflammatory process matting the stomach, duodenum and transverse colon to it. The common duct was dilated. Operative cholangiograms revealed a dilated common duct with a large stone in the hepatic duct and a smaller stone in the common duct. With removal of the stones, terminal cholangiograms showed a normal biliary tree. See Fig. 15 and 16.

Comment: This patient was obviously a poor risk. Unnecessary and prolonged exploration of the common duct would have seriously jeopardized successful surgery. The five to 10 minute time element delay, in this particular instance, saved time by having a negative terminal cholangiogram and knowing the duct was free of further obstruction.

No. 7: Mrs. P. M. This 32-year-old white female had pain, chills fever, nausea, vomiting and jaundice. The icteric index was 36, with a positive direct Vandenburg and normal liver function studies. At operation the gallbladder showed both acute and chronic inflammatory changes, with the common duct normal in size. The pancreas was markedly indurated. A low loop hepatic artery anomaly was also present. Cholangiograms were normal and pathological reports showed an acute and chronic cholecystitis with slight chronic pancreatitis.

Comment: With normal cholangiograms it was apparent that the jaundice was on an inflammatory basis, necessitating no common duct exploration.

No. 8: Mrs. F. W. This 58-year-old white female had nausea, vomiting, intermittent episodes of right upper quadrant pain and marked fatty food intolerance. Physical examination was normal except for jaundice. The icteric index was 22 with a positive direct Vandenburg. X-ray studies showed nonvisualization of the gallbladder. At operation a scarred contracted gallbladder with numerous stones was found. With the marked inflammatory process about the common duct and jaundice, we did not depend on negative cholangiograms. Common duct exploration was done and found to be negative with terminal cholangiograms confirming this and showing the duct emptying into a large duodenal diverticulum. See Fig. 17.

Comment: Certainly one could not be criticized for exploring this common duct, even though negative cholangiograms place the etiology of the jaundice on an inflammatory basis. However, the advisability of passage of probes, dilators, etc., blindly through the ampulla of Vater is questioned, and when pressure is necessary this should be highly condemned. In this particular instance, one can readily see how the production of a false passage with perforation of a duodenal diverticulum could easily occur.

No. 9: Mrs. H. L. This 36-year-old white female previously had acute pancreatitis with a serum amalyse of 795 and a serum bilirubin of 2.3 mgm. per cent. After subsidence of the acute pancreatitis the patient had periodic right upper quadrant pain. Cholecystograms revealed biliary calculi. Laparotomy revealed a thick-walled, contracted gallbladder containing stones and a diffuse induration of the pancreas with distention of the common duct. Operative cholangiogram showed a spasm of the ampulla with no stones present. In view of the pancreatitis T-tube drainage was deemed advisable. A T-tube was inserted, and cholangiograms were repeated, with amyl nitrite given to the patient just preceding these films. These showed a normal biliary tree. See Fig. 18 and 19.

No. 10: Mr. T. P. This 73-year-old white male had progressive painless jaundice. An upper gastrointestinal series was normal

302

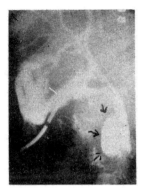

Fig. 17

with non-visualization of the gallbladder present. At operation a thick-walled gallbladder was found, containing two large calculi, which almost completely filled it. Catheter cholangiograms revealed a normal biliary tract from the junction of the cystic and common ducts to the ampulla of Vater. The common hepatic duct showed a zone of complete obstruction produced by an extrinsic scar and inflammatory process. With excision of scar and passage of dilators into the hepatic tree a free flow was obtained. A T-tube was then inserted and terminal cholangiograms were normal. See Fig. 20 and 21.

Comment: The jaundice was on the basis of obstruction by an inflammatory scar of the

common hepatic duct. It is evident that this obstruction as shown by operative cholangiography, could have been easily overlooked. With such an error the post-operative course could have been very stormy instead of uneventful.

No. 11: Mr. O. S. P. This was a 50-year-old white male with jaundice, weight loss, loss of appetite, and an enlarged liver. The thymol turbidity was 12 units, with cephalin flocculation 4 plus. A liver biopsy showed pericholangitic cirrhosis from obstruction. The patient's jaundice increased despite vigorous medical management and at the insistence of the pathologist an exploratory laparotomy was performed. At the time of operation a perfectly normal gallbladder with a hepatitis exclusively limited to the right lobe was found. Needle cholangirgraphy showed a perfectly normal ductal system. See Fig. 22.

Comment: In this group of individuals any type of extensive surgery certainly has an increased morbidity and mortality rate. Common duct exploration would have been most hazardous. Because of the findings at the time of laparotomy one feels considerably more confident in pursuing medical treatment on such a case, when adequate visualization of the ductal system reveals no evidence of obstruction.

No. 12: Mr. G. B. This was a 73-year-old white male with right upper quadrant pain, fever and recurrent jaundice. The patient

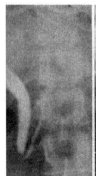

Fig. 18

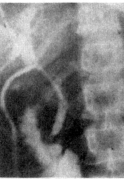

Fig. 19

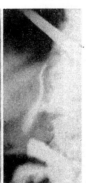

Fig. 20

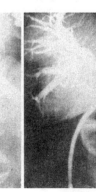

Fig. 21

had had an acute attack with apparent rupture of the gallbladder two weeks prior to admission. At operation a large subhepatic abscess was found. Grossly the gallbladder also presented a picture suggestive of adenocarcinoma. Cholangiograms showed a normal common duct. However, marked extension of the carcinomatous process in the right hepatic radical was present.

Comment: With the advent of more radical surgery, carcinomatous involvement of the gallbladder and the liver is often-times resected. In this instance cholangiograms revealed the carcinomatous process advanced well beyond the line of any resection.

No. 13: Mr. O. D. This 77-year-old white male had intermittent but progressive painless jaundice. Liver function studies were normal with preoperative x-rays showing a normal upper gastrointestinal tract and non-visualization of the gallbladder. At surgery the gallbladder was found enlarged with no stones present. The common duct was dilated and a 1 cm. nodular mass was palpated at the ampulla of Vater. Catheter cholangiograms revealed a small obstructing neoplasm at the ampulla. Following resection terminal cholangiograms showed normal emptying of the reconstructed common duct. See Fig. 23 and 24.

Comment: The prognosis in carcinoma of the common duct is vastly different from that of carcinoma of the head of the pancreas. Cholangiography aided materially in establishment of the diagnosis of duct carcinoma prior to extensive surgery.

In addition to these cases presented above, operative cholangiography has been found to be of extreme value in the biliary tract explorations of biliary atresia as reported by Swenson and Fisher. It is of infinite value also in common duct reconstruction following duct injury as reported by Hughes et al.

In examination of films following serial injection, we feel the first injection of radio-opaque media into the biliary tract is quite comparable to the first swallow of barium in an upper gastro-intestinal tract examination. We have continued using serial films with repeat films being necessary in less than two per cent of the last 106 cases. This gives information of the biliary system, both intra-and extra-hepatic, which can be obtained in no other way.

Over-all Results With Routine Operative Cholangiography By Type

Needle Cholangiography—44 cases

8 non-diagnostic

  18.2 per cent error

Catheter Cholangiography—106 cases

2˙ non-diagnostic-repeat films satisfactory

  1.88 per cent error

Terminal Cholangiography—45 cases

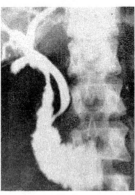 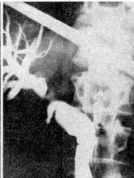 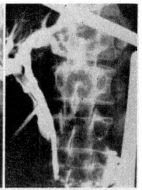

Fig. 22   Fig. 23   Fig. 24

3 repeated with diagnostic films obtained

30 per cent common duct exploration in 150 cases.

This group of cases covers a three and a half year period. The longest follow-up is 42 months. All cases of terminal cholangiography have been rechecked in six weeks with standard T-tube cholangiograms. There have been no cases of retained stones proven by these recheck cholangiograms, and no evidence of retained stones, clinically, from the remainder of this group of 150 patients.

Summary

1. A group of 50 consecutive cases of biliary tract surgery with 200 sets of cholangiograms have been presented. There was no operative mortality nor increased morbidity.

2. A description of technique, both from a radiological and surgical standpoint, has been described.

3. Pitfalls in interpretation have been presented and normal anatomical variations described.

4. Clinical usage and intrinsic value of routine operative cholangiography has been illustrated by case discussion.

5. Fallacies of the usual criteria for common duct exploration are presented.

6. The inadequacies and related dangers of blind common duct exploration are demonstrated.

7. Statistical results are presented with a diagnostic error of 1.88 per cent present in the last 106 cases.

Conclusions

With the routine use of operative cholangiography much knowledge has been obtained pertaining to both the anatomical and physiological variance that may occur within the biliary ductal system. The incidence of re-exploration of the common duct reported in the literature as 6-20 per cent make overlooked common duct stones and strictures a pertinent problem. In our opinion, an incidence of reoperation as high as one per cent constitutes a valid reason for using routine operative cholangiography. Common bile duct exploration is not easily taught to surgical residents because of several factors in judgment and technique. Routine operative cholangiograms can facilitate this training and provide a permanent, objective record to assist the young surgeon in developing and checking his judgment. We can see no valid reason why this procedure should not be more widely used by teaching institutions as well as in general surgical practice.

REFERENCES

1. Caylor, H. D.: Cholangiography in Surgery, Am. J Surg. 87:4:516, 1954.

2. Crile, George, Jr.: Errors in Surgery of the Biliary Tract, Cleveland Clin. Quart. 21:2-90 (April) 1954.

3. Cotte, G.: Sur l'exploration radiologiqu e des voies biliaires avec injection de lipiodol apres cholecystostomie ou choledocotomie. Bull. et mem Soc. Nat. de Chir. 55:863, 1929

4. Hight, D., and Lingley, Jr.: Value of Cholangiograms During Biliary Tract Surgery, New Eng. J. Med., 246:761-765, 1952.

5. Hughes, C. R., Hannan, J. R., and Melvey, B. E.: Cholangiography in Stone Stricture and Operative Injury of Biliary Ducts. J.A.M.A. 137:687, 1948.

6. Mirizi, P. L.: Cholangiografi durante las operaciones de las vias viliares. Bol. Soc. Cir. B. Aires, 16:1133, 1932.

7. Mixter, C. H. and Hermanson, L.: A Critical Evaluation of Cholangiography, Am. J. Surg., 40:223, 1938.

8. Partington, P. F. and Sacks, M.D.: Routine Use of Operative Cholangiography. S. G. and O., 87:299, 1948.

9. Primbram, B. O. C.: The Method for Dissolution of C. D. Stones Remaining after Operation. Surgery, 22:806, 1947.

10. Shatley, L. R. and Saypol, G. M : Intra-Abdominal Choledochography: Preliminary Report of Method of Detecting Stones in Common Bile Duct, Am. J. Surg. 84:229-232, 1952.

11. Sherman, C. D., Jr., and Stabins, S. J.: The Case for Operative Cholangiography, S. G. and O., 98:223, 1954.

12. Swedburg, Jr.: Routine Cholangiography at Operation for Gallstones, Act. Chir. Scandinav., 103:175, 1952.

13. Swenson and Fisher: Utilization of Cholangiograms During Exploration for Biliary Atresia, New Eng. J. Med., page 247, 1952.

14. Walters, Waltmon: Physiologic and Surgical Considerations in Treatment of Complicated Lesions of the Biliary Tract. Arch. Surg., 68:1: (January), 1954.

Both Bone Fractures of the Leg,

PRINCIPLES OF TREATMENT

CARLO SCUDERI, M.D.

One of the most common fractures of the present mode of living is the both bone fracture of the leg. Once the fundamentals of the treatment of these shaft fractures are understood, the various present methods of treatment can be rationally applied.

Pathological Physiology

In Figure I is diagramatically shown an intact tibia and fibula with the large muscle bellies of the calf. The major muscles of this group have their origin in the femur and their insertion in the bones of the foot. As long as the tibia and fibula remain intact, these muscles function without impairment. The muscle tone remains uniformly normal. However, as soon as the firm fixation of the tibia and fibula are removed, and pain is produced because of a both bone fracture of the leg, these muscles are thrown into spasm. The contraction of these muscles becomes markedly intensified and prolonged over the normal. The origin and insertion of these muscles tend to approximate one another because of the muscle contractions and the loss of bone stability as results in fractures as illustrated in Figures 4, 5, 6, and 7. Shortening and displacement inevitably occurs unlese adequate treatment is rendered.

Solitary Fracture of the Fibula

Occasionally the shaft of the fibula is fractured and the tibia remains intact. No shortening can occur, and the displacement of the fibular fracture is minimal, if at all. (Figure 2).

This particular fracture can be successfully treated without any cast in cooperative adults. Avoidance of weight bearing by the use of crutches for five to six weeks is usually all that is necessary to attain a successful result.

In children and uncooperative adults, the application of a cast from the lower third of the femur to the toes, reminds the patient that he is not to bear any weight on

THE AUTHOR

Carlo Scuderi, M.D., Chicago, presented the article, "Both Bone Fractures of the Leg—Principles of Treatment," at the 1954 meeting of the Oklahoma Academy of General Practice. Doctor Scuderi is associate professor of surgery at the University of Illinois and is also senior attending surgeon at Cook County Hospital. He is chairman of the department of orthopedic surgery at St. Elizabeth's Hospital and Columbus Hospital in Chicago and on the surgical staff of Cook County Graduate School.

the extremity . Secondly, should the patient become unruly, the cast will minimize any possible secondary trauma with resulting pain.

Solitary Fracture of The Tibia

As the tibia is the main weight bearing bone of the lower leg, fractures of the tibia alone are of a greater magnitude than solitary fractures of the shaft of the fibula. (Figure 3). However, as long as the fibula remains intact, the tibia has an excellent internal splinting and no shortening can occur. Displacement of the bones at the fracture site may occur but it is most unusual for it to be very great. Pain from this type of fracture is substantial, and for this reason, immobilization in a cast is very important. The cast should extend from the middle third of the femur to the toes. Unlimited weight bearing in this type of fracture is not advisable under four to five months in the average adult. Of course, many factors come into play, and clinical judgment must govern the merits of each particular case. In children the period of healing is much more rapid in all of the fractures discussed in this paper, and the period of immobilization should be shortened accordingly.

In certain rare occasions where a very severe local force has produced the fracture with complete displacement of the bone ends, open reduction with simple reapposition of the bone fragments may be necessary. The most common etiological cause of this type of fracture is the automobile.

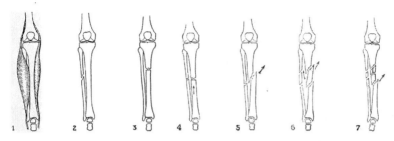

November, 1954—Volume 47, Number 11

Transverse Fractures of the Tibia and the Fibula

Occasionally the tibia and fibula are broken at the same level, in a transverse direction. (Figure 4). The ends are jagged and are locked with one another. It is very difficult for this fracture to disengage itself. No shortening can occur and only angulation will result. For this reason, the simple immobilization of the leg in a circular cast extending from the mid thigh to the toes is all that is required. Any axial deviation can be corrected by secondary wedging of the cast.

Oblique Fractures of the Tibia and the Fibula

In Figure 5, we see an oblique both bone fracture of the tibia and fibula with overriding and displacement. It is impossible to successfully reduce and maintain the reduction during the process of healing by the use of a simple cast in this type of case. Muscle spasm and contracture inevitably will pull the fragments past one another. For this reason some form of therapy is required which will counteract or prevent this shortening and displacement.

Skeletal traction will overcome the shortening and frequently the displacement, but this procedure requires a long hospital stay with the leg in traction until some evidence of beginning union takes place. This is somewhere in the vicinity of five to seven weeks.

Double pin fixation with a Steinman pin through the proximal and one through the distal fragment with reduction and immobilization in a circular cast will work very well if correctly used. Distraction of the fragments must be avoided. Once the correct alignment is attained, the patient can be permitted up and about on cruches and can be discharged to his home and treated as an out-patient.

The use of beaded wires incorporated in a cast maintain excellent reduction and fixation. In the hands of men experienced in this field, this method is most satisfactory.

The use of multiple pin fixation of the fragments with external bar stabilization should be reserved for only those cases where large skin defects prohibit the use of other methods. This method frequently leads to avoidable complications and is secondary to other methods of choice.

In the presence of good skin, and a patient in relatively good health, the author has felt that internal fixation by the use of two screws is most satisfactory. By this method immediate anatomical apposition is attained and the use of a circular cast is then necessary until a solid bony union occurs. Because of the anatomical apposition and the firm fixation, this type of treatment produces a bony union in about one-third less than the usual length of time required by most other methods.

Adequate equipment is necessary to reduce and maintain reduction during the operative procedure if success is to result. Improvised methods during the operation are frequently disastrous. The use of a constrictor and a fracture table are indispensable pieces of armamentarium.

This method has been used by the author whenever feasible for the last 18 years with a negligible number of complications or failures.

Both Bone Fractures of the Tibia and Fibula with an Intermediary Third Fragment

In Figure 6 is a complicated fracture because the intermediary fragment tends to get out of line and usually one or the other end goes on to a non-union. For this reason early adequate reduction is necessary and can only be successfully obtained by open reduction and plating on the lateral side of the tibia. The T & G stainless steel plate lends itself very readily to this type of fracture because it is long and can be overlapped one upon the other to give length and strength to the fixation. Intramedullary nailing of this type of fracture using the Rush Pin works very well in the hands of those experienced in the procedure. It requires less dissection and less time than a plate application. The author has been highly pleased with his experiences in this type of fracture using the Rush Pin.

Skeletal traction will serve to overcome the shortening but does not assure proper alignment of the third fragment. In addition distraction easily results, leading to a non-union.

Severly Communited Both Bone Fractures of the Leg

In Figure 7 is illustrated a severely communited both bone fracture of the leg. Skeletal traction is certainly indicated in this type of injury, otherwise shortening and angulation result. Double pin fixation is definitely contra-indicated. It is axiomatic "The more comminuted a fracture, the less is the indication for surgery". Any attempt at internal fixation in this type of fracture only adds to the already existing problem. This type of case requires long immobilization and protection from weight bearing and frequently requires a bone graft for a delayed or non-union.

In some cases where the tibia is markedly comminuted and the fibula has a simple fracture, plating of the fibula restores length, alignment, and gives relatively good fixation to the fracture of the comminuted tibia. This procedure works ideally when one has an associated compounding of the tibia. Less dissection is required, and the foreign body of the plate and screws are away from the damaged soft tissue.

Conclusions

1. Early adequate reduction and fixation are desirable in all cases.

2. The counteracting of the forces produced by muscle contractures must be understood and constantly kept in mind during the treatment.

3. Single fractures of the fibula or tibia, or transverse fractures of both bones of the leg can be successfully treated by casts alone.

4. Oblique both bone fractures of the leg are best treated by open reduction and internal screw fixation. Double pin fixation or beaded wires can also be used with very satisfactory results.

5. Intermediary third fragments of the tibia with displacement are best treated by internal plate fixation or intramedullary pin fixation of the Rush or Lotte type, in order to prevent shortening and also to lessen the incidence of non-union.

6. Severely comminuted both bone fractures of the leg are best treated by skeletal traction or double pin fixation.

"Medic" Is New TV Program

"Medic," a stirring, step-by-step approach to current medical, surgical and psychological problems, is a new series appearing three out of four Mondays at 8:00 p.m. on WKY-TV.

Produced as documentary dramas which are based upon authentic medical information, "Medic" has received the official endorsement of the Los Angeles County Medical Associaton.

This portrayal of the medical profession is written and supervised by James Moser, best known for his original work with the NBC Television-Radio series, "Dragnet." The triumphs and tragedies of the struggles of the medical profession for the preservation of life provide the basic theme for the 30-minute show.

WKY-TV invites comments from members of the medical profession in reference to this unusual television series.

Cortisone in

BLACK WIDOW SPIDER BITE

JOHN M. GOUDY, M.D., and H. A. MASTERS, M.D.

Cortisone has proven of value in a wide variety of allergic and toxic conditions. During a study on the use of this drug in the treatment of venomous snake bites, we received numerous inquiries about its effectiveness in black widow spider bite. We wish to report the treatment of two such cases in which we achieved good results. An additional case of spider bite, not a black widow, has been treated, and will be included in this report, since it illustrates some of the difficulties which arise in evaluating the use of cortisone in any condition.

Black widow spider bite appears to respond to a wide variety of therapeutic agents. It is characteristic of this condition that the patient appears gravely ill when first seen, but recovers very rapidly, often within 24 hours. The mortality rate is very low, considering the severity of the symptoms, being given as under six per cent and there are no reports of fatality in the recent literature.

Calcium gluconate is accepted as the standard treatment (1), but good results have been reported with neostigmine methylsulfate (2), magnesium sulfate (3), sodium thiosulfate (4), phyatromine (5), epinephrine (6), and opiates (7). Perhaps the most important point in the treatment is to avoid confusion with acute surgical conditions of the abdomen, which the condition often mimics quite closely.

Case I: The first patient was an eight month old male infant, well developed and very well nourished, who was bitten on the right leg by a black shiny spider, 24 hours before admission. Examination revealed an acutely ill infant with 105 (R) temperature, abdominal distention, and erythema and edema of the right leg, extending from the ankle to the hip. A small papule within a blanched area two centimeters in diameter marked the spider bite. The possibility of

THE AUTHORS

John M. Gowdy, M.D. and H. A. Masters, M.D., Tahlequah, wrote "Cortisone in Black Widow Spider Bite." Doctor Gowdy is medical officer in charge, Wm. W. Hastings Hospital operated by the United States Department of the Interior Office of Indian Affairs. Doctor Masters, a graduate of the University of Oklahoma School of Medicine, is in private practice in Tahlequah. He interned at University and Crippled Children's Hospitals and served his residency at St. Anthony's, Oklahoma City.

osteomyelitis was considered and ruled out by x-ray. Laboratory findings were leukocytosis and a predominance of neutrophiles.

Streptomycin and cortisone one-fourth cubic centimeters each) were given immediately, and daily thereafter for three days. After the initial injection, abdominal distention and, apparently, pain continued.

Three cubic centimeters of calcium gluconate was given intravenously four hours after admission, with immediate relief. During the next 12 hours the temperature dropped slowly to 101 (R). It rose to 104 (R) on the day following admission, then became, and remained normal. The local symptoms subsided rapidly and the patient was discharged on the fifth hospital day.

Case II: The second patient presented himself for treatment four hours after being bitten on the lower lip by a spider which he described as brown and hairy, definitely not a black widow. Examination revealed an acutely ill male 64 years of age, with pain and swelling of the lower lip and considerable edema along the mandible on the affected side. Oral temperature was 101.4, but no other signs or symptoms were present. At the time of admission, no local wound could be seen. He was placed on Benadryl (R), 100 milligrams orally four times daily, and ice packs were applied locally. Pain was controlled by aspirin, 10 grains as needed.

The following day the edema and pain were considerably lessened, but the fever persisted around 101. Beginning ulceration of the lip was noted and the patient complained of generalized aching and chilling. These symptoms persisted for the next three days. Twenty five milligrams of cortisone were given on the third day. Because of the fever and local infection, streptomycin was also given. While no definite results from cortisone could be demonstrated, the patient felt that it helped and requested another injection on the following day.

Ulceration of the lip progressed, and on the fifth day a blister developed on the mucosa beneath the external wound. Through and through perforation could not be demonstrated, although the mucosal lesion became much larger than the external ulcer. The patient made an uneventful recovery and was released on the eighth hospital day. All edema had subsided and the external wound was completely healed, although slight mucosal ulceration persisted.

Case III: The third patient was a four-year-old white male who entered the office one hour after having been bitten by a black widow spider. The spider was seen and killed by his father. On admission the boy was cramping severely and had difficulty in getting his breath. He was given 1-6 grain of morphine which gave partial relief in 30 minutes. At that time he was given 2-10 cubic centimeters of adrenalin. This had no apparent effect. He was then given 10 milligrams of hydrocortisone, orally. Within one hour following the hydrocortisone he was reasonably comfortable and fell asleep. He was asked to remain in the office five hours. At the end of that time he had awakened from the effect of the morphine and was still reasonably comfortable. He was sent home with a prescription of hydrocortisone, five milligrams of which was to be given orally twice a day. Since there was no assurance that the hydrocortisone would give continued relief from the pain and cramping, morphine was also prescribed,

Two days later he returned to the office. He had been reasonably comfortable and had not required any of the morphine. The only remaining symptom was slight aching in his legs. The dose of hydrocortisone was reduced to five milligrams once a day. If symptoms returned, he was to increase the dosage. It was reported that he had no return of symptoms and medicine was discontinued after four days treatment.

Comment

Cortisone has been shown to be of some danger in acute infections, and we are reluctant to employ it in the presence of fever without the protection of an antibiotic. Secondary infection is common in all types of spider bite and was apparently a factor in the first two cases.

The question naturally arises as to the role of cortisone in the tissue breakdown noted in Case II. This type of reaction commonly follows the bite of non-poisonous spiders and we do not feel that the cortisone was responsible. We have employed cortisone in much higher dosage following surgery with no evidence of impairment of healing.

ACTH is available in a form which can be given intravenously for more rapid action. This preparation would probably be more useful for the acute pain and abdominal cramping. It should be emphasized that the symptoms of black widow spider bite may closely mimic acute surgical conditions of the abdomen, and unnecessary operations may be performed if this fact is not remembered.

Antivenin is available for treatment, but in view of the many preparations which are effective, there is little need for its use.

REFERENCES

1. Taubenhaus, L. J.: Black Widow Spider Bite Syndrome; N. Carolina Med. J., 13;37 (Jan.) 1952.

2. Boone, J. A. and Bell, J. E.: Neostigmine Methylsulfate. An Apparent Specific for Arachnidism; J.A.M.A., 129:1016 (Dec. 8) 1945.

3. Pulido, M. A.: Comment in J.A.M.A., 130:733 (March 16) 1946.

4. Davis, P. L.: Comment in J.A.M.A., 130:733 (March 16) 1946.

5. Holloway, O. R.: Use of Physostigmine in Treatment of Black Widow Spider Bite; Ark. Med. Soc. J.; 47:75 (Sept.) 1950.

6. Couric, E. S.: Effective Treatment for Black Widow Spider Bite; S.M.J.; 45:1193 (Dec.) 1952.

7. Hale, R. E.: Comment in J.A.M.A., 130:172 (Jan. 19) 1946.

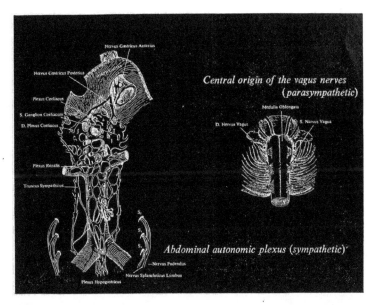

Central origin of the vagus nerves
(parasympathetic)

Abdominal autonomic plexus (sympathetic)

Control of Gastric Motility and Spasticity in Peptic Ulcer with Banthine®

"The need[1] for suppressing gastric motility and spastic states is ... fundamental in peptic ulcer therapy. Since the cholinergic nerves are motor and secretory to the stomach and motor to the intestines, agents capable of blocking cholinergic nerve stimulation are frequently used to lessen motor activity and hypermotility."

Banthine[2] "has dual effectiveness; it inhibits acetylcholine liberated at the postganglionic parasympathetic nerve endings and it blocks acetylcholine transmission through autonomic ganglia."

It has been shown[1] to diminish gastric motility and secretion significantly as well as intestinal and colonic motility.

The usual schedule of administration in peptic ulcer is 50 to 100 mg. every six hours, day and night, with subsequent adjustment to the patient's needs and tolerance. After the ulcer is healed, maintenance therapy, approximately half of the therapeutic dosage, should be continued for reasonable assurance of nonrecurrence.

Banthine® (brand of methantheline bromide) is supplied in: Banthine ampuls, 50 mg.—Banthine tablets, 50 mg.

It is accepted by the Council on Pharmacy and Chemistry of the American Medical Association. Searle Research in the Service of Medicine.

1. Zupko, A. G.: Pharmacology and the General Practitioner, GP 7:55 (March) 1953.

2. McHardy, G. G., and Others: Clinical Evaluation of Methantheline (Banthine) Bromide in Gastroenterology, J.A.M.A. 147:1620 (Dec. 22) 1951.

Association Activities

PRESIDENT'S LETTER

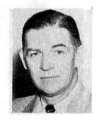

Desegregation is part of the new world social order, and of all social reforms that have taken place in the past 30 years, desegregation will probably result in the greatest benefits. It is certainly Christian in principle, and is definitely an advance in our ethical and moral thinking.

The problem of social and economic racial equality has been studied for years by the best minds of all races. In the United States prejudice and the fear of a disturbed economy have ben the most harassing stumbling blocks to the solution of the problem. Individual members of the medical profession, for the most part, have made little distinction in a man's color, creed, or economic status, but the medical profession as a whole is due some criticism for not taking an earlier and more definite lead in the solving of this problem.

Segregation of the members of our own profession has persisted until recent years, but, fortunately, this is rapidly disappearing. Several Oklahoma county societies, namely: Grady, Tulsa, Okfuskee, Okmulgee, and Muskogee have ended segregation in the past five years, which is a wise and just policy, and one for which they should be commended. At its September meeting the Oklahoma County Medical Society voted by an overwhelming majority to admit three Negro doctors as members. This lead should be followed by the remaining county societies in the state.

President

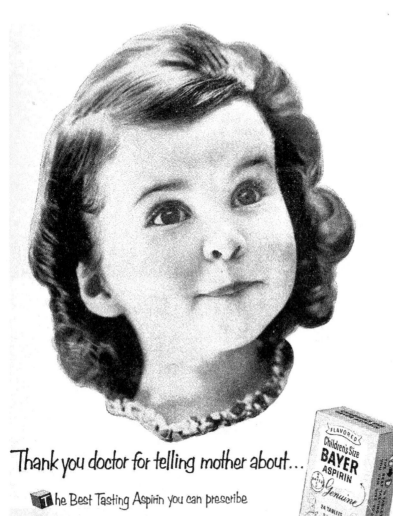

Thank you doctor for telling mother about...

The Best Tasting Aspirin you can prescribe

The Flavor Remains Stable down to the last tablet

15¢ Bottle of 24 tablets (2½ grs. each)

We will be pleased to send samples on request

THE BAYER COMPANY DIVISION of Sterling Drug Inc., 1450 Broadway, New York 18, N.Y.

Make Plans Now For AMA's Miami Meeting

Sunny skies, swaying palms and broad sandy beaches are but a few of the attractions Miami offers physicians and their wives planning to attend AMA's eighth annual Clinical Meeting Nov. 29-Dec. 2. An excellent scientific program — including lectures, exhibits, motion pictures and color television — plus a large array of technical exhibits have been lined up for AMA visitors.

This year's program stresses the practical everyday problems which face the general practitioner. The lecture program will include subjects of broad interest in the fields of medicine, surgery, pediatrics, neuropsychiatry, and obstetrics and gynecology. Motion pictures will be shown continuously, and a special evening film program has been arranged. Bringing the operating room directly into the lecture hall, color television programs will originate from the Jackson Memorial Hospital. The Scientific Exhibit will feature about 80 exhibits, and demonstrators will be on duty throughout the week to answer physicians' questions.

Lectures, both the Technical and Scientific Exhibit, motion pictures and color television Exhibits, motion pictures and color tele-at Dinner Key Auditorium. The McAllister Hotel has been selected as the headquarters for House of Delegates meetings.

Cancer Society Notes

The American Cancer Society, Oklahoma Division, wishes to announce its second annual medical and scientific meeting December 3, 1954, at the Skirvin Hotel, Oklahoma City.

A panel of outstanding authorities will read papers in the field of cancer treatment and care. The speakers and their tentative subjects are:

Claude F. Dixon, M.D. — 1. Intestinal Polyps and Their Management; 2. Cancer of the Rectum.

Herbert E. Schmitz, M.D.—1. Cancer of the Vulva; 2. Cancer of the Cervix.

David A. Wood, M.D.—1. Pathology of the Thyroid Gland; 2. Utilization of Frozen Sections in the Treatment of Cancer.

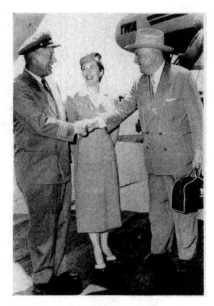

Physician Is Indian Ambassador In Europe

Charles Ed. White, M.D., Muskogee, right, is pictured pausing for a short chat with Capt. Charles Kratovil and Hostess Beth Howard prior to his departure for Geneva where he addressed the International Congress on Gynecology and Obstetrics July 26.

Doctor White made the journey as an official ambassador of the Cherokee Indian Tribe, a post last held by General Sam Houston in 1829. The official action was unanimously approved by the 12-man executive committee of the Cherokees.

The honor was conferred by Principal Chief of the Cherokees, W. W. Keeler, Vice-President of the Phillips Petroleum Company and Earl Boyd Pierce, attorney for the Cherokee Nation.

Donald B. Effler, M.D.—1. Cancer of the Esophagus and Upper End of the Stomach; 2. Cancer of the Lung.

Charles S. Cameron, M.D.—The Present Outcome of the American Cancer Society's Extensive Survey in the Relation of Tobacco Smoking and Cancer of the Lung.

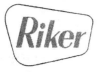

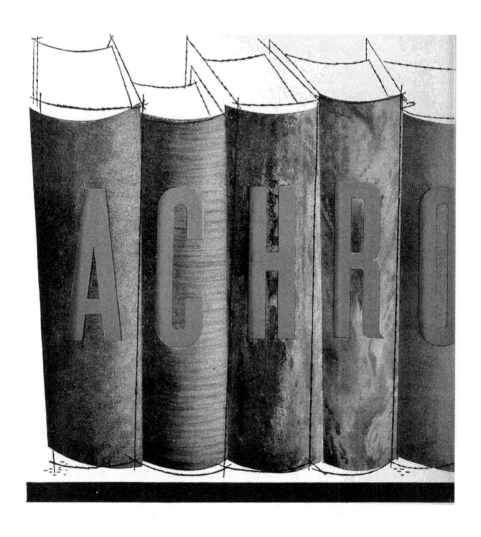

Medical history is being written today

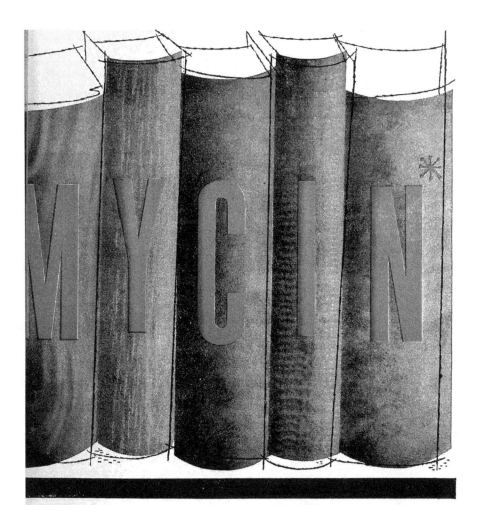

Hydrochloride
Tetracycline HCl *Lederle*

The introduction and rapid widespread adoption of ACHROMYCIN has opened a new chapter in the history of broad-spectrum antibiotics.

ACHROMYCIN fulfills the requirements of the ideal antibiotic in virtually every respect . . . wide-range antimicrobial activity, *in vivo* stability, tissue penetration, minimal toxicity.

ACHROMYCIN is truly a broad-spectrum weapon, effective against Gram-positive and Gram-negative bacteria, as well as certain mixed infections.

ACHROMYCIN is more stable and produces fewer side effects than certain other broad-spectrum antibiotics.

ACHROMYCIN provides prompt diffusion in body tissues and fluids.

ACHROMYCIN is destined to play a major role among the great therapeutic agents.

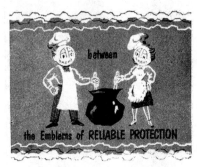
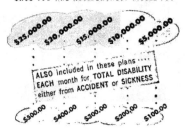
Deaths

WALTER H. MILES, M.D.
1891-1954

Walter H. Miles, M.D., director of the Oklahoma City Health Department for 28 years, died August 31 after an illness of two weeks. Born October 26, 1891 in Maquoketa, Iowa, he came to Oklahoma City in 1901 with his parents. He received a bachelor of science degree from Oklahoma University in 1916 before going on to medical school. He received his medical degree in 1918. He served in the army from 1940 to 1946 and saw duty in Africa and Sicily with the 45th, then in the winter of 1943 was assigned to public health work and served in Italy and later Austria under military government.

He was active in medical organizations, the Reserve Officers organization, American Legion, Army and Navy club, Masons, Shrine, Knights of Pythias, Lions Club and Congenial Dinner Club.

THAD C. LEACHMAN, M.D.
1874-1954

Thad C. Leachman, M.D., formerly of Woodward, died in a Richmond, Virginia, hospital August 5.

He was honored by Woodward county citizens on September 2, 1948, at a celebration attended by more than 4,000 adults he had delivered.

Doctor Leachman was born at Terre Haute, Ind. and was graduated from the University of Tennessee medical school. He began his practice at Woodward in 1904, moved for a brief time to Rogers County, Ark., then to Bellingham, Wash., and returned to Woodward in 1906 where he practiced until his retirement.

He was active in medical organizations and was a member of the Masonic lodge and a charter member of the Woodward Kiwanis club.

FREDERICK R. SUTTON, M.D.
1875-1954

Frederick R. Sutton, M.D., Bartlesville physician for 26 years, died in an Oklahoma City hospital August 11 after an extended illness. He had retired from practice in 1925 and moved to Oklahoma City.

He was born in Hartford, Kansas and came to Oklahoma in 1889. He attended medical school in Kansas City and graduated from Columbia in New York.

ALEXANDER BARKLEY, M.D.
1859-1954

Alexander Barkley, M.D., one of Oklahoma's first physicians, died in Oklahoma City September 25. He had been in ill health for some time.

Doctor Barkley was born in Beardstown, Mo. He studied medicine in St. Louis and practiced in Rigor, Mo. until 1893 when he made the Cherokee Strip run. He practiced at Pond Creek and Hobart. He retired for a short time but the shortage of doctors in World War I forced him to resume his practice. He moved to Norman in 1922 when he again retired.

THOMAS W. STALLINGS, M.D.
1877-1954

Thomas W. Stallings, M.D., a Life Member of the Tulsa County Medical Society, died July 15 after an illness of two years.

He attended Tulane University and in 1905 received his medical degree from Louisville Medical School, Louisville, Kentucky. He entered practice at Allen, Oklahoma in 1907 and later practiced in Tishomingo before moving to Tulsa in 1917.

E. E. HEADY, M.D.
1869-1954

E. E. Heady, M.D., pioneer Harper county physician, died in a Texas hospital August 6. He was born at Monticello, Ind. and began teaching school when 17 years old. He later attended the University of Louisville School of Medicine and moved to Oklahoma in 1895. He served in the medical corps in World War I. When he retired from practice in 1943, he was practicing in Goodwell.

J. W. DRIVER, M.D.
1898-1954

J. W. Driver, M.D., Perry, died September 19 following a cerebral hemorrhage.

Doctor Driver was born at Helena, Mo. He moved to Ponca City with his family as a boy and lived there until going to college. After graduation in 1933 from the Rush Medical College he began the practice of medicine at Perry.

ALONZO C. McFARLING, M.D.
1878-1954

A. C. McFarling, M.D., died July 29 in Shawnee. He was graduated from the Fort Worth School of Medicine in 1909 and had practiced in Shawnee nearly 40 years.

ANNUAL CLINICAL CONFERENCE

CHICAGO MEDICAL SOCIETY

MARCH 1, 2, 3, 4, 1955

Palmer House, Chicago

DAILY HALF-HOUR LECTURES BY OUTSTANDING TEACHERS AND SPEAKERS on subjects of interest to both general practitioner and specialist.

PANELS ON TIMELY TOPICS.

MEDICAL COLOR TELECASTS.

TEACHING DEMONSTRATIONS.

SCIENTIFIC EXHIBITS worthy of real study and h e l p f u l and time-saving TECHNICAL EXHIBITS.

The CHICAGO MEDICAL SOCIETY ANNUAL CLINICAL CONFERENCE should be a MUST on the calendar of every physician. Plan now to a t t e n d and make your reservations at the Palmer House.

Book Reviews

MANUAL OF ANTIBIOTICS 1954-55. Prepared under the editorial direction of Henry Welch, Ph.D. Cloth. $2.50. Pp. 87. Medical Encyclopedia, Inc., 30 East 60th St., N.Y. 22, N.Y. Distributed by American Pharmaceutical Association, 2215 Constitution Ave., N.W., Washington, D.C.

The flood tide of trade-names for antibiotic preparations manufactured, or distributed by, American drug houses is well mirrored in this compilation. In it are listed over 600 such names varying from the ludicrous to the sublime. For example: Biokets; Bovoc Pink-eye Powder; Cafed Nose drops, etc! All of the antibiotic drugs commercially available in the United States are listed alphabetically by their generic terms. Under these are grouped the trade-names of each manufacturer, the active ingredients and the indications for usage. Separate indices list trade-names, generic terms, and, finally, manufacturer addresses.

In his preface Doctor Welch states that it is planned to revise and keep up to date the constant flow of new trade-names for the antibiotic preparations.

The manual will be useful primarily to pharmacists, reference libraries and the fellow who misplaces the equivalent flood of three - color - product - information brochures that pours through his office door each day.   —John G. Matt, M.D.

BEYOND THE GERM THEORY. Edited by Iago Galdston, M.D., New York Academy of Medicine. Published by the Health Education Council. 1954.

This is a most interesting sort of compilation. The authors, physicians, and Ph.D.,'s have chosen a rather interesting title for the manuscript. It would seem to me after reading the book that now, according to the authors, the "term" to fear is *man.* Microscopic organisms have, so far as the writers of the book are concerned, become unimportant. "Man, science demonstrated, can in a measure fend against germs by destroying them and by neutralizing their poisons.

I would only say—really!? I am not so secure about the end results of antibiotics! Not a mention of viruses is made in the book.

The essence of the treatise is that germs are of no longer any threat or trouble to man — but instead, that man himself as a germ has become the primary problem and cause of disease.

Such philosophical ruminations as expounded by the authors could result in the development of a bizarre pseudo-scientific psychological empire!

I would like to issue an admonition to the grandchildren of the authors — watch out for other miscroorganisms, insects, other animals, and maybe plants that were not given any authority and respect at the "council table".   —Coyne H. Campbell, M.D.

Five Attend Public Relations Conference

The AMA's Public Relations Institute in Chicago September 1 and 2 attracted almost 300 state and county medical society representatives. Among those attending the "crackerbarrel institute" from Oklahoma were John McDonald M.D., John W. Records, M.D., Chairman of Oklahoma's Committee, Dick Graham, Executive Secretary, all from Oklahoma State Medical Association; Alma F. O'Donnell, Executive Secretary, Oklahoma County Medical Society; and Jack Spears, Executive Secretary, Tulsa County Medical Society.

The institute, planned primarily for lay executive and PR personnel, M.D. chairmen of PR committees, and Auxiliary PR committee women, was the most successful ever held. The two-day meeting featured experts in medical television production, direct mail promotion, AMA services, medical fees, the role of medical assistants, medical motion pictures, and inter-organizational cooperation.

Another meeting, keyed to the public relations needs of individual physicians, will be the AMA's Seventh National Medical Public Relations Conference in Miami at the McAllister Hotel, Sunday, November 28 — the day preceding the opening of the Clinical Session.

DOCTOR, WHEN YOUR PATIENTS ASK...

What have VICEROYS got that other filter tip cigarettes haven't got ?

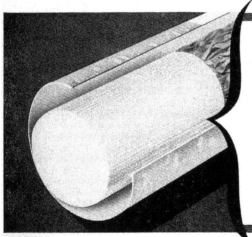

The Answer Is
20,000 FILTERS
in Every Viceroy Tip

Only Viceroy has this new-type filter. Made of a non-mineral cellulose acetate—it gives the greatest filtering action possible without impairing flavor or impeding the flow of smoke.

Smoke is also filtered through Viceroy's king-size length of rich, costly tobaccos. Thus, Viceroy smokers get *double the filtering action* . . . for only a penny or two more than brands without filters.

WORLD'S LARGEST-SELLING FILTER TIP CIGARETTE

New King-Size

Filter Tip VICEROY

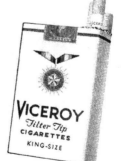

ONLY A PENNY OR TWO MORE
THAN CIGARETTES WITHOUT FILTERS

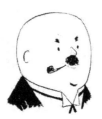

for the 3 patients in 4

with seborrheic dermatitis
of the scalp

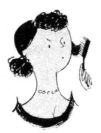

Have you prescribed SELSUN for them yet? Here are the results you can expect: complete control in 81 to 87 per cent of all seborrheic dermatitis cases, and in 92 to 95 per cent of common dandruff cases. SELSUN keeps the scalp scale-free for *one to four weeks*—relieves itching and burning after only two or three applications.

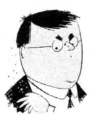

SELSUN is applied and rinsed out while washing the hair. It takes little time, no complicated procedures or messy ointments. Ethically advertised and dispensed only on your prescription. In 4-fluidounce bottles. *Abbott*

prescribe ...

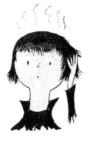

SELSUN®
SULFIDE *Suspension*

(Selenium Sulfide, Abbott)

401065

Calm AND *Relaxed*

WITH MEBARAL®

The calming influence of Mebaral is eminently helpful in

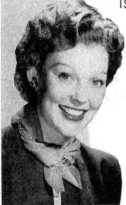

- tension and anxiety states
- nervous symptoms of the menopause
- neurasthenia
- mild psychoses
- hysteria
- hyperthyroidism
- migraine
- pruritus
- hyperemesis nervosa
- hyperemesis gravidarum
- restlessness and irritability associated with pain or infection
- cardiovascular disorders
- allergies
- alcoholism

DOSAGE:

Adults—32 mg. to 0.1 Gm.
(optimal 50 mg.), 3 or 4 times daily.

Children—16 to 32 mg.,
3 or 4 times daily.

HOW SUPPLIED:

Tablets of 32 mg. (½ grain)
Tablets of 50 mg. (¾ grain)
Tablets of 0.1 Gm. (1½ grains)
Tablets of 0.2 Gm. (3 grains)
scored for division

Winthrop-Stearns INC.
NEW YORK 18, N. Y.   WINDSOR, ONT.

Mebaral, trademark reg. U. S. Pat. Off., brand of mephobarbital

⟞⟞⟞*Have You Heard?*

HAROLD G. SLEEPER, M.D., Oklahoma City, has been elected councilor for Oklahoma of the Mid-Continent Psychiatric Association.

FRANK AUSTIN, M.D., formerly a major in the medical corps stationed at Fort Sill, has opened his office in Lawton.

ALFRED H. BUNGARDT, M.D., until recently medical director of Crippled Children's Hospital, has entered private practice in Tulsa.

C. H. SMITH, M.D., has opened his office in Duncan.

SAMUEL SEPKOWITZ, M.D., Oklahoma City, has been named pediatrician for the Oklahoma County Juvenile Court.

WILLIAM O. COLEMAN, M.D., has opened his offices in the Osler Annex, Oklahoma City.

ROBERT ZUMWALT, M.D., graduate of the University of Oklahoma School of Medicine, is now in practice at the Tecumseh Clinic.

W. P. LERBLANCE, JR., M.D., Hartshorne, has been appointed a member of the Pittsburg County Excise Board.

JACK BAXTER, M.D., Shawnee, has reported for active duty with the U. S. navy as lieutenant commander.

JACK C. MILEHAM, M.D., Chandler, has recently opened his new 23 room hospital and clinic in Chandler.

G. R. BOOTH, M.D., Wilburton, was honored by the University of Tennessee as a graduate of 1904. He was one of 47 physicians presented the Golden "T" certificate September 27.

DONALD WILLIAMSON, M.D., has joined L. M. PASCUCCI, M.D. and E. S. KERCKES, M.D. in their recently-established radiological private office, in Tulsa.

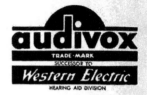

Tenth Annual

POSTGRADUATE COURSE

in

SURGERY

Four Days, January 17 to 20, 1955

Guest Instructors:

RICHARD B. CATTELL. M.D., The Lahey Clinic
DAVID M. DAVIS, M.D., Jefferson Medical College
J. ENGLEBERT DUNPHY, M.D., Harvard Medical School
DAVITT A. FELDER, M.D., University of Minnesota
JOHN H. GRINDLAY, M.D., The Mayo Clinic
CHARLES HUFNAGEL, M.D., Georgetown University
AMOS R. KOONTZ, M.D., Johns Hopkins University
CHAMP LYONS, M.D., Medical College of Alabama
EARLE B. MAHONEY, M.D., University of Rochester
K. ALVIN MERENDINO M.D., University of Washington
H. WILLIAM SCOTT, JR., M.D., Vanderbilt University
DANLEY P. SLAUGHTER, M.D., University of Illinois
HARVEY B. STONE, M.D., Johns Hopkins University
ORVAR SWENSON, M.D., Tufts College
HOWARD ULFELDER, M.D., Harvard Medical School
NATHAN A. WOMACK, M.D., University of North Carolina

✤ ✤ ✤ ✤

Also twenty members of the faculties in Surgery and Gynecology of the University of Kansas.

For program announcement and information, write:

Extension Program in Medicine

UNIVERSITY OF KANSAS SCHOOL OF MEDICINE

Kansas City 12, Kansas

Editorials

Medical Service Society of America

The Medical Service Society of America presented the General Practitioner of the Year a plaque and key at the interim session of the American Medical Association at Miami. National recognition thus comes to a young organization whose interest in the health of the public parallels our own.

The detail men are the spokesmen for the great and small pharmaceutical manufacturers who are allocating a sizeable portion of their income for research either in their own laboratories or in those of the universities or both. As such, they have the same pride of accomplishment in the successful treatment of the sick as do those of us who prescribe their products to that end.

Competition for patronage is a game which, if played fairly, must have rules—there are always scoundrels. Men with like competitive interests band together into organizations and the organization makes the rules or code of ethics for its particular members. We have done this with our medical societies. The detail men are doing this with the Medical Service Society of America.

Once the code is established by agreement among its members, an organization is free to use its force for the betterment of its members, the community as a whole or segments of it. The House of Delegates of the Oklahoma State Medical Association passed a resolution in 1949 commending the Medical Service Society for its help in developing the Medical Research Foundation.

The detail man today is a sincere, intelligent, educated man who stands ready to support the physician. His society's goal, "to promote better understanding, cooperation and relationship between its members and the professions it serves and the betterment of public health" is not idle chatter and the A.M.A.'s recognition of the Medical Service Society is a welcome one.

We Are The Middle Men

A few short years ago, the patient met his physician entirely on a person to person basis. His problem was one for which he sought help. He consulted the physician of his choice as medical advisor and friend. There was no intervening party. This situation, of course, was conducive to a good mutual understanding of trust and respect. He paid his physician from his personal funds based on an understanding of mutual agreement. Adjustment of fee was the rule instead of the exception.

I recall a piece of sage advice given to me by one of my early and experienced colleagues, to the effect that a physician was unwise to ever incur the enmity of a patient over the misunderstanding of a fee and it has been my experience that such advice was well given.

How times have changed! Such relationship has almost become extinct.

Planted now between the physician and his patient, is a mass of agents; insurance companies, employees medical associations, industrial commissions, employer's liability groups, welfare societies, government agencies. This list is endless.

All tend to bring out resentment, and such resentment materially alters the patient's recovery. Too often these agents wish to make settlements on a minimum basis and too often the patient feels he has not received that to which he is entitled. Where does the physician stand? Squarely in the cross-fire.

Our great need now, it would seem, is a positive effort on the part of the profession to secure a standard insurance contract. If we fail to do this our public relations seem destined to continual deterioration. Until this can be accomplished, an individual physician must adhere literally to the ungarnished statement of facts in his handling of these matters, explaining always to the patient that an insurance policy is a contract between the patient and the insurance company and the interpretation of its provisions is outside of his jurisdiction and responsibility.

Scientific Articles

Pertinent Medical and Physical Data on
Eye Witness Account of AN ATOMIC EXPLOSION

GIFFORD H. HENRY, M.D.

Detonation of a nominal sized atomic bomb releases energy equivalent to 20,000 tons of TNT, and the hydrogen bomb could release energies many times that amount. The atomic bomb derives its energy from the splitting of fissionable atoms, the hydrogen bomb from fusion of atomic particles into atoms of heavier atomic weight. Great as is the force from these man-made weapons, natural forces release even greater energy. Severe tropical hurricanes may expend energy equivalent to 1,000 atomic bombs, and earthquakes energy equivalent to 1,000,000 nominal sized bombs.

While all nuclear detonations are exceedingly powerful within a limited area, people can survive relatively close to the blasts provided certain precautions are observed. In the tests at the Atomic Energy Proving Grounds in Yucca Flat, Nevada in March of 1953, troops were in trenches two miles from ground zero. They were shaken up but not injured. Observers on a mountain side seven miles from the blast experienced no ill effects.

Let us consider what happens at the instant of explosion. Four forces are immediately set in motion: heat, light, blast and nuclear radiation. The observer, wearing high-density goggles, feels a transient heat wave on his face and sees a huge fireball develop on the horizon. The fireball is composed of gases heated to 1,000,000 degrees centigrade, sufficient to ignite ordinary frame structures at a distance of two miles; the intensity of its light is 100 times that of the sun. After one second the fireball attains a radius of 450 feet and rises rapidly in the air like a huge balloon. After five seconds it can be observed safely with the naked eye.

Within a few seconds a huge high-pressure wave is plainly visible moving out rapidly from the base of the formation. This shock wave travels at a progressively dimin-

THE AUTHOR

Gifford H. Henry, M.D., Tulsa, who wrote "Eye Witness Account of an Atomic Explosion," has been active as chairman of the O.S.M.A. Civilian Defense Committee. Doctor Henry served 42 months in the armed service during World War II. He was graduated from the University of Illinois and interned at the Brooklyn Navy Hospital. He served a residency in orthopedics and surgery at the Long Island College Hospital, New York.

ishing speed until at zero-plus-fourteen seconds the observer feels a strong concussion against his body and hears an ear-clicking report like a thunderclap. Reverberating rumbles echo from the surrounding mountains for several seconds.

The greater part of the nuclear radiation is released at the time of the detonation and after 90 seconds no longer constitutes a practical hazard. The remainder of the radiation is emitted by fission fragments which continue to send out radiations until attenuated by fall-out and dispersal, depending on the half-lives of the various isotopes.

The airblast may behave somewhat erratically outside the immediate area because of weather conditions. In a few instances it has cracked plaster and broken windows 80 miles from the explosion, while structures much closer exhibited no ill effects. In "Operation Doorstep," an ordinary frame house erected 3,500 feet from ground-zero immediately caught fire on the side closest to the blast, but the flames died out before the blast reached the house and demolished it. The second Civil Defense house constructed 7,500 feet from the blast did not catch fire or collapse, although it sustained severe structural damage. Pressure on the closest house was estimated at seven pounds a square inch and on the second house at two pounds a square inch. Cars and trucks placed around the test site were damaged in varying degrees. The damage consisted mainly of cracked windshields and crushed tops.

Mannequins had been placed in natural poses in various rooms of the houses. They were scattered about by the blast which blew out all the windows, blinds, sashes and doors. Those in specially prepared shelters in the basement were not moved from their positions and were apparently undamaged.

Since the nuclear device was detonated from a 300-foot tower, the immediate radiation effects were dissipated within a few minutes, but the delayed effects were somewhat remarkable. A prevailing easterly wind carried the atomic cloud over the area where the Civil Defense test structures had been erected. The radioactive fall-out from the cloud was so great in this area that everything was highly contaminated. Monitoring teams that entered the area were unable to remain because of the high level of radioactivity on the ground, so the film badges which had been placed in various locations around the test sites could not be recovered immediately. By the time the badges could be picked up, it was impossible to say how much of the fogging was due to initial radiation and how much was due to delayed radiation.

Authorities of the Civil Defense and Atomic Energy Commission emphasize that rescue parties could have entered the area long enough to accomplish their aims provided they did not remain there very long. Five men who entered the area to inspect the residence at 7,500 feet received one-third of the total allowable dosage of radiation within a few minutes. Several hours after the detonation civilian observers were permitted to approach the area until they were stopped at the 10 milliroentgen-per-hour line. Beyond that line special precautions would have been necessary. It was interesting that the intensity of radiation within the second house was only one-tenth that on the outside of the house. The inference is that houses afford considerable protection against secondary rays. The intensity of radiation dropped precipitately the first 24 hours. At zero-plus-1 hour it had fallen to five per cent, and at the end of the day it was only one-tenth of one per cent of the initial level.

Instruments for detecting radioactivity are used in the field for surveys after atomic bursts; they are used in the laboratory for experimental and clinical investigations, and for safety of personnel. In general, detection is accomplished by photographic emulsions, scintillations in fluoroscopic screens, coloring of crystals, deposition of colloids, biologic effects, and ionization in gases and vapors. Of these, the ionization instruments are the most extensively used. The Geiger-Muller tube and the ionization chamber are the two types of instruments which are most useful medically.

The number of casualties from an atomic bomb depend on weather and topography as well as on the type of burst—air, ground, or water. In Hiroshima approximately 80,-000 people were killed, 15,000 of them by radiation and burns. In Nagasaki where the terrain afforded some protection, 40,000 were killed. In a water burst, relatively few casualties would be anticipated, except from radioactive spray and tidal wave. In a ground burst, casualties would be minimized because the explosive effects would be concentrated at the earth's surface.

Effects of Nominal Sized Bomb

Radius in Miles	Deaths (%)	Surviving Casualties (%)
0 - ½	90	10
½ - 1	50	35
1 - 1½	15	40
2 - 2½	0	10
2½ - 3	0	5
3 - 3½	0	1
3½ - 4	0	0

Approximatey one-third of the injured would require extensive hospital treatment, one-third would require a moderate amount of hospital care, and one-third could be handled as out-patients.

Doubling the size of the bomb increases the radius of damage by one-fourth. At five miles distance there would be no casualties from a bomb eight times the nominal size. If several bombs were used in different areas, the casualties would multiply in direct proportion to the number of bombs. No city could begin to take care of the casualties resulting from such an attack.

Radiation effects on body tissues are considered to be the result of ionization of the body cells resulting in cell injury or death. These ion pairs are formed in living tissue by the primary or secondary impact of charged atomic particles which enter the body from an external radioactive source. Alpha particles (positively charged nuclei of helium atoms) have a range of a few centimeters in air or tissue and are easily stopped by thin shielding. Beta particles (negatively charged electrons) have a somewhat longer range in air and can penetrate one centimeter of aluminum shielding. Nevertheless, they are a hazard chiefly when absorbed internally. Gamma rays (high frequency electro-magnetic waves) travel long distances in air and can penetrate metal and concrete shielding. Neutrons have no electrical charge but are capable of inflicting severe damage to tissue within a limited range.

Effects of radiation may be acute or chronic, and may be external or internal, or a combination of both. If a person receives an internal dose of a long-lived radioactive isotope, it may cause chronic radiation illness culminating in death. Within a few hours after heavy exposure to total body radiation, the patient has symptoms consisting of anorexia, nausea, vomiting, fever, weakness and prostration. Leukopenia will develop by the second day. If he survives the first few days, diarrhea and hemorrhages appear by the end of the week. The earlier the severe symptoms appear, the worse the prognosis. If the patient survives the first six weeks, he may recover following a chronic illness complicated by hemorrhage, anemia, and ulcerations of the mucous membranes of the throat and intestinal tract. A person who has radiation illness does not himself become radioactive and is not a hazard to the personnel of medical rescue teams.

There is no effective treatment for radiation illness. Whole blood, plasma and other fluid infusions combined with antibiotics and sulfonamides constitute the first line of defense. Liver extract, vitamins, and minerals are useful adjuncts.

Let us now consider permissible levels of exposure to radiation. Using the same roentgen unit as in x-ray work, at zero to 25 roentgens there is no effect on the human body. At 25 to 50 roentgens there are possible blood changes but no serious injuries. At 50 to 100 roentgens, blood cell changes are noted, but there is no disability. At 100 to 200 roentgens there is probable injury and possible disability. At 200 to 400 roentgens injury and disability are certain and death is possible. At 400 roentgens, radiation is fatal to one-half of the persons exposed; 600 roentgens is universally fatal.

The medical observer of an atomic blast experiences the exhilaration of seeing an entirely new force in action. He is impressed with the power and beauty of the desert panorama. He is rudely shocked out of his contemplative mood when the concussion wave unexpectedly rocks him back on his heels. The force transmitted across seven miles of desert in approximately 14 seconds is indeed impressive.

When the troops arrive by helicopter from their forward trenches he is relieved to learn that simple earth barriers at two miles give adequate protection from the effects of the explosion, and that no serious radiation effects on the troops are reported.

The portion of the test which was conducted by the Civil Defense Administration officials would indicate that frame houses of standard design, if located one and one-half miles from ground zero, might partially withstand the blast and afford some protection for the occupants if they were forewarned. Basement lean-to shelters shielded the mannequins from serious damage, while dummies in the upper floors of the houses received a severe pummeling.

It is medically significant that rescue parties may enter a contaminated area to participate briefly in rescue work. Monitoring teams can determine the length of stay and the advisability of relieving teams to avoid over-exposure of personnel.

When the knowledge acquired in this and similar tests is absorbed by the medical professon, our possible task of caring for atomic casualties will be greatly simplified. The destructive power of the new weapon, great as it is, can be greatly lessened by intelligent planning and calm execution of medical relief.

BIBLIOGRAPHY

1. Behrens, Charles F. Atomic Medicine. (Textbook) Second Edition, 1953.
2. Publication AG-11-1 (2), Federal Civil Defense Administration, Superintendent of Documents, U. S. Government Printing Office, Washington, D. C., 1950.

Case Report:

CONGENITAL CYSTIC DISEASE *of the* LUNG

L. MEREI, M.D. and L. LIPNICK, M.D.

The earliest referencs to pulmonary cysts was made by Thomas Bartholinus in 1687. Medical interest however was not aroused until 1925 when Koontz drew attention to this interesting condition.

Bronchogenic multiple cysts have been reported a number of times. The case to be presented is of special interest because of its extensiveness with minimal symptoms.

THE AUTHORS

L. Merei, M.D., and L. Lipnick, M.D., of the Muskogee V. A. Hospital were co-authors of "Congential Cystic Disease of the Lung, Report of a Case." Doctor Lipnick is radiologist at the hospital.

Case Report

This 24-year-old veteran (R.D.P.) first noted hemoptysis and severe left chest pain in 1942. These symptoms occurred aboard a troop ship on the way to Alaska. On hospitalization x-rays of the lungs were made and a diagnosis of cystic lung was established. Now (1954) after 12 years, he complains of a dull pain in the left chest that bothers him more at night, shortly after retiring. Occasionally he spits up blood and is coughing. The cough appeared after the first intercurrent infection of the cysts. He coughed up a moderate amount of purulent material. The family history is not contributory.

Physical examination shows a well developed, well nourished, cooperative, well oriented patient. The findings are essentially negative except for two well healed scars on the right side of the abdomen due to previous laparotomy. As to the chest there are no abnormalities to be demonstrated.

Laboratory findings are within normal limits with a hematocrit of 51, sedimentation rate of 17, urinalysis negative, serology negative, sputum negative for tubercle bacilli, WBC 7,000, RBC 4,900,000 hemoglobin 14.9. There was no fever on admission or at any time during his stay in the hospital. X-ray examination on March 16, 1954, shows "ring shadows and crescent shadows

in the right upper lobe and in almost the entire left lung. The oval cystic radiolucent areas are seen from the level of the 1st to the 4th anterior ribs, in the right lung. Similar oval radiolucencies are seen from the left infraclavicular region to the left base as far down as the left dome of the diaphragm. On April 8th a bronchogram was done and it showed numerous grape-like sacs filled with lipiodol arising from the bronchi in all the lobes of both lungs, from the apices to the bases." Bronchoscopic examination was done on April 16, 1954, and was negative. No treatment was given as patient was admitted mainly for establishing a definite diagnosis.

Pulmonary cysts may be congenital and acquired. A simple classification of congenital cystic disease of the lung is according to cell type.

A. Bronchogenic cell type.
  1. Solitary
  2. Multiple

B. Alveolar cell type.
  1. Solitary (balloon cyst and pneumatocele)
  2. Multiple

C. Bronchogenic and alveolar type combined.

The most plausible pathogenesis of congenital cystic disease according to Klosk, Bernstein and Parsonnett, is of altered development. "The lungs are formed from the lung buds whose ends become lobulated at about the fourth week of embryonic life, there being three lobules formed on the right and two on the left. These lobulations undergo dichotomous branching, the terminal portions of the branches becoming expanded to form atria. At about the sixth month the alveoli are formed as evaginations from the latter. If the process is arrested early, during early subdivisions, large solitary cysts may be formed. If the process is arrested later in embryonic development, multiple cysts will result."

Another factor may be an arrest in the development of the bronchiole in the tube stage. From the clinical and pathological point of view, congenital cystic disease falls in two main groups. The first is the large solitary cyst which may occupy one or more lobes, often displacing the heart and mediastinum to the contralateral side. Such cysts compress the surrounding parenchyma and are usually found in infancy and early childhood. They give symptoms of cyanosis and dyspnea accompanied by physical signs of tension pneumothorax. These solitary cysts are lined by a layer of columnar and

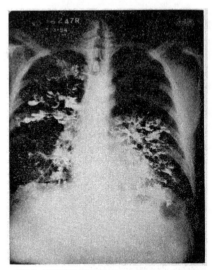

Fig. 2. Bronchogram: There are numerous grapelike sacs filled with lipiodol arising from the bronchi in all the lobes and in both lungs from the apices to the bases. The appearance is that of cystic lung disease or congenital sac called cystic bronchiectasis. In the erect films air fluid levels are seen in these sac like structures.

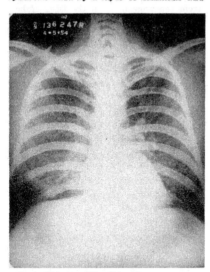

Fig. 1. Plain Chest Film (PA): There are numerous ring and crescent shadows in the upper half of the right lung field and throughout the left lung having the appearance of cysts. The cyst walls are thin. In numerous areas of the left lung the cysts are closely packed. The hilar vascular trunks are thickened. Heart is normal in size.

cuboidal epithelium, and a layer of connective tissue. No doubt all these cysts communicate with a bronchus, but this communication may be difficult to demonstrate grossly. The second form of congenital cystic disease is one in which the lung parenchyma is replaced by areas of cystic degeneration ranging from multiple miliary cysts scattered throughout lung parenchyma to large multilocular or unilocular cysts occupying one or more lobes. These cystic cavities are lined by cuboidal and columnar epithelium which may be thrown into folds by intraluminary proliferation. Between these two extremes intermediate forms may be encountered giving the lung tissue a spongy appearance. In such instances it is made up of clusters of thin-walled cavities varying in size from 1 to 3 cm. These cavities communicate freely with bronchi and are lined with ciliated or nonciliated epithelium. They show the usual architecture of a bronchus—smooth muscle, cartilaginous rings and mucous glands in the cavity wall. Radiographically this form of cystic disease is characterized by the honeycomb appearance of pulmonic fields. The lung structure shows a large number of thin-walled, sharply defined annular shadows without accompanying interstitial parenchymal infiltration. This roentgen appearance is especially diagnostic when the lesions are in the upper lobes and bilateral.

There are certain features in which the congenital malformation differs from acquired bronchiectasis. In congenital cystic disease of the small diffuse type, the upper lobes are most often the site of the lesion. Whereas, in acquired bronchiectasis the dependent portions of the lung, particularly the basilar segments of the lower lobes and lingular segments of the upper lobe, are most frequently involved. In the congenitally malformed lung the cystic areas in many instances are of a uniform size compared to both tubular and saccular dilatations seen in acquired bronchiectasis.

The diagnosis of the congenital cystic disease of the lung is usually not difficult when its possibility is kept in mind. In those cases where symptoms are produced by overdistention of the cyst with air, the conditions most frequently confused are spontaneous pneumothorax and diaphragmatic hernia. When fluid is present, empyema may be suspected. Following superimposed infection in a case of cystic disease of the lung a misdiagnosis of lung abscess, bronchiectasis, tuberculosis or pneumonitis may occur. Symptomatology is dependent upon disturbances of intrathoracic pressure by over distension of the cysts or of suppurative disease following infection of the cysts. Dyspnea, cough with moderate expectoration, chest pain and cyanosis can occur from resulting changes in pulmonary physiology. Complications such as mediastinal herniation and fatal asphyxia are not uncommon with large cysts. Other common symptoms are: hemoptysis, ranging from severe hemorrhage to slight streaking; cough; moderate expectoration; wheezing; pain in the chest; cardiac palpitation; and repeated febrile attacks. In addition, obstruction of neighboring bronchioles may predispose to bronchiectasis with added symptoms. The presence of congenital cystic disease of the lung, however, does not exclude co-existing diseases such as lung abscess, tuberculosis, empyema, carcinoma of the lung, etc.

Diagnosis of congenital cystic disease should be based upon careful chronological history of symptoms. Physical examination, especially of the chest, may be of help. Radiographic inspections provide the best means of clinical diagnosis.

Clinically congenital cystic disease divides itself into an asymptomatic group (discovered by routine x-ray inspections), and a group with symptoms which require the patient to seek medical aid. The presence of a bronchial communication leading to each cyst with alternating periods of drainage and obstruction ultimately results in an infection and distention. Active therapy therefore must be instituted in all cases including the asymptomatic. Results are especially good if the complications are minimal or absent. The most common complication is superimposed infection by secondary invaders. Antibiotics reduce infections and complications of cystic disease to a minimum. Optimum therapy is to remove the cystic areas if the distribution is not so wide spread as to preclude surgery. Depending upon the extent of involvement simple excision of the cyst, lobectomy or pneumonectomy, may be done. Age is no contraindication for small infants withstand pulmonary surgery better than adults.

Resume

A case of congenital polycystic disease of the lungs is presented. Clinical roentgenologic pictures of the disease are shown. The differential diagnosis between this disease and other diseases of the lungs is based on clinical and roentgenological evidence. The disease rarely manifests itself until it is associated with secondary infection.

REFERENCES

Reviewed in the Veterans Administration and published with approval of the Chief Medical Director. The statements and conclusions published by the authors are the result of their own study and do not necessarily reflect the opinion or policy of the Veterans Administration.

For Oklahoma ---

A MEDICAL EXAMINERS SYSTEM

HOWARD C. HOPPS, M.D.

THE AUTHOR

Howard C. Hopps, M.D., professor and chairman of the department of pathology at the University of Oklahoma School of Medicine who wrote "A Medical Examiners System for Oklahoma." The article is being published simultaneously in the Bar Association *Journal* and the *Journal* of O.S.M.A.

Of the many relationships which exist between medicine and the law, none is more important than those activities which have as their common purpose the protection of society against the wilful and wanton destruction of human life, and the recognition of public hazards which threaten human life.

The procedure by which legal investigation is accomplished when homicide is known or suspected is normally divided into two phases: 1) inquestual or the obtaining and appraisal of evidence, 2) judicial, culminating in a trial by jury of the accused. The initial phase is primarily medical and is activated by the finding of a dead body. Whose corpse is it? When did death occur? How was it caused? The quality of justice will depend upon the promptness and competence with which this investigation is conducted.

Although the United States boasts the best medical service and the most skilled medical care of any nation in the world, our system of medicolegal investigation is one of the poorest. In many states, as in Oklahoma, the responsibility for the medicolegal examination rests not with specially trained medical personnel, but with a Justice of the Peace whose training and experience is most apt to be in law. This system is the relic of a bygone age, dating back to the early history of England at which time the coroner (crown's man—representative of the king) served to protect the king's interests in the recovery of buried treasure, in the matter of game poaching, fines levied and collected for miscellaneous crimes including murder, in collecting property in case of suicide, etc.

We should adjust our laws to fit modern times rather than to continue with this outmoded practice. Determination of the cause of death, time and manner of death, identification of the dead, etc., are among the most difficult problems in medicine and require the services of those specially trained in certain phases of pathology, chemistry, serology, etc. It requires also a well equipped laboratory where complex chemical, photographic, serologic and tissue examinations can be skillfully performed.

What are the purposes of medicolegal investigation? These fall into four major categories:

1. To determine if death is related to public welfare; unrecognized hazards to public health must be brought to light.
2. To insure that crime shall not pass unrecognized; to recognize those apparently natural deaths which are in fact homicides.
3. To provide evidence useful in apprehending and in convicting criminals whose acts have resulted in death of their victim—this includes hit and run drivers, rapists, etc.
4. So that innocent persons will not be punished; this includes proper recognition of those deaths which suggest an effect of violence, but which are actually the result of natural causes.

What is the need of a medical examiners system in Oklahoma? On the basis of statistics gathered in those states with a well functioning medical examiners system, it is estimated that there occurs in the State of Oklahoma each year:

1. Approximately 450 deaths from suicide or homicide.
2. Approximately 1800 accidental deaths caused by mechanical injury or poisoning.

3. Approximately 2200 unexpected deaths of obscure causation or deaths of persons who were not attended by a physician.

In addition to those many cases concerned with criminal acts, there are numerous cases of civil liability which could be more efficiently and much more judiciously handled with a properly functioning medical examiners system. Under the present conditions in our state, a medicolegal autopsy is a costly procedure, often difficult to arrange. As a result, this special service is used to limited extent and principally by corporations and insurance companies in cases where it will be of primary benefit to them. This is only natural. Furthermore, the evidence so procured is often presented and evaluated in a somewhat prejudiced fashion since it was obtained by and for persons with prejudiced interests. Every individual, regardless of his legal knowledge and financial status, should have the opportunity to secure that complex medical evidence and objective expert medical analysis which would come about as a matter of course with a proper medical examiners system.

What questions may be answered by a proper medicolegal examination?

1. What is the identity of the body or part thereof?
   a. Is it of human origin?
   b. Whose is it?
2. Was death from unnatural causes and if so was it:
   a. Accidental?—If so does it represent a hazard to public health?
   b. Deliberate?—If so was it:
      1) Self-inflicted, i.e. suicide?
      2) Inflicted by another person or persons, i.e. homicide?
3. Can the circumstances in which homicide occurred be reconstructed?
   a) Nature of the instrument or poison, etc., responsible.
   b) Method of its application or use.
   c) Position and activities of victim and assailant at and just before the injury.
   d) Length of time elapsed between injury and death.
   e) Physical capacity of the victim after injury.
   f) In the case of multiple wounds, order of occurrence and relation of each to death.
   g) Existence of extenuating circumstances, e.g. pre-existing disease.
4. Can evidence be provided to determine the identity of the assailant and establish his guilt?
   a) Through recovery and identification of portions of the assailant from the victim.
   b) Through recovery and identification of portions of the victim from the assailant.
   c) From recognition of specific peculiarities concerning the manner of injury or nature of injury.

To answer these questions effectively and to serve the general purposes of a medicolegal investigation we must provide the necessary legislation to enact and support a medical examiners system. Such a system, in contrast to the present one in which Justices of the Peace act as coroners, would place this state among that enlightened group which has recognized and met this important responsibility.

In conclusion, I should like to quote from Gradwohl's famous essay on The Office of Coroner, "Thus we have at present an officer known as a coroner, created by statute or constitution, a quasi-magistrate, a conservator of the peace throughout his county, holding inquests in sudden deaths, issuing subpoenas, administering oaths to jurors, acting as marshal or sheriff when such officers cannot act, conducting post-mortem examinations himself or designating some other person to do so, making chemical and microscopic examinations of parts of the bodies of deceased individuals, or causing someone else equally skilled or unskilled, as the case may be, to do the same; in short, performing the duties of judge, advocate, physician, pathologist, bacteriologist, toxicologist! The system is absurd on the face of it. Since the time of Erasmus, we have had no pantologists; therefore it is easy to understand that the incumbent of this office is never qualified to perform all the duties for which he is elected by the people and charged by the constitution of the state to carry out."

Association Activities

PRESIDENT'S LETTER

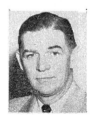

For some time past there has been a varying amount of interest in and speculation about the advisability of securing a permanent home for the offices of our organization. Last spring the Council asked that the president appoint a committee to be known as the Building Committee to study the problem. Members of this committee are Dr. Paul Champlin of Enid, Dr. Alfred Sugg of Ada, Dr. John McDonald of Tulsa, Dr. W. A. Howard of Chelsea, Dr. C. E. Northcutt of Ponca City, and the present president and president-elect of the O.S.M.A.

This committee met recently and after weighing the pros and cons decided to recommend to the House of Delegates, in December, that a lot in a suitable location be purchased, and a structure be built to house the offices of the State Association. The committee will also recommend the limiting of the cost of lot and structure to $100,000. It is hoped that by the time the House of Delegates meets in December that data can be furnished as to possible location and cost of property, and also the cost of financing the project.

Our present location is quite temporary, and suitable renting elsewhere is difficult to find, as well as expensive. The committee unanimously agreed that the Association could well afford to finance such a project as has been outlined.

I wish you all a Merry Christmas and a Happy New Year!

President

Amebiasis[1] a "Poorly Reported" Disease

Until serious complications arise,
amebiasis may pass unrecognized and
patients receive only symptomatic treatment.

Although amebiasis is a disease with serious morbidity and mortality, statistics on its incidence[1] are incomplete because its manifestations are not commonly recognized and consequently not reported.

"Vague symptoms[2] referable to the gastrointestinal tract, such as indigestion or indefinite abdominal pains, with or without abnormally formed stools, may result from intestinal amebiasis. Not infrequently in cases in which such symptoms are ascribed to psychoneurosis after extensive x-ray studies have been carried out, complete relief is obtained with antiamebic therapy."

To prevent possible development of an incapacitating or even fatal illness and to eliminate a reservoir of infection in the community, diagnosing and treating[3] even seemingly healthy "carriers" and those having mild symptoms of amebiasis is advised.

Early diagnosis[1] is important because infection can be rapidly and completely cleared, with the proper choice of drugs and due consideration for the principles of therapy. For treatment of the bowel phase these authors find Diodoquin "most satisfactory."

For chronic amebic infections, Goodwin[4] finds Diodoquin to be one of the best drugs at present available.

Diodoquin, which does not inconvenience the patient or interfere with his normal activities, may be used in the treatment of acute or latent forms of amebiasis. If extraintestinal lesions require the use of emetine, Diodoquin may be administered concurrently. It is a well tolerated and relatively nontoxic orally administered amebacide, containing 63.9 per cent of iodine.

Diodoquin (diiodohydroxyquinoline), available in 10-grain (650 mg.) tablets, reduces the course of treatment to twenty days (three tablets daily). Treatment may be repeated or prolonged without

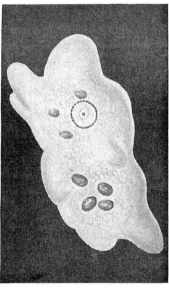

Endamoeba histolytica (trophozoite).

serious toxic effect. It is accepted by the Council on Pharmacy and Chemistry of the American Medical Association. G. D. Searle & Co., Research in the Service of Medicine.

1. Hamilton, H. E., and Zavala, D. C.: Amebiasis in Iowa: Diagnosis and Treatment, J. Iowa M. Soc. *43*:1 (Jan.) 1952.

2. Goldman, M. J.: Less Commonly Recognized Clinical Features of Amebiasis, California Med. *76*:266 (April) 1952.

3. Weingarten, M., and Herzig, W. F.: The Clinical Manifestations of Chronic Amebiasis, Rev. Gastroenterol. *20*:667 (Sept.) 1953.

4. Goodwin, L. G.: Review Article: The Chemotherapy of Tropical Disease: Part I. Protozoal Infections, J. Pharm. & Pharmacol. *4*:153 (March) 1952.

Cancer In Oklahoma

Through a grant-in-aid from the National Cancer Institute, the University of Oklahoma School of Medicine (Department of Preventive Medicine) plans to review certain environmental factors present in patients, on whom the diagnosis of cancer has been made.

Surveys of cancer in 10 major cities have failed to consider occupational exposures of work materials or avocational contactants to which a cancer patient was exposed through hobbies, maintenance farming, "second job," radiation therapy, habits of tobacco, alcohol, or drug addiction, unusual health practices, climate factors, or family tendency.

This current investigation, being conducted under the direction of Dr. Jean Spencer Felton, Associate Professor (Industrial Medicine) will be limited to patients known presently to have the disease, or who have died during the period of the study. It does not represent a survey of old records, but will be a day-to-day compilation of data relating to the newly diagnosed condition.

The research plan envisions the contacting of private practitioners, health departments, hospitals, tumor clinics, voluntary and official health agencies, and physicians in industry for assistance in assembling the information. Contacts will be made in person, by letter, and through report forms. It is hoped that each case of cancer becoming recognized within Oklahoma—a state of both industrial and agricultural activities—will be made known to the research team.

On receipt of all pertinent data, statistical evaluations will be conducted to determine rates, and possible identification of exposure factors common to the type, location, portal of entry of incitants, or duration of the malignant growth.

Oklahoma medicine has an opportunity here to contribute vital understandings of the cancer problem, to the world. The University believes that this project will give information relative to the occupational cause of cancer, and the possible carcinogenicity of industrial materials heretofore un-

American Medical Association Directory To Be Ready Soon

The new, 19th Edition of the AMERICAN MEDICAL DIRECTORY is now in galley form, and it is expected that the book will be ready for delivery about the middle of 1955. The previous edition was issued in 1950. Since that time, it has not been possible to publish a new edition because changes in the membership structure of the American Medical Association made it difficult to obtain an accurate list of members.

Within the next few weeks, a directory information chart will have been mailed to every physician in the United States, its dependencies, and Canada, requesting information to be used in compiling the new Directory. Physicians receiving an information card should fill it out and return it promptly regardless of whether any change has occurred in any of the points on which information is requested. It is urged that physicians also fill out the right half of the card, which requests information to be used exclusively for statistical purposes. Even if a physician has sent in similar information recently, he should mail the card promptly to the Directory Department of the American Medical Association to insure an accurate listing of his name and address. There is no charge for publishing the data, nor are physicians obligated in any way.

It provides full information on medical schools, specialization in the fields of medical practice, memberships in special medical societies, tabulation of medical journals and libraries, and statistics on the distribution of physicians and hospitals in the United States.

---

recognized as cancer-productive. In essence, this study may determine with some exactitude, the role of work in the increased incidence of cancer. It is hoped that all who are in medicine will aid in the program. Additional details will be forwarded to each physician as the research planning progresses.

Those who are interested can address the School of Medicine at 801 N. E. 13th Street, Oklahoma City 4, Oklahoma.

when patients need hormones

℞

PRESCRIBE

Schering

SCHERING HORMONES

SUPERIOR
QUALITY
Schering's high standards and quality control assure products of uniform action and clinical efficacy.

MINIMUM
COST
With hormones produced by Schering, the physician is certain of unquestioned quality at minimum cost.

Special
bonus offers
now available—
See your dealer.

Book Review

ENDOCRINE TREATMENT IN GEN-
ERAL PRACTICE. Edited by Max A.
Goldzieher, M.D. and Joseph W. Goldzieher, M.D. Cloth. $8.00, Pp 474. Spring-
er Publishing Company, Inc., 44 East
23rd., New York 10, New York.

This is a very well written introduction
to almost all of the many phases of endocrine treatment. The chapters on growth,
normal and abnormal, on aging, and all of
the chapters that have to do with general
metabolism and nutrition are well and in-
terestingly written. The disorders of the
organ systems were presented in a slightly
different form than usual and the chapters
dealing with these are of much interest.
The portion of the book dealing with fer-
tility and infertility; particularly the male
infertility, was of marked interest; however, the separation into male and female
sections eliminates the Huhner test as an
index to determine which member of the
couple should be stressed in the work up.
This is important, because sterility is not a
gynecological or urological problem, but is
a partnership problem. Pregnancy, abortion
and other complications of pregnancy, are
well discussed. Guides to the uses and dosage
of ACTH and Cortisone are given, as well
as those of all the other hormones in clinical use. The section on disorders of resistance is very useful and gratifying as
was the section on neoplastic disease. The
enclosed section of diet prescription sheets
is well worth noting and adapting to one's
own practice. There is a useful index of
currently available hormone preparation.
Certainly this is a book that can be recommended to all general practitioners and
to most specialists because it covers so completely today's knowledge of the general in-
ter-related activities of the endocrine se-
cretions, and presents in detail how and
when they should be used in the daily practice of medicine. —Herbert S. Orr, M.D.

Have You Heard?

BLAIR POINTS, M.D., a graduate of the first
University of Oklahoma School of Medicine
class, has retired as Veterans Administration
disability rating specialist, in Oklahoma City.

DAVE B. LHEVINE, M.D., Tulsa, spoke on
"Radioactivity" at a meeting of the Sand
Springs Rotary club earlier this fall.

E. B. THOMASSON, M.D. has reopened his
office in Durant following a recent illness.

CURTIS BERRY, M.D., Norman, has been
named to the Board of Education of that city.

E. W. KING, M.D., Bristow, has been elected
chief of staff of the new Bristow Memorial
Hospital.

ROBERT ALLEN, M.D., Bartlesville, attended
the recent meeting of the Pan-Pacific Surgical Association in Honolulu, Hawaii.

DON J. WILSON, M.D., formerly of Gaines-
ville, Texas, has opened his office in Marietta.

ROBERT H. FURMAN, M.D., Oklahoma City,
was recently guest speaker at a meeting of
the McAlester Rotary Club.

J. HOYLE CARLOCK, M.D., Ardmore, represented the O.S.M.A. on the recent Oklahoma
Industrial Tour.

CARY W. TOWNSEND, M.D., Oklahoma City,
was recently honored on his 75th birthday
with a surprise party given by the physicians
and their employees on his floor in the Medical Arts Building.

P. D. CASPER, M.D. and W. H. PORTER, M.D.
have recently moved into their new clinic in
Del City. The clinic will provide Del City
with its first fully equipped laboratory service and emergency room, as well as provide
working quarters for three doctors and a
dentist.

ELMER HESS, M.D., President-Elect of the
A.M.A., paid a brief visit to Oklahoma City
in November when he delivered the annual
C. B. Taylor lectureship at the medical school.

HOWARD A. BENNETT, M.D., Oklahoma City, presented a paper in Cincinnati recently to the American Society of Anesthesiologists on "The Intercostal Nerve Block in Upper Abdominal and Chest Surgery."

FORMAL OPENING OF THE NEW MEDICAL CENTER in Pauls Valley was held recently. Physicians associated in the clinic are Ray H. Lindsey, M.D., J. N. Byrd, Jr., M.D., J. A. Graham, M.D., R. E. Spence, M.D., and John M. Moore, M.D. The 36 room clinic is housed in a red brick building of modern construction.

McCURTAIN COUNTY MEMORIAL HOSPITAL has opened in Idabel. Built at a cost of $260,000, the new hospital contains 16 patient rooms, operating room, delivery room, emergency room, Laboratory, x-ray room, kitchen, business office, lobby, employees dining room, nursery, ward room, and power and utility areas.

GILBERT L. HYROOP, M.D., Oklahoma City, attended the one week meeting of the American Society of Plastic and Reconstructive Surgery held in October at Miami, Fla.

New Director Named For Cancer Society of Oklahoma

Clark Sudduth, formerly director of public relations and campaign of the Texas Division of the American Cancer Society, is the new executive director of the Oklahoma Division of the American Cancer Society.

Mr. Sudduth was born and reared in Louisiana, is a graduate of the University of Houston and in addition to his experience with the Cancer Society, has held positions as newspaper reporter, industrial magazine editor and public relations counselor.

The Cancer Society has also appointed a new field representative. He is David Steen, former Executive Secretary of the Oklahoma Advisory Health Council.

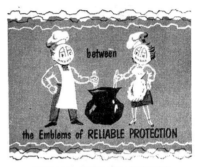
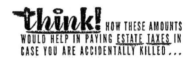
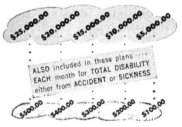

Announcements

Oklahoma Academy of General Practice
Biltmore Hotel, Oklahoma City, February 14-15, 1955.

Oklahoma State Medical Association
May 9-10-11, 1955, Cimarron Ballroom, Tulsa. House of Delegates Sunday, May 8, Mayo Hotel.

American Medical Association
June 6-10, 1955, Atlantic City, New Jersey.

Medical Technology Course
University of Kansas Medical Center, January 10-11-12, 1955. (Program elsewhere in this issue.)

American Psychiatric Association
Regional research meeting, Galveston, Texas, February 18-19 1955. Those desiring to present papers are requested to contact Dr. Martin L. Towler, 112 North Blvd., Galveston, Texas. Theme will be "The Physiologic Basis, Values, Limitations, and Hazards of Pharmacologic Products Recently Introduced in the Treatment of Psychiatric Disorders."

Ophthalmology and Otolaryngology Seminar
University of Florida, Miami, Florida. For further information contact Shaler Richardson, M. D., Jacksonville, Fla. The Sans Souci Hotel, Miami Beach, will be headquarters. Ophthalmology lectures will be presented January 17, 18, 19 and otolaryngology lectures will be given January 20, 21 and 22.

American Board of Obstetrics and Gynecology
Next scheduled examinations will be held Friday, February 4, 1955. Case abstracts numbering 20 should be sent to the secretary, Robert L. Faulkner, M.D., 2105 Adelbert Road, Cleveland 6, Ohio, as soon as possible after receiving notification of eligibility of the Part I written examination.

General Practice Review
Six day general practice review to be offered at the University of Colorado Medical Center, Denver, during the week of January 17-22, 1955. Detailed program and complete information may be obtained by writing to: Office of Graduate and Postgraduate Medical Education, University of Colorado Medical Center, 4200 East Ninth Ave., Denver 20, Colo.

University of Oklahoma Medical School Postgraduate Conferences
Conferences are held on the third Thursday of each month in Room 220 of the Medical School at 7:30 p.m. There is no registration fee or other charge. Schedule is as follows:

January 20—Diffuse Pulmonary Disease. Moderator: James F. Hammarsten, M. D. Panel: To be announced.

February 17—Newer Knowledge of the Thyroid in Health and Disease. Moderator: Stewart G. Wolf, M. D. Panel: Leonard P. Eliel, M. D., Robert P. Howard, M. D., and Henry H. Turner, M. D.

March 17—Practical and Theoretical Aspects of Management of Coronary Artery Disease. Moderator: Robert H. Furman, M. D. Panel: To be announced.

April 21—Mechanism of Ascites. Moderator: Edward M. Schneider, M. D. Panel: J. R. Colvert, M. D., Leonard P. Eliel, M. D., and Robert H. Furman, M. D.

May 19—Therapy of Hypertension. Moderator: William W. Schottstaedt. Panel: To be announced.

American College of Surgeons
First sectional meeting of 1955 will be held at Galveston January 17, 18, 19. Surgeons who are not Fellows of the College may also attend these sessions. Registration fee is $5.00. The meeting is designed for surgeons living in Texas, Arizona, New Mexica, Oklahoma and Louisiana and their guests. Further information may be obtained from Robert M. Moore, M. D., Professor of Surgery, University of Texas Medical Branch, Galveston. He is chairman of the committee on arrangements.

Medical and Surgical Conference
Temple division of the University of Texas Postgraduate School of Medicine announces its forthcoming medical and surgical conference to be held March 7, 8, and 9, 1955 to be presented by members of the staff of Scott and White Clinic. Registration forms are available from the office of the Assistant Dean, University of Texas Postgraduate School of Medicine, The Temple Division, Temple, Texas.

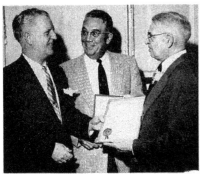

Wilkie Hoover, M.D. (left), President of the Tulsa County Medical Society, presents a Life Membership plaque to Paul Grosshart, M.D. (center) and James W. Rogers, M.D., Tulsa physicians who retired last year. The presentation was made at the October 11th meeting of the Society at the Blue Cross Plan building. Plaques were presented in absentia to Bunn Harris, M.D., Jenks; W. J. Trainor, M.D., former Tulsan now of Wilmington, Ohio; C. E. Calhoun, M.D., Sand Springs; and Clarence C. Hoke, M.D., Tulsa.

Technology Course Offered

The University of Kansas School of Medicine announces its Sixth Annual Postgraduate Course in Medical Technology, January 10, 11 and 12, 1955, to be presented at K. U. Medical Center, Kansas City 12, Kansas.

The course will deal with subjects in hematology, bacteriology, mycology, serology, chemistry and miscellaneous laboratory procedures. In addition to didactic lectures, the program will be highlighted by demonstrations, a discussion of the selection and care of laboratory glassware, films on "Phase Microscopy" and "The Normal Kidney," and a symposium as the closing feature of each day's program.

The distinguished guest faculty includes: Norman F. Conant, Ph.D., Professor of Mycology and Associate Professor of Bacteriology, Duke University School of Medicine, Durham, N.C.; Eugene Hildebrand, M.D., Pathologist, Mercy Hospital, Denver, Colo.; J. N. McConnell, Sales Manager, Scientific Products Division, American Hospital Supply Corporation, Evanston, Ill.; and Franklin R. Miller, M.D., Hematologist, The Snyder Clinic, Winfield, Kans.

The course is open to all serving in medical laboratories upon payment of the $12.00 enrollment fee.

Medical Societies Around the State

Tulsa County

Fall meetings of the Tulsa County Medical Society have featured addresses by Robert P. Glover, M.D., Philadelphia, who spoke on "The Present Status of Surgery for Stenotic Valvular Heart Disease," Conrad G. Collins, M.D., New Orleans, whose paper was on "Management of Pelvic Abscesses," and Capt. Carroll P. Hungate, Olathe, Kans. who spoke on "The Medical Aspects of Civil Defense." John L. Bach, Chicago, director of press relations for the A.M.A. was guest speaker at the annual Tulsa County Medical Society press, radio, television dinner.

East Central

The October meeting of the East Central Oklahoma Medical Society was held at the Muskogee General Hospital when James S. Hammersten, M.D., Assistant Professor of Medicine, University of Oklahoma School of Medicine and chief of the medical service at the Oklahoma City V.A. Hospital was guest speaker. Twenty-one members of the society attended the meeting.

Kay-Noble-Pawnee-Payne-Osage

Physicians from Kay, N o b l e , Pawnee, Payne and Osage counties met for a district meeting in Pawhuska recently. Speakers were Bruce Hinson, M.D., O.S.M.A. President, and Executive Secretary Dick Graham. Divonis Worten, M.D. received a Life Membership certificate at the meeting.

Jefferson County

At a banquet and program sponsored jointly by the Jefferson County Medical Society and the Waurika Chamber of Commerce, D. B. Collins, M.D., Waurika, was honored for his 50 years' service as a physician. He was presented with an O.S.M.A. 50 Year Pin. Presentation was made by E. S. Lain, M.D.

Woodward County

Three pioneer Woodward County physicians recently received Life Membership certificates. They were H. L. Johnson, M.D., who spent 30 years as assistant superintendent and superintendent at the Western State Hospital, Fort Supply; and C. W. Tedrowe, M.D. and O. A. Pierson, M.D., both of Woodward. Joe L. Duer, M.D., vice-councilor, made the presentations.

☰ Deaths

FLOYD E. WARTERFIELD, M.D.
1870-1954

Floyd E. Warterfield, M.D., Muskogee resident for 44 years, died November 10 after a long illness.

He was graduated from the University of Arkansas School of Medicine and opened his practice at Bokoshe, Indian Territory. He came to Muskogee in 1910 after practicing in Holdenville since 1900. His specialty was urology.

He was active in the Indian Territory Medical Association and later in the Oklahoma State Medical Association. In 1948 he received a 50 Year pin. He was also active in a number of lodges and had received all degrees of York Rite Masonry in Muskogee.

H. E. HUSTON, M.D.
1893-1954

H. E. Huston, M.D., 61 year old retired physician, died in his sleep September 26 at his home on Honey Creek Bay near Grove.

Doctor Huston had practiced in Alfalfa county before illness forced his retirement in 1940. After resting and apparently recuperating, he went to Kiowa, Kans. in 1951 where he operated a hospital and conducted his practice but ill health again forced him to retire.

He was active in Grand Lake area activities, taught a Sunday school class at the Methodist Church, was a veteran of World War I, a Mason, Rotarian, member of American Legion and several medical organizations.

WILLIAM EDWARD CRAVENS, M.D.
1864-1954

William Edward Cravens, M.D., retired Hugo physician, died October 8 at the home of a daughter in Tulsa after several weeks' illness.

Doctor Cravens was born in Fort Smith and was a graduate of Baylor Medical School. He had practiced in Hugo and Wink and Odessa, Texas.

A. W. COFFIELD, M.D.
1869-1954

A. W. Coffield, M.D., Drumright, died following a heart attack October 5.

Doctor Coffield was born August 10, 1869 near Paris, Ark. He attended medical school at Atlanta, Ga., Louisville, Ky. and Kansas City, Mo. He opened his first office at Lehigh, Indian Territory and came to Drumright in 1912.

JAMES BURNETT HAMPTON, M.D.
1880-1954

James Burnett Hampton, M.D., retired physician, died at the home of his daughter in Duncan October 11.

Doctor Hampton was born August 24, 1880 in Leitchfield, Ky. He had practiced in Miami for 39 years before moving to Duncan in 1949.

R. J. SHULL, M.D.
1878-1954

R. J. Shull, M.D., pioneer Choctaw county physician, died November 5 at his home in Hugo.

Doctor Shull was born December 22, 1878 at Winchester, Va. He received his medical degree from the University of Louisville in 1900 and moved to Hugo soon after he graduated. He served also as a medical corps captain in World War I, was a resident physician at Oklahoma A. and M. College and spent four years as a member of the staff of Indian hospitals at Talihina and Claremore. He was a member of the Hugo Elks Lodge and the First Presbyterian church.

Doctor Lull Explains
AMA Legislative Policy

Before leaving for the World Medical Association meeting in Rome, George F. Lull, M.D., Secretary-manager of the A.M.A. penned a concise article on the present legislative policy of the American Medical Association for publication in the "Washington Insurance Newsletter," edited by Al Goldsmith. The article was published in that newsletter of October 2. Since the subject holds so much interest for doctors generally, the article is reproduced herewith in full:

As a guest writer, appreciative of the opportunity to make use of these columns, I should like to outline the general philosophy underlying the legislative policies of the American Medical Association. Then I should like to discuss briefly the A.M.A. position on some of the specific proposals which have attracted major attention during the 83rd Congress.

To begin with, the A.M.A holds as a basic premise that this nation's unparalleled scientific and socio-economic progress in the field of medical care is a direct result of the traditional American system calling for solution of problems by voluntary methods rather than by governmental direction. At the same time, the A.M.A. also recognizes that there are certain areas of activity in which government action may be either necessary or desirable to protect the public health or to promote the most efficient mobilization of medical resources.

The A.M.A., therefore, is willing to support any sound legislative proposal which it believes would aid in the expansion and improvement of the nation's medical system while at the same time avoiding the dangers of government control over either the recipients or suppliers of medical service.

However, the Association will continue to oppose any legislative proposals which it believes would impede the nation's medical progress, undermine the free practice of medicine and lead either directly or indirectly to government regulation of physicians, patients, hospitals, medical schools, medical insurance plans or any other elements in the country's existing medical care system.

With this general background in mind, it should be emphasized that the A.M.A. endorsed the principles and objectives of the Eisenhower health program and gave active support to most of the specific proposals in that program. For example, the Hill-Burton Act amendments, designed to promote the construction of rehabilitation centers, nursing homes, diagnostic and treatment centers and hospitals for the chronically ill, were supported and suggestions were made for improving the legislation. The same was true of the proposals for revamping the public health grants-in-aid program.

Unfortunately, however, those controversial items which the A.M.A. opposed received considerably more attention, both in and out of Congress, than the many bills which the Association supported. Therefore, I should like to outline briefly the reasons for our opposition to the Administration's reinsurance proposal and to two of the proposed changes in the Social Security Act.

Reinsurance

The stated purpose of the reinsurance proposal is to "encourage and stimulate private initiative in making good and comprehensive health services generally accessible on reasonable terms." While in complete agreement with that objective, the A.M.A. opposed the reinsurance bills for these reasons:

1. The mechanism suggested would not accomplish the stated purpose of the bills.

2. The phenomenal progress of the health insurance industry makes federal intervention not only unnecessary but a dangerous intrusion into a successful area of private enterprise.

3. "Reinsurance" would not make health insurance more attractive to persons who can afford to pay premiums and have not done so. It would not make health insurance available to the indigent unless the government provides a subsidy for the purpose of selling insurance at less than the cost of servicing the contract.

4. The program, without subsidy, would not make health insurance available to any

(Continued on Page 346)

accepted

ACH

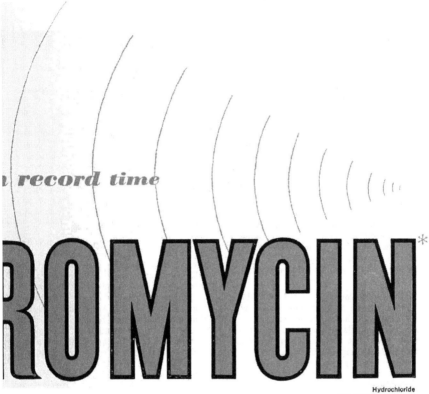

record time

ROMYCIN

Hydrochloride
Tetracycline HCl <u>Lederle</u>

ACHROMYCIN, new broad-spectrum antibiotic, has set an unusual record for rapid acceptance by physicians throughout the country. Within a few months of its introduction, ACHROMYCIN is being widely used in private practice, hospitals and clinics. A number of successful clinical tests have now been completed and are being reported.

ACHROMYCIN has true broad-spectrum activity, effective against Gram-positive and Gram-negative organisms, as well as virus-like and mixed infections.

ACHROMYCIN has notable stability, provides prompt diffusion in body tissues and fluids.

ACHROMYCIN has the advantage of minimal side reactions.

LEDERLE LABORATORIES DIVISION *AMERICAN Cyanamid COMPANY* Pearl River, New York

*REG. U.S. PAT. OFF.

DR. LULL EXPLAINS

(Continued from Page 343)

additional groups or geographic areas that voluntary insurers cannot reach.

5. Most insurance authorities agree that the extent of health insurance liability is such that a federal reinsurance program is absolutely unnecessary.

6. The bills would give the Secretary of the Department of Health, Education and Welfare an extensive but unjustified regulatory control over the nation's health insurance industry.

Social Security Amendments

The A.M.A. took a position on only two provisions in the bill to amend the Social Security Act —(1) the proposed compulsory coverage of physicians under Title II of the Act and (2) the so-called "waiver of premium" section to preserve the insurance rights of individuals with extended total disability. The Association opposed those two provisions, which were of direct medical interest, but took no position on the bill as a whole, which would be outside its province.

Compulsory Coverage—The A.M.A. House of Delegates on at least three occasions in the recent past has expressed strong opposition to compulsory coverage, but it has made clear that it does not oppose voluntary coverage for any physicians who might desire it. We oppose compulsory coverage because: (a) most physicians' do not retire until after the age of 74 and therefore would not benefit; (b) group treatment does not apply logically to physicians, whose lives and training emphasize individual activity,

and (c) there is no sound reason for compulsory coverage of a group against their expressed wishes.

The Jenkins-Keogh Bills—as an alternative to compulsory coverage under Social Security, the A.M.A. actively supports the Jenkins-Keogh bills, which would provide tax deferment benefits designed to stimulate the establishment of retirement pension plans by self-employed persons and by many employed persons not now covered by company plans. In the opinion of the A.M.A., these bills will provide for the development of a voluntary pension program which is equitable, free from compulsion and attuned to the retirement needs of physicians. Moreover, these bills will eliminate certain discriminations and inequities which exist under present tax laws by extending the tax deferment privilege to the country's ten million self-employed and also to millions of employees who work for companies without private pension plans.

Waiver of Premium— This section of the Social Security amendments provides a waiver of Social Security taxes for those totally and permanently disabled, with the disability to be determined by medical examinations carried out under government regulations. The A.M.A. opposed this section because it could become an entering wedge for the regimentation of the medical profession by creating a mechanism for the adoption of a federal cash permanent and total disability benefit program which in turn could lead to a full-fledged system of compulsory sickness insurance. This section, therefore, cannot be appraised solely as an isolated, detached effort to provide some measure of aid to disabled workers.

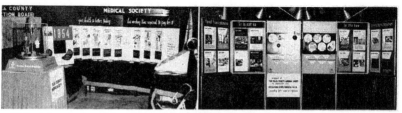

Pictured above are views of the exhibits at the Tulsa State Fair held in September. Exhibits were sponsored jointly by the Tulsa County Medical Society and the Oklahoma State Medical Association.

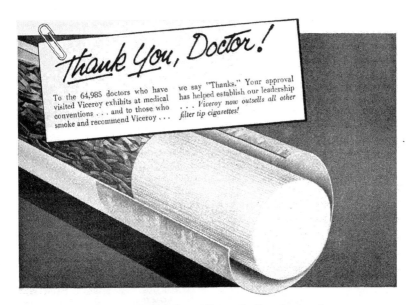

Thank You, Doctor!

To the 64,985 doctors who have visited Viceroy exhibits at medical conventions . . . and to those who smoke and recommend Viceroy . . . we say "Thanks." Your approval has helped establish our leadership . . . *Viceroy now outsells all other filter tip cigarettes!*

NEW VICEROY GIVES SMOKERS

20,000 FILTERS

in every Viceroy Tip

Only Viceroy has this new-type filter. Made of a non-mineral cellulose acetate—it gives the greatest filtering action possible without impairing flavor or impeding the flow of smoke.

Smoke is also filtered through Viceroy's king-size length of rich costly tobaccos. Thus, Viceroy smokers get *double the filtering action* . . . for only a penny or two more than brands without filters.

WORLD'S LARGEST-SELLING FILTER TIP CIGARETTE

New King-Size Filter Tip **VICEROY**

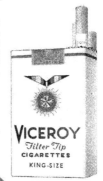

VICEROY *Filter Tip* CIGARETTES KING-SIZE

ONLY A PENNY OR TWO MORE THAN CIGARETTES WITHOUT FILTERS

Index to Contents

The use of the Index will be greatly facilitated by remembering that articles are often listed under more than one heading. Scientific articles may be found under the name of the author and the various phases of the subject discussed as well as under the listing of Scientific Articles. Editorials and deaths are listed under the special headings as well as alphabetically.

Pages Included in Each Issue.

Key to Abbreviations

(S)—Scientific Article
(E)—Editorial
(SA)—Special Article
(BR)—Book Reviews
(TC)—Therapeutic Conference
(CR)—Case Report
(ABS)—Abstract
(D)—Deaths
(PIC)—Picture
(GN)—General News
(CPC)—Clinical Pathologic Conference

atopic
dermatitis...

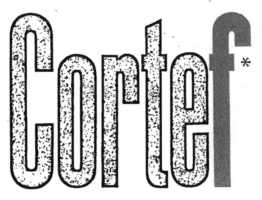

acetate ointment

In 5 Gm. tubes of 1.0% and 2.5% concentration

*Trademark for Upjohn's brand of hydrocortisone (compound F)

Upjohn *The Upjohn Company, Kalamazoo, Michigan*

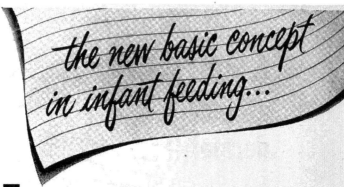

the new basic concept in infant feeding...

Lactum

MEAD'S |LIQUID| FORMULA FOR INFANTS

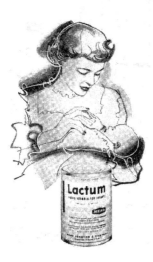

Conforming in every respect to the latest and most scientific evidence on infant feeding, Lactum provides a clinically proved cow's milk formula, with demonstrated nutritional advantages, plus new convenience made possible by its ready-to-use liquid form.

Outstanding among Lactum's nutritional benefits is its generous milk protein content—providing a more-than-ample margin of safety above the Recommended Daily Allowance. Its natural milk fat not only supplies an effectively utilized source of calories but permits a uniformly smooth, perfectly homogenized formula. Supplementary carbohydrate (Dextri-Maltose) is incorporated for caloric adequacy and protein sparing.

Both in formulation and in manufacture, Lactum reflects Mead Johnson and Company's long experience in developing more effective products for infant feeding to meet the changing needs of the medical profession.

Lactum's time-saving convenience is welcomed by today's busy young mothers. They merely add 1 part Lactum to 1 part water for a formula supplying 20 calories per fluid ounce.

MEAD JOHNSON & COMPANY · EVANSVILLE, INDIANA, U.S.A.

Volume 47 • Number 12 • December, 1954

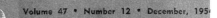

the

journal

OF THE OKLAHOMA STATE MEDICAL ASSOCIATION

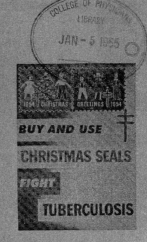

1954 CHRISTMAS GREETINGS 1954

BUY AND USE

CHRISTMAS SEALS

FIGHT

TUBERCULOSIS

PUBLISHED MONTHLY
UNDER DIRECTION OF THE COUNCIL

from the literature...

"The value of CHLOROMYCETIN in the treatment of infections due to most bacteria, the pathogenic rickettsiae, and many of the large viruses has now been well established."[1]

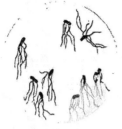

in typhoid fever

"Our experience...and many others all show that chloramphenicol [CHLOROMYCETIN] has an established place in the treatment of typhoid fever."[2]

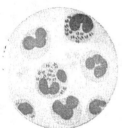

in meningitis

"At the present time chloramphenicol [CHLOROMYCETIN] is recognized as a potent antibiotic whose ease of administration and prompt diffusion into serum and spinal fluid makes it a particularly useful agent in the treatment of many forms of purulent meningitis."[3]

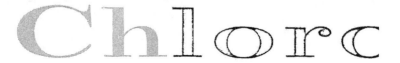

(1) Yow, E. M.; Taylor, F. M.; Hirsch, J.; Frankel, R. A., & Carnes, H. E.: J. Pediat. 42:151, 1953. (2) Dodd, K.: J. Arkansas M. Soc. 10:174, 1954. (3) Hanbery, J. W.: Neurology 4:301, 1954. (4) Miller, G.; Hansen, J. E., & Pollock, B. E.: Am. Heart J. 47:453, 1954. (5) Keefer, C. S., in Smith, A., & Werner, P. L.: Modern Treatment, New York, Paul B. Hoeber, Inc., 1953, p. 65.

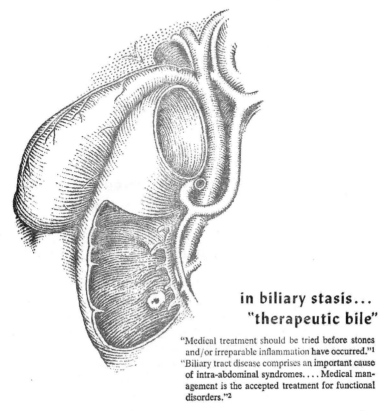

in biliary stasis...
"therapeutic bile"

"Medical treatment should be tried before stones and/or irreparable inflammation have occurred."[1]

"Biliary tract disease comprises an important cause of intra-abdominal syndromes.... Medical management is the accepted treatment for functional disorders."[2]

Decholin® and Decholin Sodium®
(dehydrocholic acid, *Ames*)   (sodium dehydrocholate, *Ames*)

"... increase the volume output of a bile of relatively high water content and low viscosity."[3]

Decholin Tablets, 3¾ gr. (0.25 Gm.), bottles of 100, 500, 1000 and 5000. *Decholin Sodium*, 20% aqueous solution, ampuls of 3 cc., 5 cc. and 10 cc.; boxes of 3, 20 and 100.

1. Segal, H.: Postgrad. Med. *13*:81, 1953. 2. O'Brien, G. F., and Schweitzer, I. L.: M. Clin. North America *37*:155, 1953. 3. Beckman, H.: Pharmacology in Clinical Practice, Philadelphia, W. B. Saunders Company, 1952, p. 361.

AMES COMPANY, INC.
Elkhart, Indiana

Ames Company of Canada, Ltd., Toronto

53754

A protein margin of safety

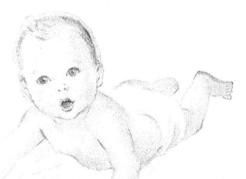

- **for greater nitrogen retention**
- **for firmer muscle mass**

LIQUID

POWDERED

LACTUM

NUTRITIONALLY SOUND FORMULA FOR INFANTS

In the bottle-fed infant, a higher protein intake, with greater nitrogen retention, results in firmer muscle mass, better tissue turgor and better motor development.[1] A protein intake that does not maintain positive nitrogen balance "cannot be considered optimal or even safe for any length of time."[2]

During the first year of life, the infant's nourishment is derived primarily from his formula. Hence it is especially important that the formula be generous in protein. The usual Lactum® feedings provide 2 Gm. protein per pound of body weight—25% more than the Recommended Daily Allowance of 1.6 Gm. per pound (3.5 Gm. per kilogram).

Gm.
PROTEIN

Gm.
PROTEIN

Lactum formula
for a 10 lb. infant

Recommended
Daily Allowance
for a 10 lb. infant

1. Jeans, P. C., in A.M.A. Handbook of Nutrition, Philadelphia, Blakiston, 1951, pp. 275-298. 2. Stare, F. J., and Davidson, C. S., in The Proteins, American Medical Association, 1945.

MEAD JOHNSON & COMPANY • EVANSVILLE, INDIANA, U.S.A.